Dr. R. C. Harris

L-Carnitine and its role in medicine:
From function to therapy

L-Carnitine and its role in medicine: From function to therapy

edited by

R. Ferrari, S. DiMauro and G. Sherwood

ACADEMIC PRESS
Harcourt Brace Jovanovich, Publishers
London   San Diego
New York   Boston   Sydney   Tokyo   Toronto

ACADEMIC PRESS LIMITED
24–28 Oval Road
London NW1 7DX

United States Edition published by
ACADEMIC PRESS INC.
San Diego, CA 92101

A catalogue record for this book is available from the British Library
ISBN 0-12-253940-0

Typeset by Photo·graphics, Honiton, Devon
and printed in Great Britain by Mackays of Chatham plc, Chatham, Kent

Contents

IIIb PERIPHERAL VASCULAR DISEASE

IIIc RENAL DIALYSIS

IIId DIABETES

List of Contributors

S. Ahmad, Scribner Kidney Center, University of Washington, 2150 North 107th Street, Seattle, Washington 98133, USA.

Corrado Angelini, Regional Center for Neuromuscular Diseases, Neurological Clinic 1, University of Padova, Padova, Italy.

Maria Bakas, Metabolic Research and Analysis, Inc., Fresno, California, USA.

Roberta Barbato, Centro per la Studi della Fisiologia Mitocondriale, C.N.R. e Dipartimento di Chimica Biologica, Università di Padova, Padova, Italy.

M. Bennett, The Kimberley H. Courtwright and Joseph W. Summers Metabolic Disease Center, Baylor University Medical Center, 3500 Gaston Avenue, Dallas, Texas 75246, USA.

E. Bertini, Departments of Metabolism and Cardiology, Bambino Gesu' Children's Hospital, Istituto di Ricovero e Cura a Carattere Scientifico, Rome, Italy.

M. Bevilacqua, Departments of Metabolism and Cardiology, Bambino Gesu' Children's Hospital, Istituto di Ricovero e Cura a Carattere Scientifico, Rome, Italy.

G. Biase, Università degli Studi di Bari, Istituto di Malattie Dell' Apparato Cardiovascolare 70124 Bari, Italy.

Loran L. Bieber, Department of Biochemistry, Michigan State University, East Lansing, Michigan, USA.

Eric P. Brass, Department of Medicine and Pharmacology, Case Western Reserve University, Cleveland, Ohio 44106, USA.

G. Brevetti, Department of Medicine, II Medical School, University of Naples 'Federico II', Naples, Italy.

A. B. Burlina, Department of Paediatrics, University of Padova, Padova, Italy.

V. Calabrese, Istituto di Chimica Biologica, Università di Catania Viale Andrea Doria, No. 6, 95100 Catania, Italy.

Franco B. S. Carrara, Division of Biochemistry and Genetics, Istituto Nazionale Neurologico 'Carlo Besta', Milano, Italy.

N. J. Dhalla, Division of Cardiovascular Sciences, St Bonniface General Hospital Research Center and Department of Physiology, Faculty of Medicine, University of Manitoba, Winnipeg, Canada, R2H 2A6.

Ian M. C. Dixon, Division of Cardiovascular Sciences, St Bonniface General Hospital Research Centre and Department of Physiology, Faculty of Medicine, University of Manitoba, Winnipeg, Canada, R2H 2A6.

M. Di Biase, Università degli Studi di Bari, Istituto di Malattie Dell' Apparato Cardiovascolare 70124 Bari, Italy.

Stefano DiDonato, Division of Biochemistry and Genetics, Istituto Nazionale Neurologico 'Carlo Besta', via Celoria II, 20133 Milano, Italy.

Fabio Di Lisa, Centro per la Studio della Fisiologia Mitocondriale, C.N.R. e Dipartimento di Chimica Biologica, Università di Padova, Padova, Italy.

S. DiMauro, The H. Houston Merritt Clinical Research Centre for Muscular Dystrophy and Related Diseases, Columbia University, New York, NY 10032, USA.

M.-L. Dubelaar, Department of Physiology, University of Limburg, Maastricht, The Netherlands.

C. Fernandez, Servizio di Cardiologia Ambulatoriale, USL 61, Palermo, Italy.

Roberto Ferrari, Cattedra di Cardiologia, Università degli Studi, P. le Spedali Civili, 1, 25123 Brescia, Italy.

Eckart Fleck, Klinik für Innere Medizin, Kardiologie, Deutsches Herzzentrum Berlin, Augustenburger Platz 1, 1000 Berlin 65, Germany.

G. M. Gagliardi, Departments of Metabolism and Cardiology, Bambino Gesu' Children's Hospital, Istituto di Ricovero e Cura a Carattere Scientifico, Rome, Italy.

Barbara Garavaglia, Division of Biochemistry and Genetics, Istituto Nazionale Neurologica 'Carlo Besta', Milan, Italy.

F. de Giuli, Cattedra di Cardiologia, Università degli Studi di Brescia, Brescia, Italy.

D. E. Hale, Division of Endocrinology and Diabetes, Department of Pediatrics, The University of Pennsylvania School of Medicine, The Children's Hospital of Philadelphia, 34th Street and Civic Center Boulevard, Philadelphia, PA 19104, USA.

Charles Hoppel, Department of Veterans Affairs, Medical Center, 10701 East Boulevard, Cleveland, OH 44106, USA.

W. C. Hülsmann, Department of Cardiology, Thorax Centre, PO Box 1738, 3000 DR Rotterdam, The Netherlands.

K. Jue, University of California, San Francisco and Valley Children's Hospital, Fresno, California, USA.

Janos Kerner, Sigma Tau Laboratories, Pomezia, Italy.

Peter K. Kosolcharoen, Department of Cardiology, William S. Middleton Memorial Veterans Hospital, University of Wisconsin, Madison, WI, USA.

L. Linn, Metabolic Research and Analysis, Inc., Fresno, California, USA.

Gary D. Lopaschuk, Departments of Pediatrics and Pharmacology, The University of Alberta, Edmonton, Canada, T6G 2S2.

R. Lorefice, Istituto di Chimica Biologica, Università di Catania Viale Andrea Doria No. 6, 95100 Catania, Italy.

Andrea Martinuzzi, Regional Centre for Neuromuscular Diseases, Neurological Clinic 1, University of Padova, Padova, Italy.

Roberta Menabò, Centro per la Studio della Fisiologia Mitcondriale, C.N.R. e Dipartimento di Chimica Biologica, Università di Padova, Padova, Italy.

Milan Novak, Department of Pediatrics, University of Miami School of Medicine, Miami, Florida, USA.

Grzegorz Opala, Metabolic Research and Analysis, Inc., Fresno, California, USA.

E. Pasini, Cattedra di Cardiologia, Università degli Studi di Brescia, Brescia, Italy.

Ashvin K. Patel, Cardiology Section, William S. Middleton Memorial Veterans Hospital, University of Wisconsin, Madison, WI 53705, USA.

Duna Penn, University of Chicago, Department of Pediatrics, Box 107, 5825 South Maryland Avenue, Chicago, IL 60637, USA.

Sergio Perna, Department of Medicine, II Medical School, University of Naples 'Federico II', Naples, Italy.

Vera Regitz, Klinik für Innere Medizin, Kardiologie, Deutsches Herzzentrum Berlin II, Augustenburger Platz 1, 1000 Berlin 65, Germany.

Marco Rimoldi, Division of Biochemistry and Genetics, Istituto Nazionale Neurologico 'C. Besta', Milano, Italy.

N. Rizza, Istituto di Chimica Biologica, Università di Catania Viale Andrea Doria N° 6, 95100 Catania, Italy.

V. Rizza, Istituto di Chimica Biologica, Università di Catania Viale Andrea Doria N° 6, 95100 Catania, Italy.

Paolo Rizzon, Università degli Studi di Bari, Istituto di Malattie Dell' Apparato Cardiovascolare, 70124 Bari, Italy.

G. Sabetta, Departments of Metabolism and Cardiology, Bambino Gesu' Children's Hospital, Istituto Ricovero e Curo a Carattere Scientifico, Rome, Italy.

Eberhard Schmidt-Sommerfeld, University of Chicago, Department of Pediatrics, Box 107, 5825 South Maryland Avenue, Chicago, IL 60637, USA.

Kanu R. Shah, Division of Cardiovascular Sciences, St Bonniface Hospital Research Centre and Department of Physiology, Faculty of Medicine, University of Manitoba, Winnipeg, Canada, R2H 2A6.

G. Sherwood, Medical Director, Metabolic Division, Center Baylor, 35000 Gastin Avenue, Dallas, Texas 75246, USA.

Austin L. Shug, Division of Neurology, University of Wisconsin, Madison, USA.

Noris Siliprandi, Centro per la Studio della Fisiologia Mitocondriale, C.N.R. e Dipartimento di Chimica Biologica, Università di Padova, Padova, Italy.

Anne Szabo, Metabolic Research and Analysis, Inc., Fresno, California, USA.

I. Tein, The Division of Pediatric Neurology, Columbia University, New York, NY 10032, USA.

James H. Thomsen, Cardiology Section, University of Wisconsin, Madison, WI, USA.

Carol K. Vance, University of California, San Francisco and Valley Children's Hospital, Fresno, California, USA.

W. Hugh Vance, Metabolic Research and Analysis, Inc., Fresno, California, USA.

Lodovica Vergani, Regional Centre for Neuromuscular Diseases, Neurological Clinic I, University of Padova, Padova, Italy.

C. Dionisi Vici, Departments of Metabolism and Cardiology, Bambino Gesu' Children's Hospital, Istituto di Ricovero e Cura a Carattere Scientifico, Rome, Italy.

O. Visioli, Cattedra di Cardiologia, Università degli Studi, Spedali Civili, P. le Spedali Civili, 1, 25123 Brescia, Italy.

Susan C. Winter, University of California, San Francisco and Valley Children's Hospital, Fresno, California, USA.

Howard Winter, Metabolic Research and Analysis, Inc., Fresno, California, USA.

Elinor M. Zorn, University of California, San Francisco and Valley Children's Hospital, Fresno, California, USA.

Foreword

During the past decade, it has become increasingly evident that L-carnitine is intimately involved in many different aspects of medicine. The precise nature of this involvement is the subject of ongoing investigation being conducted in clinics and laboratories worldwide. The purpose of this book is to provide for the clinician an introductory overview of the role of carnitine in medicine as it is understood today. Any advances in our understanding to be made in the future might then be better placed in context.

The book is divided into three sections. After a general introduction to the basic aspects of carnitine metabolism, the involvement of carnitine in the clinical aspects of paediatric medicine and adult medicine are discussed. Each section is preceded by an overview of the ensuing chapters on selected topics.

The editors wish to acknowledge and thank the individual authors for their time and effort and Sigma Tau for their continuing support.

R Ferrari
S DiMauro
G Sherwood

PART I

INTRODUCTION TO L-CARNITINE

Role of carnitine: an overview
S. DiMauro

In the 18 years since the first report of carnitine deficiency in humans (Engel and Angelini, 1973), knowledge of the role of carnitine deficiency/insufficiency in human pathology has expanded dramatically. The initial cases of apparently isolated lipid storage myopathy have been followed by descriptions of patients, usually children, with multisystem disorders dominated by liver or heart dysfunction. Also, the initial descriptive terms 'myopathic' and 'systemic' carnitine deficiency have been replaced by a physiopathologically more meaningful distinction between primary and secondary carnitine deficiencies.

The important role of carnitine in intermediary metabolism, particulary regarding its limited biosynthesis, helps to explain how carnitine deficiency may occur as a secondary event in diverse pathological situations affecting different organs. The enlargement of the clinical spectrum has raised opportunities and, occasionally, controversies on the therapeutic efficacy of this natural compound.

Although this book is primarily directed at clinicians, formulation of intelligent pathogenetic hypotheses and instituting rational therapies require knowledge of some basic aspects of L-carnitine. Therefore, in this first section, we have considered five important topics. Dr Hoppel

1

L-Carnitine and Its Role in Medicine:
From Function to Therapy. ISBN 0-12-253940-0

offers an overview of the several critical functions of carnitine in intermediate metabolism. The chapter by Dr Brass deals with transport. This is a crucial feature for a molecule that can be synthesized by only a few tissues: in most tissues it has to cross two membrane barriers, the cell membrane and the inner mitochondrial membrane. Central to any clinical evaluation of carnitine deficiency/insufficiency is a reliable and sensitive methodology for the detection of carnitine and its esters: this is discussed by Dr Di Lisa in the third chapter. Any rational replacement therapy has to be based on knowledge about absorption, tissue distribution, and excretion of L-carnitine: this is the subject of Dr Rizza's chapter on pharmacokinetics. Finally, as an introduction to the more specific clinical sections that follow, Dr DiDonato offers a critical and concise overview of both primary and secondary carnitine deficiencies.

Part Ia

Basic aspects of carnitine

I

THE PHYSIOLOGICAL ROLE
OF CARNITINE

Charles Hoppel

Carnitine (3-hydroxy-4-N-trimethylammoniobutanoate) is present in biological materials as free carnitine (in relatively high concentration) and as acylcarnitines, which are metabolic products of reactions utilizing acyl CoA catalysed by carnitine acyltransferases. The acyl groups in the acylcarnitines range from short-chain (acetyl) to long-chain (such as palmitoyl). The water-soluble acyl groups in rat tissues and in blood and urine have been identified as acetyl-(predominant) and other acylcarnitines to a lesser extent (Choi and Bieber, 1977). The long-chain acylcarnitines have not been characterized. It is generally assumed that all roles of carnitine can be ascribed to its function as a substrate for carnitine acyltransferase reactions. However, there may be functions of carnitine and acylcarnitines which do not depend on this metabolic system.

In 1955 Friedman and Fraenkel demonstrated that, in liver, acetylcarnitine was formed from acetyl CoA and carnitine. Fritz (1955) showed that carnitine could stimulate fatty acid oxidation in liver. Work in the early 1960s (Bremer, 1962; Fritz and Yue, 1963) showed that acylcarnitines were substrates for oxidation by mitochondria. These

5

L-Carnitine and Its Role in Medicine:
From Function to Therapy. ISBN 0–12–253940–0

observations have stimulated a great amount of research activity in many laboratories over the past three decades which has provided a good framework for understanding the physiological role of carnitine.

Table 1 outlines the known and possible physiological roles of carnitine and provides the focus for this chapter. The obligate role of carnitine in mitochondrial oxidation of long-chain fatty acids is the best characterized system. The existence of carnitine acyltransferases with substrate specificities different from the long-chain transferase system involved in mitochondrial fatty acid oxidation, and the presence of acylcarnitines in tissues, led to a search for a function for the shorter-chain acylcarnitine systems. The suggestion of a buffering effect of carnitine on the acyl CoA/CoASH ratio in the cell and, in particular, in mitochondria has gained acceptance. The mechanism for this buffering is through mass action as the system appears to be at steady-state and near equilibrium (the equilibrium constant for the carnitine acyltransferases is close to 1).

An extension of this buffering concept, also involving the carnitine acyltransferase system, proposes a scavenger role for carnitine. When acyl CoAs accumulate in either mitochondria or tissues, the laws of mass action favour the formation of acylcarnitines. Acylcarnitines can leave cells via the carnitine transport system, enter the circulation and then be excreted in the urine. As long as free carnitine is available the ratio of acylcarnitine to carnitine will reflect the acyl CoA to CoA ratio. If the acyl group is a compound that cannot be further metabolized then this may be a means of eliminating that compound.

The involvement of carnitine in intracellular communication by transporting acyl groups from one compartment to another is an attractive concept, but still has not been demonstrated unequivocally. An intercellular transport function of acylcarnitines also has been

TABLE I.
Physiological roles of carnitine

I.	Mitochondrial long-chain fatty acid oxidation
2.	Buffering of the mitochondrial acyl CoA/CoA couple
3.	Scavenger system for acyl groups
4.	Peroxisomal fatty acid oxidation, intracellular communication
5.	Branched-chain amino acid metabolism
6.	Membrane stabilization

proposed but this awaits documentation. The stabilization of the mitochondrial membranes by carnitine probably represents the removal of disruptive acyl CoAs from the membranes as acylcarnitines.

CARNITINE ACYLTRANSFERASES

Carnitine is a substrate for a series of reactions catalysed by carnitine acyltransferases (Table 2). The basic, reversible reaction is:

$$\text{Acyl CoA} + \text{Carnitine} \rightleftharpoons \text{Acylcarnitine} + \text{CoA}$$

There are three groups of transferases distinguished primarily by their substrate specificities (Bieber, 1988). The trivial names for each of the groups have been in common usage but as pointed out by Bieber (1988) the substrate specificity differs depending on the source of the carnitine acyltransferase. The question of how many carnitine acyltransferases exist within a cell has not been resolved. Enzymes have been purified from each of the groups and detailed molecular studies are being done.

The subcellular localization of the carnitine acyltransferases is also still unsettled but there is a consensus that the enzymes are widely distributed within the cell. Table 3 outlines the localization of the groups within the cell. The role of carnitine is mediated through the carnitine acyltransferases and it is important to review some selected data on these enzymes.

TABLE 2.
Carnitine acyltransferases

Substrate	Enzyme group
Short-chain acyl groups	Carnitine acetyltransferase (CAT)
Medium-chain acyl groups	Carnitine octanoyltransferase (COT)
Long-chain acyl groups	Carnitine palmitoyltransferase (CPT)

TABLE 3.
Subcellular localization of carnitine acyltransferases

Enzyme	Location
Carnitine acetyltransferase (CAT)	Mitochondria
	Peroxisomes
	Microsomes
Carnitine octanoyltransferase (COT)	Peroxisomes
	Microsomes
Carnitine palmitoyltransferase (CPT)	Mitochondria

Carnitine acetyltransferase

Carnitine acetyltransferase (CAT) activity has been demonstrated in mitochondria, peroxisomes and microsomes and the enzyme has been purified from many sources (Bremer, 1983; Bieber, 1988). The submitochondrial localization in mitochondria is on the inner membrane facing the matrix (Edwards et al, 1974). Miyazawa et al (1983a; 1983b) used mRNA from liver to translate both mitochondrial and peroxisomal CAT. Their data suggest that both enzymes (M_r 67 500) are formed from a larger precursor of M_r 69 000. In addition, antibodies against the two CAT activities show cross-reactivity. In the yeast *Candida tropicalis*, Ueda et al (1984) showed that the peroxisomal and mitochondrial CATs have different subunit sizes but that common larger precursors are modified to form the peroxisomal and mitochondrial enzymes. The enzymes isolated from mammalian sources show a broad substrate range with maximal velocity with propionyl CoA, while the activity with acetyl CoA and butyryl CoA is somewhat less. Mouse liver peroxisomal CAT has low apparent K_m values for acetyl CoA and carnitine whereas the apparent K_m values for the reverse reaction are higher (Farrell et al, 1984). This is in contrast to the apparent K_m values for acetyl CoA and carnitine for most of the other CAT enzymes.

Carnitine octanoyltransferase

Carnitine octanoyltransferase (COT) activity is found in microsomes and peroxisomes associated with specific proteins that have been purified. In mitochondria the COT activity is associated with mitochondrial CAT and carnitine palmitoyltransferase (CPT) and the existence of a separate enzyme has not been demonstrated (Clarke and Bieber, 1981). COT has been purified from rat liver (Miyazawa et al, 1983c) and the M_r (66 000) of the translated product was the same as the mature enzyme. The enzyme had a broad substrate specificity with the highest activity with hexanoyl CoA, but there was activity with the longer-chain acyl derivatives. COT with M_r 60 000 has also been purified from mouse liver peroxisomes. The mouse enzyme also had a broad substrate specificity with maximal activity with hexanoyl CoA. The carnitine acyltransferase activity in purified intact peroxisomes, using decanoyl CoA and palmitoyl CoA as substrates, is inhibited by malonyl CoA (Derrick and Ramsay, 1989). This acyltransferase showed maximal activity with decanoyl CoA and myristoyl CoA as substrates in both intact peroxisomes and mitochondria. This substrate specificity observed in the intact peroxisome differs from that seen using the purified enzyme from either mouse or rat liver. A further observation is that the microsomal carnitine acyltransferase, using decanoyl CoA as substrate, was inhibited by malonyl CoA (Lilly et al, 1990). In microsomes the velocity is 10 times faster with decanoyl CoA as substrate compared with palmitoyl CoA. These very interesting observations raise questions concerning the regulation of the synthesis of acylcarnitines in both organelles.

Carnitine palmitoyltransferase

Carnitine palmitoyltransferase has been described as an exclusively mitochondrial enzyme (Hoppel and Brady, 1985). Kopec and Fritz (1971, 1973) purified two forms of CPT from calf liver. The enzyme was a dimer of M_r 150 000, and one of the forms catalysed an irreversible reaction and was extremely labile. A protein was purified from rat liver with a native M_r of 280 000–320 000, with subunits of 69 200 (Miyazawa et al, 1983c). The M_r of the precursor of CPT was 71 600 (Ozasa et al, 1983). The enzyme showed broad substrate specificity with maximal activity with myristoyl CoA. In subcellular distribution studies it was confined to the mitochondria (Miyazawa et al, 1983c). These authors showed that CAT, COT and CPT were immunologically different.

Clarke and Bieber (1981) purified CPT from beef heart mitochondria and found that the native enzyme migrated as part of a detergent micelle of M_r 510 000 but had a subunit M_r of 67 000. This enzyme showed highest activity with decanoyl CoA as substrate. Ramsay et al (1987) described the purification of a soluble CPT from bovine liver mitochondria in a monomeric form of 63500. This enzyme was most active with myristoyl CoA and palmitoyl CoA. Subsequently, Ramsay (1989) concluded that the soluble CPT was probably peroxisomal in origin. This same conclusion was reached by Healy et al (1988). Thus the issue of how many CPTs exist in the cell has become more complicated.

Using a different approach, the mitochondrial CPT system has been probed using inhibitors (Declercq et al, 1987) and detergents, as well as an antibody directed at CPT (Woeltje et al, 1987). These authors concluded that there are two immunologically distinct CPTs in rat liver mitochondria. They were not able to purify CPT-1, but they identified it as a protein which binds radioactive tetradecylglycidyl CoA and has a subunit M_r of about 90000. Murthy and Pande (1990) have described the preparation of a soluble malonyl CoA sensitive CPT that behaves similarly to the M_r 90000 protein. A separation of CPT activity and malonyl CoA binding was reported by Lund and Woldegiorgis (1986) but they were unable to recombine the enzyme with the malonyl CoA binding components. However, Lund (1987) was able to extract a labile malonyl CoA sensitive CPT from the membrane residues. Recently, Kerner and Bieber (1990) were able to isolate a malonyl CoA-sensitive CPT in the form of a complex, and separate the CPT activity from inhibition. A CPT has been purified to homogeneity from rat liver mitochondria and antibodies against this protein precipitated all the CPT activity in sonicated mitochondria (Brady and Brady, 1987a, 1987b).

There is a great deal of uncertainty concerning the CPT system. Are the mitochondria that exhibit CPT activity? Are there two separate proteins in medium-chain acyltransferases located in the peroxisomal and microsomal fractions of liver and CPT activities, in fact one and the same? Since these enzymes are critical to the physiological role of carnitine the answers will be of great importance in understanding this complex system.

ROLE OF CARNITINE IN MITOCHONDRIAL LONG-CHAIN FATTY ACID OXIDATION

Process of carnitine stimulation

The best described function of carnitine in cellular metabolism is in the mitochondrial oxidation of long-chain fatty acids. The steps involved in the role of carnitine in this process, using palmitate as an example, are outlined in Table 4. The activation of the long-chain fatty acid (palmitate) to form palmitoyl CoA occurs in the endoplasmic reticulum (microsomal fraction) and on the outer surface of the mitochondrial outer membrane via a long-chain acyl CoA synthetase. The palmitoyl CoA must then pass through the outer membrane into the intermembrane space of the mitochondria. How this movement of acyl CoAs occurs is not known but the data of Clouet et al (1989) suggest that this step may be important. While palmitoyl CoA is the substrate for β-oxidation in the mitochondrial matrix, the inner membrane is impermeable to it.

In the seminal studies discussed above from the laboratories of Fritz and Bremer, a framework for the understanding of the role of carnitine developed. The palmitoyl CoA present between the outer and inner boundary membranes is converted to palmitoylcarnitine by an 'outer' CPT (variously called CPT_o, CPT-I, CPT-1, CPT-A and overt CPT). The location of this CPT activity is still uncertain. The enzymic activity was originally described by Hoppel and Tomec (1972) and by Brosnan et al (1973) as localized on the outer surface of the inner membrane. The work of Murthy and Pande (1987a, 1987b) has placed this CPT

TABLE 4.

Steps involved in the role of carnitine in mitochondrial long-chain fatty acid metabolism (palmitate used as an example)

1. Activation of palmitate to form palmitoyl CoA (microsomal acyl CoA synthetase and outer surface of mitochondrial outer membrane).

2. Transfer of palmitoyl CoA through the mitochondrial outer membrane into the intermembrane space.

3. Transfer of palmitoyl group from CoA to carnitine. (Carnitine palmitoyltransferase—various authors refer to this as CPT-I, CPT-1, CPT-A, CTP_o [outer and overt].) Localized either to the inner surface of the outer membrane or outer surface of inner membrane.

4. Translocation of the palmitoylcarnitine through the inner membrane. (Carnitine–acylcarnitine translocase is an antiport system whereby palmitoylcarnitine is transported into the matrix in exchange for carnitine.)

5. Transfer of palmitoyl-group matrix palmitoylcarnitine to palmitoyl CoA using matrix CoA, releasing carnitine. (Carnitine palmitoyltransferase (variously called CPT-II, CPT-2, CPT-B, CPT_i [inner or latent].)

6. Palmitoyl CoA then enters the β-oxidation pathway at long-chain acyl CoA dehydrogenase.

activity on the inner surface of the outer membrane. Both of these locations have the enzyme facing the same compartment.

The palmitoylcarnitine is transported across the mitochondrial inner membrane via a carnitine acylcarnitine translocase which is an antiport system with carnitine from the matrix exchanging with the palmitoylcarnitine. This translocase was initially described by Ramsay and Tubbs (1974, 1975) and Pande (1975) and the protein has now been purified (Indiveri et al, 1990). The matrix palmitoylcarnitine is a substrate for the inner CPT using matrix CoASH to form palmitoyl CoA in the matrix and release carnitine. The palmitoyl CoA then can enter the β-oxidation pathway at the long-chain acyl CoA dehydrogenase. Thus, carnitine is an obligate in the transfer of the long-chain acyl group across the mitochondrial inner membrane to the site of β-oxidation.

Control of fatty acid oxidation

In a landmark study on the control of hepatic fatty acid oxidation, McGarry et al (1977) observed that malonyl CoA was a specific and reversible inhibitor. The model of malonyl CoA inhibition in the regulation of fatty acid oxidation and ketone production was reviewed by McGarry and Foster (1980). A further refinement of the model was presented by McGarry et al (1989). The rate of fatty acid synthesis is increased in the fed state whereas the rate of fatty acid oxidation is low. Under these conditions, malonyl CoA (the product of acetyl CoA carboxylase and the first intermediate in fatty acid synthesis) inhibits the outer CPT and decreases fatty acid oxidation. Although conditions associated with accelerated ketogenesis in the liver are accompanied by an increased intrahepatic content of carnitine (McGarry et al, 1975; Brass and Hoppel, 1978), this increase in liver carnitine alone is not sufficient to account for the accelerated ketogenesis. The key to the development of the ketotic state occurs with an increase in the ratio of glucagon to insulin which activates adenylyl cyclase with the consequent increase in cAMP. In addition to the decrease in malonyl CoA there is increased delivery of fatty acids to the liver and an increase in carnitine transport into the hepatocyte. Also contributing to the effect are the decreased sensitivity to malonyl CoA of both the outer CPT and oxidation of palmitate during fasting (Ontko and Johns, 1980; Cook et al, 1980; Bremer, 1981; Saggerson and Carpenter, 1981, 1983). In hyperthyroidism in rats the mitochondrial outer CPT activity increases, and it shows a decreased sensitivity to malonyl CoA

(Stakkestad and Bremer, 1983). In addition, Pande and Parvin (1980) have observed that thyroxine treatment increases the hepatic content of carnitine.

ROLE OF CARNITINE IN THE BUFFERING OF THE ACYL CoA/CoA RATIO

The changes in carnitine metabolism during alterations in metabolic state suggested that the CAT system was near equilibrium and that it buffers the tissue content of acetyl CoA (Pearson and Tubbs, 1967). Mass action ratios were determined by Kondrup and Grunnet (1973) and these were felt not to reflect the direction of hepatic metabolism. The interaction between carnitine and the CoA pool has been studied by injecting carnitine in doses sufficient to increase tissue carnitine in fed and fasted rats. The production of acylcarnitine after injection was characteristic of the metabolic state of the rat. The acylcarnitine to carnitine ratio is different in fasted rats compared with controls and the difference was maintained or accentuated after carnitine administration. This supports the idea that the state of the hepatic carnitine pool reflects, and results from, the metabolic state of the liver, rather than that changes in the carnitine pool cause changes in hepatic metabolism (Brass and Hoppel, 1980b). Brass and Hoppel (1980a) have shown that in isolated rat liver mitochondria carnitine did not change the rates of oxidative metabolism of palmitoylcarnitine, despite increasing acetylcarnitine formation. The data were also consistent with the concept that the carnitine pool does not cause major changes in the mitochondrial CoASH pool or in mitochondrial oxidative metabolism of palmitoylcarnitine.

Metabolic studies in humans have shown that short-chain acylcarnitines increase with fasting (Hoppel and Genuth, 1980) while free carnitine decreases. These changes are accentuated in diabetic ketosis (Genuth and Hoppel, 1979). The increase in plasma acylcarnitines during these ketotic conditions was largely due to insulin deficiency as demonstrated during acute hormonal effects in thin and obese subjects. The corresponding decrease in free carnitine in plasma was attributable both to insulin deficiency and glucagon excess (Genuth and Hoppel, 1981).

The efflux of acylcarnitine from mitochondria has been quantitated by Lysiak et al (1986) and shown to depend on the substrate and source of mitochondria. The effect of the addition of carnitine on the intramitochondrial acyl CoAs was determined by Lysiak et al (1988) and these acyl CoAs were shown to decrease with a concomitant increase in CoA. This was dependent on the tissue and substrate. They interpreted the data to demonstrate that carnitine can modulate the short-chain acyl CoA/CoA ratio rather than merely reflecting the state of metabolism. Thus, by mass action this system can move acyl groups as acylcarnitine derivatives from one compartment to another.

Carnitine in branched-chain amino acid metabolism

Carnitine stimulates the oxidation of branched-chain amino acids (Paul and Adibi, 1978; Bremer, 1983). When mitochondria are exposed to branched-chain, α-oxo acids, branched-chain acylcarnitines are readily formed (Lysiak et al, 1986). The question of whether carnitine directly stimulates branched-chain amino acid oxidation seems to be answered in the negative with the production of the acylcarnitines reflecting the metabolic state. Thus, these effects are similar to the buffering effect of carnitine on other metabolic processes. Hokland and Bremer (1988) showed that branched-chain hydroxy acids are metabolized by the perfused kidney. The hydroxy acids and acylcarnitines are preferentially excreted in the urine. A high kidney content of carnitine increases the excretion of acylcarnitines in the urine. Guder and Wagner (1990) have demonstrated that proximal renal tubule cells readily formed acylcarnitines and may be a major source of urinary acylcarnitine. In the liver, Hokland (1988) has shown that when branched-chain acylcarnitines are formed there is a net loss of carnitine from the liver.

Carnitine as a scavenger for acyl groups

An extension of the buffering effect occurs when there is a block in the metabolism of an acyl CoA or when an acyl CoA is formed which cannot be further metabolized. Such may be the case for the 2-methyloctanylcarnitines which were identified in human urine by Kerner and Bieber (1985). Brass and Beyerinck (1988) showed that the accumulation of propionyl CoA in hepatocytes resulted in the inhibition of metabolism. Carnitine can partially reverse this inhibition and the effect is accompanied by the formation of propionylcarnitine and increasing the amount of CoA. Other chapters in this book will discuss the use of carnitine as a therapeutic agent.

Exercise as an example of a physiological state

Long et al (1982) noted a relationship between the concentration of carnitine and the oxidation of long-chain fatty acids in various tissues. In muscle homogenates, the concentration of carnitine that gives half-maximal rates of oxidation is about 20 times higher than that needed in liver. These data suggest that the kinetics of skeletal muscle mitochondrial CPT should be sufficiently different from that observed with liver mitochondrial CPT. Interestingly, under low-intensity exercise for 30 min (where fatty acid oxidation might be expected) there was no change in skeletal muscle carnitine (Hiatt et al, 1989). However, when the same work-load is applied for 90 min, there is a progressive increase in plasma acylcarnitine concentration with decreasing free carnitine (Carlin et al, 1986). During intense muscular contractions for 4 min there was an increase in skeletal muscle acetylcarnitine with a corresponding decrease in free carnitine (Harris et al, 1987). When the exercise is conducted for 30 min at a work-load between the lactate threshold and maximal capacity, the muscle short-chain acylcarnitine concentration is 5.5 times greater while free carnitine content decreases by 60% (Hiatt et al, 1989). However, these changes were not reflected in the plasma or urine. Similar results were obtained by Sahlin (1990) in studying incremental exercise work-loads. Carter et al (1981) showed that high-intensity, short-duration exercise in rats increased the proportion of skeletal muscle acetylcarnitine within the acylcarnitine fraction and lowered acetyl CoA content. All these data are consistent with the hypothesis that the increased acetylcarnitine to carnitine ratio reflects the increased production of acetyl CoA from increased pyruvate generation during intense exercise.

ROLE OF CARNITINE IN PEROXISOMAL FATTY ACID OXIDATION

The β-oxidation system of peroxisomes is distinct from that in the mitochondria. A characteristic of the peroxisomal system is that the process leads to chain-shortening of long-chain fatty acids and β-oxidation of fatty acyl groups is not complete. During peroxisomal oxidation of palmitate (Bartlett et al, 1990) and linoleic acid (Diczfalusy et al, 1990) intermediates of fatty acid oxidation have been described. Vamecq et al (1989) have shown that dicarboxyloyl CoAs formed in the endoplasmic reticulum (microsomes) are oxidized by a peroxisomal enzyme. Thus, the products of peroxisomal β-oxidation are chain-shortened fatty acyl CoAs and acetyl CoA. Since peroxisomes contain CAT and COT activity a rigorous search has been conducted to define the contribution of carnitine to β-oxidation (Bieber et al, 1982; Bremer, 1983; Bieber, 1988). Direct evidence of a role is still not available. Using isolated hepatocytes, Leighton et al (1989) investigated the fate of the acetyl CoA units from peroxisomal β-oxidation. They found that free acetate release could account for all the acetyl CoA produced in peroxisomes but only a small proportion in mitochondria. In a set of innovative experiments, Buechler and Lowenstein (1990) demonstrated that peroxisomes in intact hepatocytes oxidize long-chain fatty acids by a carnitine-dependent mechanism. They used a combination of inhibitors to show that 2-bromo-fatty acids are metabolized in both peroxisomes and mitochondria.

OTHER ROLES OF CARNITINE PROBABLY DEPENDENT ON CARNITINE ACYLTRANSFERASES

Membrane stabilization

A progressive decrease in membrane potential and respiratory control occurs when rat liver mitochondria are aged in vitro. If the rat is treated with carnitine before isolating mitochondria from the liver, or if the isolated liver mitochondria are aged in the presence of carnitine, a protective effect is observed (DiLisa et al, 1986). There is a much higher membrane potential and the mitochondria show better respiratory control in the treated groups compared with the non-treated rats. This effect has been attributed to the removal of long-chain acyl CoAs from the mitochondrial membranes. Direct confirmation of this very interesting observation has not yet been published.

OTHER ROLES OF CARNITINE NOT DEPENDENT ON CARNITINE ACYLTRANSFERASES

A number of effects of acylcarnitines that do not appear to be mediated by carnitine acyltransferase action have been described. Spedding and

Mir (1987) demonstrated that palmitoylcarnitine shifted to the left the Ca^{2+} concentration–response curves in K^+-depolarized taenia preparations from the guinea pig caecum. Palmitoylcarnitine seems to interact selectively with the Ca^{2+} channel. The calcium-antagonist effects of calcium-channel blockers (nifedipine, diltiazem and verapamil) were reduced whereas the lipophilic class III calcium antagonists were resistant.

In rat heart mitochondria, palmitoylcarnitine promoted Ca^2 efflux due to a direct action on the Na^+–Ca^{2+} antiporter system (Baydoun et al, 1988). These changes in mitochondrial handling of calcium occur at lower concentrations of palmitoylcarnitine than the effect of the calcium channel.

Miotto et al (1989) showed that isovalerylcarnitine inhibited the proteolysis that occurs with amino acid deprivation in the perfused liver. This effect is reasonably specific for isovalerylcarnitine.

Fritz and Burdzy (1989) demonstrated that carnitine and acylcarnitines inhibited the aggregation of erythrocytes elicited by clusterin or fetuin. This effect occurred with both L-carnitine and D-carnitine, and also acylcarnitine with both carnitine isomers.

Acknowledgements

I thank S. Ingalls and P. Minkler for help with the manuscript.

REFERENCES

Bartlett K, Hovik R, Eaton S et al (1990) *Biochem. J.* 270: 175–180.
Baydoun AR, Markham A, Morgan RM & Sweetman AJ (1988) *Biochem. Pharmacol.* 37: 3103–3107.
Bieber LL (1988) *Annu. Rev. Biochem.* 57: 261–283.
Bieber LL, Emaus R, Valkner K & Farrell S (1982) *Fed. Proc.* 41: 2858–2862.
Brady LJ & Brady PS (1987a) *Biochem. J.* 241: 751–757.
Brady PS & Brady LJ (1987b) *Biochem. J.* 246: 641–649.
Brass EP & Beyerinck RA (1988) *Biochem. J.* 250: 819–825.
Brass EP & Hoppel CL (1978) *J. Biol. Chem.* 253: 2688–2693.
Brass EP & Hoppel CL (1980a) *Biochem. J.* 188: 451–458.
Brass EP & Hoppel CL (1980b) *Biochem. J.* 190: 495–504.
Bremer J (1962) *J. Biol. Chem.* 237: 3628–3632.
Bremer J (1981) *Biochim. Biophys. Acta* 665: 628–631.
Bremer J (1983) *Physiol. Rev.* 63: 1420–1480.
Brosnan JT, Kopec B & Fritz IB (1973) *J. Biol. Chem.* 248: 4075–4082.

Buechler KF & Lowenstein JM (1990) *Arch. Biochem. Biophys.* 281: 233–238.
Carlin JI, Reddan WG, Sanjak M & Hodach R (1986) *J. Appl. Physiol.* 61: 1275–1278.
Carter AL, Lennon DLF & Stratman FW (1981) *FEBS Lett.* 126: 21–24.
Choi YR & Bieber LL (1977) *Anal. Biochem.* 79: 413–418.
Clarke PRH & Bieber LL (1981) *J. Biol. Chem.* 256: 9861–9868.
Clouet P, Niot I & Bezard J (1989) *Biochem. J.* 263: 867–873.
Cook GA, Otto DA & Cornell NW (1980) *Biochem. J.* 192: 955–958.
Declercq PE, Falck JR, Kuwajima LM et al (1987) *J. Biol. Chem.* 262: 9812–9821.
Derrick JP & Ramsay RR (1989) *Biochem. J.* 262: 801–806.
Diczfalusy U, Alexson SEH, Sisfontes L et al (1990) *Biochim. Biophys. Acta* 1043: 182–188.
DiLisa F, Toninello A, Bobyleva-Fuarriero V et al (1986) *Topics in Aging Research in Europe* 7: 103–110.
Edwards YH, Chase JFA, Edwards MR & Tubbs PK (1974) *Eur. J. Biochem.* 46: 209–215.
Farrell SO, Fiol CJ, Reddy FK & Bieber LL (1984) *J. Biol. Chem.* 259: 13089–13095.
Friedman S & Fraenkel G (1955) *Arch. Biochem. Biophys.* 59: 491–501.
Fritz IB (1955) *Acta Physiol. Scand.* 34: 367–385.
Fritz IB & Burdzy K (1989) *J. Cell. Physiol.* 140: 18–28.
Fritz IB & Yue KTN (1963) *J. Lipid Res.* 4: 279–288.
Genuth SM & Hoppel CL (1979) *Diabetes* 28: 1083–1087.
Genuth SM & Hoppel CL (1981) *Metabolism* 30: 393–401.
Guder WG & Wagner S (1990) *J. Clin. Chem. Clin. Biochem.* 28: 347–350.
Harris RC, Foster CVL & Hultman E (1987) *J. Appl. Physiol.* 63: 440–442.
Healy MJ, Kerner J & Bieber LL (1988) *Biochem. J.* 249: 231–237.
Hiatt WR, Regensteiner JG, Wolfel EE & Brass EP (1989) *J. Clin. Invest.* 84: 1167–1173.
Hokland BM (1988) *Biochim. Biophys. Acta* 961: 234–241.
Hokland BM & Bremer J (1988) *Biochim. Biophys. Acta* 961: 30–37.
Hoppel CL & Brady L (1985) *The Enzymes of Biological Membranes* 2: 139–175.
Hoppel CL & Genuth SM (1980) *Am. J. Physiol.* 238: E409–E415.
Hoppel CL & Tomec RJ (1972) *J. Biol. Chem.* 247: 832–841.
Indiveri C, Tonazzi A & Palmieri F (1990) *Biochim. Biophys. Acta* 1020: 81–86.
Kerner J & Bieber LL (1985) *Prep. Biochem.* 15: 237–257.
Kerner J & Bieber LL (1990) *Biochemistry* 29: 4326–4334.
Kondrup J & Grunnet N (1973) *Biochem. J.* 132: 373–379.
Kopec B & Fritz IB (1971) *Can. J. Biochem.* 49: 941–948.
Kopec B & Fritz IB (1973) *J. Biol. Chem.* 248: 4069–4074.
Leighton F, Bergseth S, Rortveit T et al (1989) *J. Biol. Chem.* 264: 10347–10350.
Lilly K, Bugaisky GE, Umeda PK & Bieber LL (1990) *Arch. Biochem. Biophys.* 280: 167–174.
Long CS, Haller RG, Foster DW & McGarry JD (1982) *Neurology* 32: 663–666.
Lund H (1987) *Biochim. Biophys. Acta* 918: 67–75.
Lund H & Woldegiorgis G (1986) *Biochim. Biophys. Acta* 878: 243–249.
Lysiak W, Toth PP, Suelter CH & Bieber LL (1986) *J. Biol. Chem.* 261: 13698–13703.
Lysiak W, Lilly K, DiLisa F et al (1988) *J. Biol. Chem.* 263: 1151–1156.
McGarry JD & Foster DW (1980) *Annu. Rev. Biochem.* 49: 395–420.
McGarry JD, Mannaerts GP & Foster DW (1977) *J. Clin. Invest.* 60: 265–270.

McGarry JD, Robles-Valdes C & Foster DW (1975) *Proc. Natl. Acad. Sci. USA* 72: 4385–4388.

McGarry JD, Woeltje KF, Kuwajima M & Foster DW (1989) *Diabetes/Metab. Rev.* 5: 271–284.

Miotto G, Venerado R & Siliprandi N (1989) *Biochem. Biophys. Research Commun.* 158: 797–802.

Miyazawa S, Ozasa H, Furuta S et al (1983a) *J. Biochem.* 93: 439–451.

Miyazawa S, Ozasa H, Furuta S et al (1983b) *J. Biochem.* 93: 453–459.

Miyazawa S, Ozasa H, Osumi T & Hashimoto T (1983c) *J. Biochem.* 94: 529–542.

Murthy MSR & Pande SV (1987a) *Proc. Natl Acad. Sci. USA* 84: 378–382.

Murthy MSR & Pande SV (1987b) *Biochem. J.* 248: 727–733.

Murthy MSR & Pande SV (1990) *Biochem. J.* 268: 599–604.

Ontko JA & Johns ML (1980) *Biochem. J.* 192: 959–962.

Ozasa H, Miyazawa S & Osumi T (1983) *J. Biochem.* 94: 543–549.

Pande SV (1975) *Proc. Natl Acad. Sci. USA* 72: 883–887.

Pande SV & Parvin R (1980) *Biochim. Biophys. Acta* 617: 363–370.

Paul HS & Adibi SA (1978) *Am. J. Physiol.* 234: E494–E499.

Pearson DJ & Tubbs PK (1967) *Biochem. J.* 105: 953–963.

Ramsay RR (1989) *Biochem. J.* 249: 239–245.

Ramsay RR & Tubbs PK (1974) *Biochem. Soc. Trans.* 2: 1285–1286.

Ramsay RR & Tubbs PK (1975) *FEBS Lett.* 54: 21–25.

Ramsay RR, Derrick JP, Friend AS & Tubbs PK (1987) *Biochem. J.* 244: 271–278.

Saggerson ED & Carpenter CA (1981) *FEBS Lett.* 129: 225–228.

Saggerson ED & Carpenter CA (1983) *Biochem. J.* 210: 591–597.

Sahlin K (1990) *Acta Physiol. Scand.* 1318: 259–262.

Spedding M & Mir AK (1987) *Br. J. Pharmacol.* 92: 457–468.

Stakkestad JA & Bremer J (1983) *Biochim. Biophys. Acta* 750: 244–252.

Ueda M, Tanaka A, Horikawa S et al (1984) *Eur. J. Biochem.* 138: 451–457.

Vamecq J, Draye J-P & Brison J (1989) *Am. J. Physiol.* 256: G680–G688.

Woeltje KF, Kuwajima M, Foster DW & McGarry JD (1987) *J. Biol. Chem.* 262: 9822–9827.

2

CARNITINE TRANSPORT

E.P. Brass

Carnitine is ubiquitous in mammalian tissues; its role in fatty acid oxidation and metabolic homeostasis is well understood and critical for normal cellular function. The normal physiological functions of carnitine are dependent on a complex, integrated series of transport systems that ensure adequate carnitine content in tissues, and appropriate distribution of the carnitine in intracellular compartments. The need for this transport system is based on several features of normal carnitine homeostasis:

1. Carnitine is a quaternary amine and thus would not be expected to diffuse readily through lipid membranes.
2. The liver is the dominant site for carnitine biosynthesis, yet carnitine is required by all tissues.
3. Carnitine is a dietary constituent and absorption from the gastrointestinal tract is potentially important.
4. The carnitine content of tissue is much greater than that in plasma and hence a concentration gradient must be established and maintained (Table 1).
5. As a small, water-soluble molecule in plasma, carnitine is readily filtered by the renal glomerulus and reabsorption is required to prevent excessive urinary carnitine losses.
6. Carnitine must function in the mitochondrial matrix as well as the extramitochondrial space, and thus must cross the permeability barrier of the inner mitochondrial membrane.

21

L-Carnitine and Its Role in Medicine:
From Function to Therapy. ISBN 0–12–253940–0

Each of these requirements is met by one or more cellular carnitine transport systems. Taken together, these systems provide a basis for understanding carnitine homeostasis and the fate of exogenously administered carnitine as a therapeutic agent.

CELL MEMBRANE CARNITINE TRANSPORT

Carnitine influx

Carnitine uptake into cells has been investigated using isolated cells, perfused tissues and in vivo. These experimental strategies have identified saturable transport systems with structural specificity.

TABLE I.
Total carnitine content of plasma, tissue and urine in man*

Compartment	Total carnitine content	Reference
Plasma	46 μM	Hoppel and Genuth (1980)
Liver	6 nmol mg^{-1} protein	DeSousa et al (1988)
	0.94 μmol g^{-1} wet weight	Boudin et al (1976)
Heart	1.26 μmol g^{-1} wet weight	Suzuki et al (1982)
	5.7 μmol g^{-1} non-collagenous protein	Pierpont et al (1989)
	0.63 μmol g^{-1} weight†	Hoppel (1990)
Kidney	0.52 μmol g^{-1} wet weight†	Hoppel (1990)
Skeletal muscle— vastus lateralis	25.6 μmol g^{-1} non-collagenous protein	Cederblad et al (1976)
	4.21 μmol g^{-1} wet weight	Lennon et al (1986)
Sperm	1100 pmol 10^{-6} sperm	Golan et al (1986)
Urine	125 μmol day^{-1}	Hoppel (1990)

*Values are for adults on their usual diets.
†Autopsy samples.

Tissues differ in the properties of the transport systems (Table 2) and are discussed individually below. It is important to recognize that, in general, experimental studies have used radiolabelled carnitine uptake as a measure of transport. This methodology would not distinguish between unilateral influx and carnitine exchange with an intracellular molecule (i.e. carnitine, acylcarnitine or butyrobetaine) unless specific controls were performed. Earlier studies should be viewed with this in mind.

Intestine

Dietary carnitine provides an important source of the compound for the body (Feller and Rudman, 1988). As carnitine is a quaternary amine, carrier-mediated absorption from the gastrointestinal lumen was postulated. Further, as an adverse carnitine concentration gradient from the lumen into the enterocyte might exist, active transport was also anticipated in early studies. Thus, Shaw et al (1983) using everted rat intestinal rings and sacs demonstrated a saturable component for ^{14}C-carnitine uptake. Transport of carnitine was decreased by inhibition of metabolic activity by anoxia, dinitrophenol and cyanide, suggestive of an active transport process. Carnitine uptake was inhibited when sodium was removed from the medium, and was also inhibited by D-carnitine and acetylcarnitine. Anatomically, carnitine transport was demonstrated in the duodenum and jejunum, but not the ileum. Kinetically, the transport system was best described as a two compartment system with K_ms of 200 and 300 μM. In common with other studies of carnitine transport a large, non-saturable component of carnitine uptake, presumably representing passive diffusion was demonstrable. At physiological pH carnitine forms a zwitterion with net neutral charge, potentially permitting passive diffusion. This apparent passive diffusion may reflect cell damage in the in vitro systems or reflect the high carnitine concentrations used to establish complete saturation plots. However, the significance of diffusion of carnitine as a mechanism for carnitine uptake is presumed to be small under physiological conditions, but may assume importance during administration of carnitine therapeutically.

Several laboratories have studied the intestinal transport of carnitine since the publication of Shaw and colleagues. Gross and Henderson (1984) characterized a saturable carnitine transport system in rat upper jejunum. This transport system also mediated uptake of D-carnitine and acetylcarnitine, and these compounds inhibited carnitine uptake. Gudjonsson et al (1985a,b) used segmented perfusion techniques and

TABLE 2.

Characteristics of tissue carnitine uptake

Tissue	K_m	Characteristics	Inhibition	Reference
Intestine	200 μM	Na-dependent, active	Dinitrophenol	Shaw et al (1983)
	1000 μM	Partially saturable	—	Gundjonssen et al (1985b)
	6 μM	Facilitated transport, Na-dependent	D-Carnitine	Gross et al (1986)
	—	No transport system	—	Li et al (1990)
Liver	5 mM	Active	Butyrobetaine K_m and $K_i = 0.8$ mM	Christiansen and Bremer (1976)
	4 mM	Na-dependent	Dinitrophenol, cyanide	Kispal et al (1987a)
Kidney	55 μM	Na-dependent	Butyrobetaine, D-carnitine	Rebouche and Mack (1984)
Heart	4.8 μM	Temperature-dependent	Fluoride, N-ethylmaleimide	Bohmer et al (1977)
	60 μM	Na-independent	Dinitrophenol, D-carnitine	Bahl et al (1981)
	24 μM	—	Mersalyl, D-carnitine	Vary and Neely (1982a)
Skeletal muscle	60 μM	Na-dependent	Dinitrophenol	Rebouche (1977)
	2 μM	—	—	Rebouche and Engle (1982)
Fibroblasts	6 μM	Temperature-dependent	N-ethylmaleimide, D-carnitine	Carnicero et al (1982)
	3 μM	—	—	Stanley et al (1990)

intraluminal administration of carnitine to characterize intestinal carnitine absorption. These systems are more physiological but require uptake into the intestine and efflux into the blood, and hence are more complex. Gudjonsson demonstrated partially-saturable uptake of carnitine with a K_m of 1000 μM in jejunum and 1300 μM in ileum. A significant amount of the ^{3}H-carnitine administered intraluminally was esterified when identified in blood. This suggested rapid esterification in passage through the intestinal mucosa, or in the liver with release of acylcarnitine. A role for intestinal transport in an enterohepatic circulation of carnitine was also postulated by the authors.

Recent studies have raised additional questions concerning intestinal carnitine transport. Gross et al (1986) used guinea-pig enterocytes to define a temperature- and sodium-dependent transport system for carnitine. However, no concentration gradient for carnitine was established, and esterification was required for cellular carnitine accumulation. This suggested a facilitated transport system, rather than active transport. The transport system had a low K_m (6 μM) and was inhibited by D-carnitine and butyrobetaine. Importantly, isolated enterocytes will lose their normal polarity and luminal transport would not be distinguishable from a blood-orientated system. Most recently, Li et al (1990) have found no evidence of a carnitine transport system in intestinal brush border vesicles.

Therapeutically, orally administered carnitine is given in quantities far in excess of physiological/nutritional amounts. Systemic bioavailability, reflecting intestinal absorption and hepatic first-pass elimination, is relatively low with values of 5–20% reported (Harper et al, 1988; Segre et al, 1988; Hoppel et al, 1990). This low bioavailability suggests that intestinal absorption represents a barrier to oral delivery of carnitine to systemic tissues.

Liver

The liver plays a unique role in carnitine homeostasis. Once dietary or orally administered carnitine is absorbed, the liver will be exposed to the carnitine via the portal vein prior to systemic distribution or elimination. Additionally, the liver is the major source of butyrobetaine hydroxylation to form carnitine in the final step of carnitine biosynthesis. Thus hepatic carnitine transport will be critical for whole body carnitine homeostasis.

Christiansen and Bremer (1976) demonstrated saturable uptake of carnitine by isolated rat hepatocytes with a K_m of 5.6 mM. This transport was temperature-dependent, occurred against a concentration gradient and was inhibited by dinitrophenol. Butyrobetaine was transported with a K_m of 0.5 mM, and inhibited carnitine transport with a K_i of 0.8 mM. Both butyrobetaine and carnitine uptake were inhibited by several compounds with equal K_is indicating a single transport system was involved in the uptake of the compounds. Thus, this transport might be considered a butyrobetaine transporter involved in carnitine biosynthesis, with carnitine as an alternative substrate of secondary importance under physiological conditions. Extracellular acetylcarnitine is utilized for hepatic metabolic processes (Farrell et al, 1986) but neither octanoyl- nor palmitoylcarnitine are efficiently metabolized by isolated hepatocytes (Brass, 1989).

Carnitine uptake by perfused rat liver has demonstrated properties similar to those in hepatocytes, with a K_m of 4 mM and partial inhibition by cyanide and dinitrophenol (Kispal et al, 1987a). Carnitine transport was sodium-dependent and inhibited by lithium. The perfused rat liver preferentially transported some acylcarnitines over carnitine from the perfusate. Hepatic carnitine content per gram is altered by fasting (Pearson and Tubbs, 1967; McGarry et al, 1975; Brass and Hoppel, 1978) and diabetes (McGarry et al, 1975), and potential regulation of hepatic carnitine uptake has been studied in the perfused liver system (Kispal et al, 1987b). Liver isolated from fasted rats demonstrated a lower K_m for carnitine uptake than liver from fed rats (2.59 mM vs 4.2 mM) with the maximal rate of transport unchanged. This change in K_m resulted in increased rates of carnitine uptake at equivalent perfusate carnitine concentrations in the physiological range. Glucagon increased carnitine uptake in livers from fed or fasted rats, while insulin decreased carnitine transport when added to perfusions of livers from fasted rats. The mechanism of glucagon and insulin action on carnitine transport is unknown, and may be secondary to altered cellular metabolism induced by the hormones. The physiological importance of the regulation of hepatic carnitine uptake in vivo has yet to be elucidated.

Kidney

Carnitine is a water-soluble, non protein-bound molecule and is readily filtered by the renal glomerulus. This results in a filtered carnitine load of 4 μmol min^{-1} or 5760 μmol day^{-1}, in contrast to the 125 μmol day^{-1} typically excreted in man. Thus, a renal tubule transport system is essential to prevent excess urinary carnitine losses. Rebouche and Mack (1984) demonstrated saturable carnitine transport in rat renal brush border membrane vesicles. Transport was sodium-dependent with a K_m of 55 μM. This K_m is consistent with the renal threshold of approximately 80 μM observed in the isolated rat kidney (Gross and Henderson, 1984). Reabsorption of carnitine by the kidney was inhibited by D-carnitine, butyrobetaine and acylcarnitines (Rebouche and Mack, 1984).

In man, the renal reabsorption of carnitine results in a fractional carnitine excretion of less than 5% (Bernardini et al, 1985). In Fanconi's syndrome, the fractional excretion is markedly increased to 20–30% (Ohtani et al, 1984; Bernardini et al, 1985; Steinmann et al, 1987). Fractional excretion of acylcarnitines is greater than for carnitine in Fanconi's syndrome (Steinmann et al, 1987), but this may reflect renal production and secretion of acylcarnitines (Hokland and Bremer, 1986). The mechanism of the renal carnitine wasting in Fanconi's syndrome is unknown, but results in hypocarnitinaemia and altered systemic carnitine homeostasis (Bernardini et al, 1985).

Heart

Myocardial tissue is dependent on fatty acid oxidation as an energy source, and hence cellular carnitine availability is critical for normal cardiac function. Human heart cells in culture transported carnitine in a saturable, temperature-dependent manner with a K_m of 4.8 μM (Bohmer et al, 1977). Transport of carnitine was inhibited by fluoride, N-ethylmaleimide and butyrobetaine, but not by cyanide or dinitrophenol (Bohmer et al, 1977; Molstad et al, 1977). In contrast, carnitine transport by adult rat myocytes demonstrated a K_m of 60 μM and inhibition by nitrophenol as well as butyrobetaine and D-carnitine (Bahl et al, 1981). Carnitine transport by rat myocytes was stimulated by treatment with dibutyryl-cAMP and β-adrenergic agonists (Bahl et al, 1981) in a manner analogous to that caused by glucagon in the liver (Kispal et al, 1987b).

Regulation of myocardial carnitine transport has been studied by Vary and Neely in the perfused rat heart (Vary and Neely, 1982a,b). In this system, transport of carnitine demonstrated a K_m of 24 μM and was inhibited by mersalyl and D-carnitine. Anoxia did not inhibit carnitine uptake, suggesting that ATP was not required. Addition of palmitate to the perfusate stimulated carnitine uptake by 60%, with the rate of carnitine transport related to the tissue palmitoylcarnitine content (Vary and Neely, 1982b). Altered myocardial carnitine content has been noted in a number of disease states (Suzuki et al, 1982; Pierpoint et al, 1989). Recently, El Alaoui-Talibi and Moravec (1989) have reported an increase in the K_m for carnitine in volume overloaded rat hearts (from 83 μM to 125 μM). However, whether changes in myocardial carnitine transport represent primary mechanisms in these disorders, or reflect secondary processes remains to be clarified.

Skeletal muscle

Skeletal muscle carnitine uptake has been studied in cultured muscle cells (Rebouche and Engel, 1982), in muscle strips (Rebouche, 1977) and in vivo (Rebouche, 1990; Miller et al, 1990). Carnitine transport in muscle strips was sodium-dependent and saturable with a K_m of 60 μM. In contrast, cultured muscle cells demonstrated a high affinity transport with a K_m of 1.9 μM, as well as a lower affinity component with a K_m of 80 μM. The relevance of these transport kinetics for in vivo carnitine handling was recently summarized by Rebouche (1990). Reviewing a series of studies he emphasized that skeletal muscle carnitine content was only dependent on plasma carnitine concentrations at low ($<$70 μM) concentrations. This was consistent with saturation of muscle uptake at higher carnitine concentrations.

Fibroblasts

Fibroblasts are a readily available source of human tissue, and have proved valuable in the diagnosis of a number of inherited metabolic disorders. Fibroblasts contain a saturable, temperature-dependent carnitine transport system (Carnicero et al, 1982) with a high affinity (K_m = 6–8 μM). Transport was inhibited by N-ethylmaleimide and D-carnitine. In at least some patients with a defect in carnitine transport, the defect is expressed in the patient's fibroblasts (Stanley et al, 1990).

Discussion and summary

Carnitine transport systems for influx from extracellular fluids have been identified and characterized in all tissues in which carnitine plays a physiological role. Most data suggest that these systems are sodium-dependent, active transport mechanisms, but definitive observations are not available. Kinetically, the liver carnitine uptake system is strikingly different from that in kidney, heart or skeletal muscle. This distinction has been further demonstrated in the cases of primary carnitine deficiency reported by Stanley et al (1990). These cases demonstrated low carnitine concentrations in plasma, liver and muscle. Following carnitine therapy, urinary carnitine fractional excretions were approximately one, indicating no reabsorption. With aggressive therapy liver carnitine content, but not muscle carnitine content, could be returned to near normal. Fibroblasts from the patients demonstrated defective carnitine uptake. Thus, the transport of carnitine into liver was unaffected, while muscle, fibroblasts and kidney transport were impaired.

The properties of normal tissue carnitine uptake will have a major influence on the fate of carnitine administered therapeutically in the absence of a primary carnitine transport defect. The limited ability of carnitine to transverse the intestine to the blood contributes to a low systemic bioavailability after oral carnitine administration (Harper et al, 1988; Segre et al, 1988; Hoppel et al, 1990). Once the carnitine has reached the systemic circulation, carnitine delivered to the kidney in excess of the reabsorption maximum will be eliminated in the urine. Thus, particularly after intravenous administration, the majority of the carnitine reaching the blood is rapidly eliminated (Harper et al, 1988). Uptake into tissues by the transport systems discussed above will be determined by the K_m and V_{max} of the transport and the plasma carnitine concentration. The normal plasma carnitine concentration is sufficient almost completely to saturate transport into skeletal muscle and heart, and hence these compartments are relatively refractory to administration of carnitine (Rebouche, 1990; Miller et al, 1990). However, the liver transport system has a high K_m and the hepatic carnitine content is readily increased by exogenous carnitine (Brass and Hoppel, 1980; Miller et al, 1990). The capacity of liver to increase its carnitine content may also contribute to the low systemic bioavailability of carnitine, as the absorbed carnitine reaches the liver through the portal circulation prior to reaching the systemic circulation.

Carnitine efflux

A second component of tissue carnitine homeostasis is efflux of carnitine from tissue to plasma. While the concentration gradient will favour carnitine efflux under physiological conditions, the plasma membrane represents a permeability barrier.

Rebouche (1977) reported that carnitine efflux from rat extensor digitorum longus was biphasic. One component of the efflux appeared to be leakage from damaged muscle. However, the second component was markedly inhibited when the temperature was decreased from 37° C to 0° C, suggesting a biochemically-mediated efflux. Sandor and colleagues have characterized carnitine efflux more extensively using the perfused rat liver (Sandor et al, 1985). Importantly, by loading the liver with carnitine, they demonstrated that carnitine efflux was saturable with respect to tissue carnitine content (K_m = 0.27 mM). Efflux was not energy-dependent, nor was it inhibited by oubain (Sandor et al, 1985). However, efflux but not influx was inhibited by mersalyl, indicating that these two transport systems were independent (Sandor et al, 1985). Further, hepatic carnitine efflux was subject to regulation, as carnitine export was decreased in livers from fasted animals as compared with controls (Sandor et al, 1985). Hokland (1988) confirmed efflux of carnitine from the perfused liver and demonstrated that isovalerylcarnitine and acetylcarnitine were transported out of the liver at rates 2.5 and 2.0 times, respectively, that of carnitine. Efflux of acylcarnitines from tissue may represent a mechanism for eliminating poorly metabolizable acyl moieties, or to facilitate interorgan transport of acyl groups. Carnitine is also present in bile (Hamilton and Hahn, 1987), suggesting that export of carnitine from the hepatocyte through the canalicular membrane is also possible.

Carnitine and acylcarnitines in urine might arise from carnitine filtered but not reabsorbed, or from efflux of carnitines from renal tubular cells. Hokland and Bremer (1986) using the isolated rat kidney demonstrated that significant amounts of carnitine and acylcarnitines present in urine were generated from renal metabolism. For example, when the kidney was perfused with carnitine and α-ketoisocaproate, branched-chain acylcarnitines comprised 21% of the urinary carnitine vs. 3% in the perfusate. The appearance of products of renal carnitine metabolism in the urine has important implications for interpreting the urinary carnitine pool as reflecting systemic metabolism. Additionally, the excretion of renal carnitine and acylcarnitines in urine implies that absolute carnitine reabsorption in the tubule has been underestimated as the urinary carnitine is not simply filtered, non-reabsorbed carnitine.

Carnitine exchange

Several early observations suggested that carnitine might cross tissue plasma membranes by mechanisms not readily explained by the influx or efflux mechanisms discussed above. While studying carnitine transport in the rat extensor digitorum longus, Rebouche (1977) noted that when the muscle was preincubated with ³H-carnitine, efflux of tritium was accelerated by adding 50 μM carnitine to the extracellular fluid, though Hokland (1988) failed to demonstrate a similar increase in carnitine efflux in the perfused liver. Calvin and Tubbs (1976) demonstrated that a carnitine–acetylcarnitine exchange system contributed to carnitine transport in sperm. This exchange, which also carried butyrobetaine, was analogous to the carnitine–acylcarnitine translocase of mitochondria (see below). In vivo, following intravenous administration of carnitine to rats there is a rapid (<5 min) appearance of acylcarnitines in the plasma (Brass and Hoppel, 1980). Observations of this type suggested that extracellular carnitine could enter tissues in exchange for intracellular carnitine or acylcarnitines.

Molstad (1980) systematically characterized the ability of carnitine, and structurally similar compounds, to stimulate the release of ^{3}H-carnitine from human heart cells in culture. Extracellular L-carnitine (100 μM) stimulated carnitine efflux by 50–200%. Betaine, D-carnitine, butyrobetaine and acetylcarnitine also increased the rate of carnitine efflux. Sartorelli and colleagues have pursued these observations in the rat heart slice model (Sartorelli et al, 1985a,b). They demonstrated that carnitine and acetylcarnitine were exchanged between the intra- and extracellular compartments (Sartorelli et al, 1985a,b). This exchange was inhibited by both N-ethymaleimide and mersalyl, but not by fluoride, cyanide or azide (Sartorelli et al, 1985a). Additionally, the exchange reaction functioned with both carnitine and butyrobetaine (deoxycarnitine) as substrates (Sartorelli et al, 1985b). An intracellular butyrobetaine–extracellular carnitine exchange might have physiological importance as the precursor for carnitine biosynthesis; butyrobetaine, generated in muscle, would exchange with the final biosynthetic product, carnitine. Butyrobetaine would then be available to the liver for hydroxylation. The authors also noted (Sartorelli et al, 1985b) that the intracellular–extracellular butyrobetaine gradient might provide the energy for carnitine influx through the exchange, and would explain equivocal results in some studies attempting to document unidirectional active transport. However, any model in which the exchange system plays a major role in muscle carnitine accumulation must be reconciled with the report of Stanley et al (1990) in which a patient with an apparently selective defect in unilateral carnitine transport had extremely low muscle carnitine content. The K_m for exchange with butyrobetaine across heart plasma membrane was 20 μM for carnitine and 39 μM for acetylcarnitine (Siliprandi et al, 1989). When carnitine was in the intracellular compartment, acetylcarnitine and propionylcarnitine promoted exchange with K_ms of 13 μM and 60 μM respectively.

The carnitine exchange mechanism appears to be functional in vivo. Following administration of carnitine to rats, butyrobetaine urinary excretion was increased (Sartorelli et al, 1989). Conversely, when butyrobetaine was administered intraperitoneally to rats, urinary carnitine excretion was increased and carnitine content in heart, skeletal muscle and kidney (but not liver) were decreased (Sartorelli et al, 1989). As discussed above, when carnitine is administered intravenously the majority of the carnitine is recovered in the urine (Harper et al, 1988; Miller et al, 1990). However, when ^{14}C-carnitine was injected in doses to yield plasma concentrations of approximately 500 μM, the specific activity of the urinary carnitine (after correction for basal excretion rates) was only 72% of that in the injection solutions (Miller et al, 1990). This suggested that the urinary excretion of endogenous, intracellular carnitine excretion was enhanced by high plasma carnitine concentrations. These in vivo observations are also consistent with carnitine–carnitine or butyrobetaine exchange between tissues and plasma. The exchange mechanism may also contribute to the tissue depletion of carnitine that occurs following administration of D-carnitine in vivo (Negaro et al, 1987; Sartorelli et al, 1989).

While there is good evidence supporting carnitine exchange systems in tissues, the role of exchange system in normal carnitine homeostasis remains unclear. The exchange system could contribute to either net carnitine accumulation (i.e. carnitine–butyrobetaine exchange) or exchange of carnitine for accumulating acylcarnitines without net change in total carnitine content. The dynamics of the reactions will depend on the relative carnitine, butyrobetaine and acylcarnitine contents in tissue and plasma, and their quantitative impact determined by the kinetics of the unidirectional transporters under the same conditions. Further research is required to define these relationships.

INTRACELLULAR CARNITINE TRANSPORT

Mitochondrial translocase

Fatty acid β-oxidation occurs primarily in the mitochondrial matrix. Long-chain acylcarnitines generated outside of the mitochondrial inner membrane must thus transverse this membrane. In the matrix, the conversion of the acylcarnitine to the acyl CoA will generate intramitochondrial carnitine. Thus, a mechanism must exist for acylcarnitine mitochondrial transport, and for carnitine to leave the matrix to replenish the cytosolic carnitine pool.

Ramsay and Tubbs (1974) using ox-heart mitochondria loaded with ^{14}C-carnitine demonstrated that incubation with extramitochondrial carnitine or acetylcarnitine increased the efflux of radioactivity without changing the mitochondrial carnitine content. The mitochondrial carnitine–acylcarnitine translocase has been subsequently well characterized (Pande, 1975; Ramsay and Tubbs, 1975, 1976; Pande and Parvin, 1976). The translocase is temperature (Pande, 1975), but not energy-dependent (Pande and Parvin, 1976). The system is saturable with respect to extramitochondrial carnitine with K_ms of 5.3 mM and 1.0 mM reported in ox-heart (Ramsay and Tubbs, 1976) and rat-heart (Idell-Wenger, 1981) mitochondria respectively. There is no cation requirement, but the system is inhibited by mersalyl and N-ethylmaleimide (Pande and Parvin, 1976). Undirectional carnitine transport across the inner mitochondrial membrane has also been described (Pande and Parvin, 1980a). Unidirectional transport occurs down a concentration gradient, and while the rates are slow, the process in inhibited by the same inhibitors active against translocase-mediated exchange.

An important aspect of mitochondrial carnitine transport is its potential regulation in intact cells. Mitochondrial translocase activity can be increased by increasing the intramitochondrial carnitine content (Pande and Parvin, 1979). This may explain the increase in translocase activity observed in liver mitochondria isolated from fasted (Pande and Parvin, 1979), diabetic (Pande and Parvin, 1979) and clofibrate-treated rats (Pande and Parvin, 1980b). Additionally, the cellular distribution of carnitine can be altered. With ischaemia, the percentage of total myocardial carnitine present in the mitochondria increases from 8% to 25% (Idell-Wenger et al, 1978). The mechanism for this net transfer of carnitine into mitochondria is unknown.

Thus, the mitochondrial translocase has a key role in normal carnitine function. Many of its properties are analogous to those of the plasma membrane carnitine–carnitine exchange system discussed above. In the case of sperm, the properties of 'cellular exchange' were similar to that in isolated mitochondria indicating that mitochondrial compartmentalization may confuse the interpretation of cellular exchange experiments, or that two similar exchange systems exist in the plasma and inner mitochondrial membranes.

FUNCTION OF CARNITINE TRANSPORT IN VIVO

As discussed above, cells contain a network of transport systems for carnitine which function in concert to maintain carnitine's concentration at its sites of action. The properties of these systems determine many of the characteristics of in vivo carnitine homeostasis and the fate of exogenous carnitine. The efflux and influx kinetics will determine the steady-state tissue carnitine content at a given plasma concentration. These parameters also contribute to the tissue's individual turnover characteristics (Table 3). Both kidney and liver have significant net carnitine efflux systems, and these compartments have turnover times one order of magnitude lower than heart or skeletal muscle. The slow turnover of muscle carnitine and the effectiveness of renal reabsorption result in a slow whole-body turnover.

FUTURE DIRECTIONS

As the components of the carnitine transport system have been identified, including influx, efflux and exchange systems, questions have been raised regarding regulation and the relative importance of these components under physiological and pathophysiological conditions. Of particular importance is the relative role of unidirectional vs. exchange plasma membrane systems. It is attractive to speculate that as carnitine is imported to tissues that butyrobetaine or poorly metabolized, accumulating acylcarnitines might be exported, but evidence for this function is lacking.

Understanding of the transport system is also critical for therapeutic considerations. How can carnitine best be delivered to a specific tissue? What is the best way to enhance tissue acylcarnitine elimination in conditions such as propionic acidaemia? Can carnitine influx be

TABLE 3.
Turnover of endogenous carnitine in the rat

Compartment	Turnover	Reference
Kidney	0.4 h	Brooks & McIntosh (1975)
Liver	1.3 h	Brooks & McIntosh (1975)
Heart	21 h	Brooks & McIntosh (1975)
	60 h	Vary & Neely (1982a)
Quadriceps muscle	100 h	Brooks & McIntosh (1975)
Whole rat	7% per day	Cederblad & Lindstedt (1976)
	355 h	Mehlman et al (1969)

stimulated and efflux inhibited? Are there advantages of acylcarnitine administration as a method to increase intracellular carnitine content from a transport perspective? As the intracellular carnitine pool is near equilibrium with respect to the acylcarnitine–carnitine distribution (Brass and Hoppel, 1980), once the acylcarnitine was imported by the cell carnitine would rapidly be generated. The foundation to address these provocative and important issues has now been developed as the mechanisms of carnitine transport have been delineated over the past 20 years, and the tools for experimental approaches provided by analytical and biochemical advances.

REFERENCES

Bahl J, Navin T & Manian AA (1981) Circ. Res. 48: 378–385.
Bernardini L, Rizzo WB, Dalakas M et al (1985) J. Clin. Invest. 75: 1124–1130.
Bohmer T, Eiklid K & Jonsen J (1977) Biochim. Biophys. Acta 465: 627–633.
Boudin G, Mikol J, Guillard A & Engel AG (1976) J. Neurol. Sci. 30: 313–325.
Brass EP (1989) Biochim. Biophys. Acta 1003: 209–212.
Brass EP & Hoppel CL (1978) J. Biol. Chem. 252: 2688–2693.
Brass EP & Hoppel CL (1980) Biochem. J. 190: 495–504.
Brooks DE & McIntosh JEA (1975) Biochem. J. 148: 439–445.
Calvin J & Tubbs PK (1976) J. Reprod. Fert. 48: 417–420.
Carnicero HH, England S & Seifter S (1982) Arch. Biochem. Biophys. 215: 78–88.
Cederblad G & Lindstedt S (1976) Arch. Biochem. Biophys. 175: 173–180.
Cederblad G, Bylund AC, Holm J & Schersten T (1976) Scand. J. Clin. Lab. Invest. 36: 547–552.
Christiansen RZ & Bremer J (1976) Biochim. Biophys. Acta 448: 562–577.
De Sousa C, Leung NWY, Chalmers RA & Peters TJ (1988) Clin. Sci. 75: 437–440.
El Alaoui-Talibi Z & Moravec J (1989) Biochim. Biophys. Acta 1003: 109–114.
Farrell S, Vogel J & Bieber LL (1986) Biochim. Biophys. Acta 876: 175–177.
Feller AG & Rudman D (1988) J. Nutr. 118: 541–547.
Golan R, Shalev DP, Wasserzug O et al (1986) J. Reprod. Fert. 78: 287–293.
Gross CJ & Henderson LM (1984) Biochim. Biophys. Acta 772: 209–219.
Gross CJ, Henderson LM & Savaiano DA (1986) Biochim. Biophys. Acta 886: 425–433.
Gudjonsson H, Li BUK, Shug AL & Olsen WA (1985a) Am. J. Physiol. 248: G313–G319.
Gudjonsson H, Li BUK, Shug AL & Olsen WA (1985b) Gastroenterology 88: 1880–1887.
Hamilton JJ & Hahn P (1987) Can. J. Physiol. Pharmacol. 65: 1816–1820.
Harper P, Elwin CE & Cederblad G (1988) Eur. J. Clin. Pharmacol. 35: 69–75.
Hokland BM (1988) Biochim. Biophys. Acta 961: 234–241.
Hokland BM & Bremer J (1986) Biochim. Biophys. Acta 886: 223–230.
Hoppel CL (1990) In Hommes FA (ed.) Techniques in Diagnostic Human Biochemical Genetics. A Laboratory Manual, pp 309–326. New York: Allen R. Liss.

Hoppel CL & Genuth SM (1980) *Am. J. Physiol.* 238: E409–E415.
Hoppel C, Floyd R, Albers L et al (1990) *Clin. Res.* 38: 833A.
Idell-Wenger JA (1981) *J. Biol. Chem.* 256: 5597–5603.
Idell-Wenger JA, Grotyohann LW & Neely JR (1978) *J. Biol. Chem.* 253: 4310–4318.
Kispal G, Melegh B, Alkonyi I & Sandor A (1987a) *Biochim. Biophys. Acta* 896: 96–102.
Kispal G, Melegh B & Sandor A (1987b) *Biochim. Biophys. Acta* 929: 226–228.
Lennon DLF, Shrago E, Madden M et al (1986) *Am. J. Clin. Nutr.* 43: 234–238.
Li BUK, Bummer PM, Hamilton JW et al (1990) *Dig. Dis. Sci.* 35: 333–339.
McGarry JD, Robles-Valdez C & Foster DW (1975) *Proc. Natl Acad. Sci. USA* 72: 4385–4388.
Mehlman MA, Kader MMA & Therriault DG (1969) *Life Sci.* 8: 465–472.
Miller LG, Ruff LJ & Brass EP (1990) *FASEB J.* 4: A801.
Molstad P (1980) *Biochim. Biophys. Acta* 597: 166–173.
Molstad P, Bohmer T & Eiklid K (1977) *Biochim. Biophys. Acta* 471: 296–304.
Negaro CE, Ji LL, Schauer JE et al (1987) *J. Appl. Physiol.* 63: 315–321.
Ohtani Y, Nishiyama S & Matsuda I (1984) *Neurology* 34: 977–979.
Pande SV (1975) *Proc. Natl Acad. Sci. USA* 72: 883–887.
Pande SV & Parvin R (1976) *J. Biol. Chem.* 251: 6683–6691.
Pande SV & Parvin R (1979) *J. Biol. Chem.* 254: 5423–5429.
Pande SV & Parvin R (1980a) *J. Biol. Chem.* 255: 2994–3001.
Pande SV & Parvin R (1980b) *Biochim. Biophys. Acta* 617: 363–370.
Pearson DJ & Tubbs PK (1967) *Biochem. J.* 105: 953–963.
Pierpoint MEM, Judd D, Goldenberg IF et al (1989) *Am. J. Cardiol.* 64: 56–60.
Ramsay RR & Tubbs PK (1975) FEBS. Lett. 54: 21–25.
Ramsay RR & Tubbs PK (1976) *Eur. J. Biochem.* 69: 299–303.
Rebouche CJ (1977) *Biochim. Biophys. Acta* 471: 145–155.
Rebouche CJ (1990) *Biochim. Biophys. Acta* 1033: 111–113.
Rebouche CJ & Engel AG (1982) *In Vitro* 18: 495–500.
Rebouche CJ & Mack DL (1984) *Arch. Biochem. Biophys.* 235: 393–402.
Sandor A, Kispal G, Melegh B & Alkonyi I (1985) *Biochim. Biophys. Acta* 835: 83–91.
Sartorelli L, Ciman M & Siliprandi N (1985a) *Ital. J. Biochem.* 34: 275–281.
Sartorelli L, Ciman M, Mantovani G & Siliprandi N (1985b) *Ital. J. Biochem.* 34: 282–287.
Sartorelli L, Mantovani G & Ciman M (1989) *Biochim. Biophys. Acta* 1006: 15–18.
Segre G, Bianchi E, Corsi M et al (1988) *Arzneim. Forsch. Drug. Res.* 38: 1830–1834.
Shaw RD, Li BUK, Hamilton JW, Shug AL & Olsen WA (1983) *Am. J. Physiol.* 245: G376–G381.
Siliprandi N, Sartorelli G, Ciman M & DiLisa F (1989) *Clin. Chim. Acta* 183: 3–12.
Stanley CA, Treem WR, Hale DE & Coates PM (1990) *Prog. Clin. Biol. Res.* 321: 457–464.
Steinmann B, Bachmann C, Colombo JP & Gitzelmann R (1987) *Pediatr. Res.* 21: 201–204.
Suzuki Y, Masumura Y, Kobayashi A et al (1982) *Lancet* i: 116.
Vary TC & Neely JR (1982a) *Am. J. Physiol.* 242: H585–H592.
Vary TC & Neely JR (1982b) *Am. J. Physiol.* 243: H154–H158.

3

METHODS FOR CARNITINE ASSAY

F. Di Lisa, L.L. Bieber, J. Kerner,
R. Menabò, R. Barbato and N. Siliprandi

Until a biological role for carnitine was recognized, standard organic chemistry methods were used for the separation of quaternary amines, followed by crystallization of the isolated carnitine. The biological interest occurred when it was discovered that carnitine is an essential factor for normal growth of the mealworm, *Tenebrio molitor*. This led to the introduction of a biological assay (Carter et al, 1952), but it obviously lacked specificity and precision. Subsequently, the role of carnitine in fatty acid oxidation (Fritz, 1955) and the occurrence of carnitine acetylation (Friedman and Fraenkel, 1955) were demonstrated. To gain further insight into carnitine functions, several methods were developed. Besides chromatographic techniques (Friedman et al, 1955), other procedures were developed for carnitine assay, but many of them were either difficult to master or lacked specificity. For example, in the bromophenol blue reaction (Friedman, 1958), all reactive quaternary compounds other than carnitine must be removed prior to colorimetric determination and the complete conversion of carnitine to its ethyl ester is essential for full colour development. The conversion of carnitine to its periodide derivative (Christianson et al, 1963) showed low recovery when applied to tissue extracts. Nevertheless, several

37

L-Carnitine and Its Role in Medicine:
From Function to Therapy. ISBN 0–12–253940–0

procedures proved to be reliable and were used to measure the activity of the first isolated and partially purified carnitine acetyl transferase (CAT, EC 2.3.1.7) (Fritz et al, 1963). CAT activity was shown by:

1. hydroxamate formation, the so-called Hestrin's reaction (1949) used by Friedman and Frenkel (1955) to quantitatively measure acetylcarnitine;
2. NADH(H$^+$) production utilizing the citrate-condensing system (Ochoa et al, 1951);
3. changes in absorbancy at 232 nm, caused by thioester formation (Beinert et al, 1953);
4. the reaction of the -SH group of coenzyme A (CoA) released from acyl CoA derivatives with 5,5'-dithiobis-(2-nitrobenzoic acid) (DTNB) (Ellman, 1959).

This latter method and the purified CAT used in the enzymatic determination of Marquis and Fritz (1964) represent a breakthrough in the evolution of carnitine assays. Subsequently CAT was crystallized (Chase et al, 1965). The commercial availability of the enzyme (Boehringer Mannheim, Germany and Sigma Chemical, USA) was of great importance to carnitine investigations especially at the clinical level.

The most sensitive method is the so-called 'radioisotopic' or 'radioenzymatic' assay first developed by Cederblad and Lindstedt (1972). However, due to the intrinsic difficulties and the higher cost associated with the handling of radioisotopes, less sensitive spectrophotometric procedures are routinely used in clinical laboratories. Automated spectrophotometric methods have also been described (Seccombe et al, 1976; Cederblad et al, 1986).

Since several pathological states and iatrogenic disorders are associated with the production and the excretion of specific carnitine esters (Roe et al, 1986; Siliprandi et al, 1989), the simple assay of free and total carnitine is no longer satisfactory. The need for sensitive, specific and possibly direct assay of carnitine esters has been recognized. With the exception of acetylcarnitine for which specific enzymatic assays have been described (see later), at present only intricate chromatographic methods allow the separation, and eventually the quantification, of the various carnitine esters of a given sample. When the problem is related to the exact identification of the chemical structure of 'non-physiological' acylcarnitines, such as valproylcarnitine (Millington et al, 1985) or pivaloylcarnitine (Vickers et al, 1985; Melegh et al, 1987), mass spectrometry must be employed. Indeed this powerful technique allowed the initial characterization of disease-specific acylcarnitines (Millington et al, 1984).

STRATEGIES FOR CARNITINE DETERMINATION

In biological systems, carnitine is present as the unesterified carnitine molecule and as acylcarnitines in which an acyl group is esterified through carnitine's hydroxyl group (Bremer, 1983) (Figure 1).

When carnitine is quantified, carnitine and acylcarnitines must be distinguished in order to evaluate correctly the state of the carnitine pool. Several methods have been employed to separate carnitine and acylcarnitines prior to analysis. The most common is the perchloric acid (PCA) fractionation (Pearson et al, 1969). The deproteinization of biological samples with PCA separates the total carnitine content into an acid-soluble fraction and an acid-insoluble fraction which may be removed by centrifugation. Free carnitine and short-chain acylcarnitines remain in the soluble fraction, while long-chain acylcarnitines are precipitated with its protein. The designation of a fraction as long-chain and short-chain acylcarnitine is rather arbitrary. It does not account for the medium-chain acylcarnitines and the partial solubility of some acylcarnitines which can partition into both the long-chain

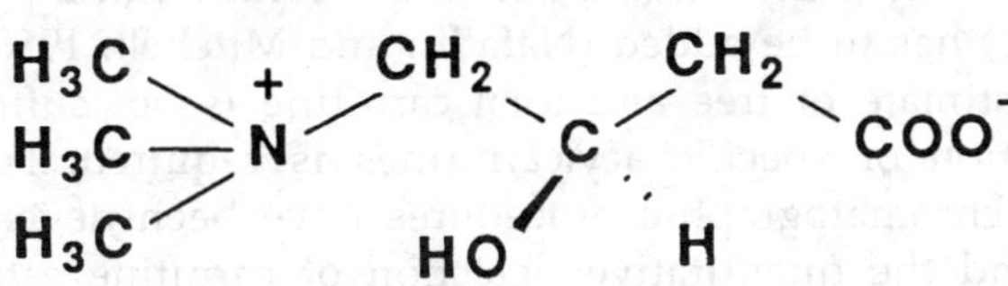

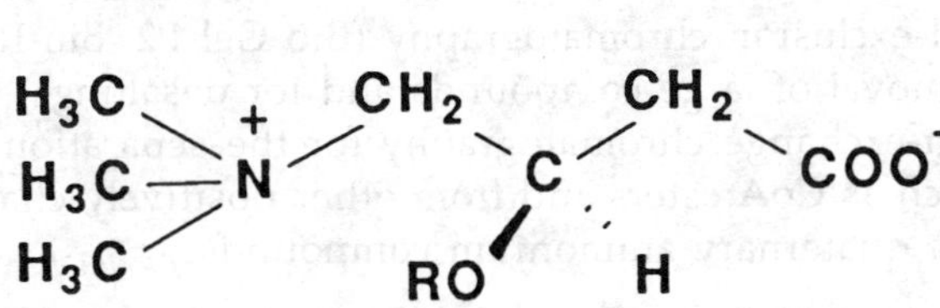

FIGURE 1. Chemical structure of free (a) and esterified (b) carnitine. R, acyl residue [e.g. $C(O)-(CH_2)_n-CH_3$].

and the short-chain acylcarnitine fractions. Inadequate washing of the protein precipitate containing the long-chain acylcarnitine fraction can also cause significant quantitative errors (Fishlock et al, 1984).

After PCA deproteinization, both the supernatant and the pellet can be alkalinized thus releasing free carnitine from its ester linkage to the acyl group. Total carnitine can then be estimated. The alkaline conditions, produced by KOH addition, necessary for the complete release of carnitine from short-chain acyl groups are milder than those used for the acid-insoluble esters. After either PCA or KOH treatment, samples have to be neutralized prior to assay. From the combined acidification and subsequent alkalinization shown in Figure 2, three different values can be obtained, namely free carnitine (A), total acid-soluble carnitine (B) and total acid-insoluble carnitine (C). The difference B − A gives the amount of short-chain acylcarnitines.

Many substances are present in both the pellet and the supernatant fluid after PCA deproteinization which can compromise the carnitine assay. Potential sources of error are: (i) thiol groups for the colorimetric methods, (ii) Coenzyme A (CoA) esters for the radioenzymatic procedures, (iii) metals and high salt concentrations for the activity of carnitine acetyltransferase. Precautions and measures will be described and discussed in the following sections. In order to reduce the salt content, e.g. in urines, extraction with organic solvents (20 volumes of 3:2 chloroform:methanol) appears to be a useful measure (Cederblad et al, 1980). To avoid bacterial contamination of urine during a 24-hour collection, thymol (5 ml of a 10% solution in 2-propanol per litre of urine) has to be added (Nafatlin and Mitchell, 1958).

An estimate of free and total carnitine is not sufficient when the recognition of specific acylcarnitines is required. For this purpose several chromatographic procedures have been developed for separation and the quantitative detection of carnitine esters (Bieber and Kerner, 1986). For these methods, different sample pretreatments have been described to achieve an acceptable degree of purity before the assay. Basically, three separation principles have been applied:

1. solvent extraction to remove salts and other molecules;
2. gel-exclusion chromatography (Bio-Gel P2, Bio-Rad, USA) for removal of large compounds and for desalting;
3. ion-exchange chromatography for the separation from anions such as CoA esters and from other positively-charged species, i.e. quaternary ammonium compounds.

For example, all of these procedures have been utilized for the isolation of α-methyloctanoylcarnitine (Kerner and Bieber, 1985).

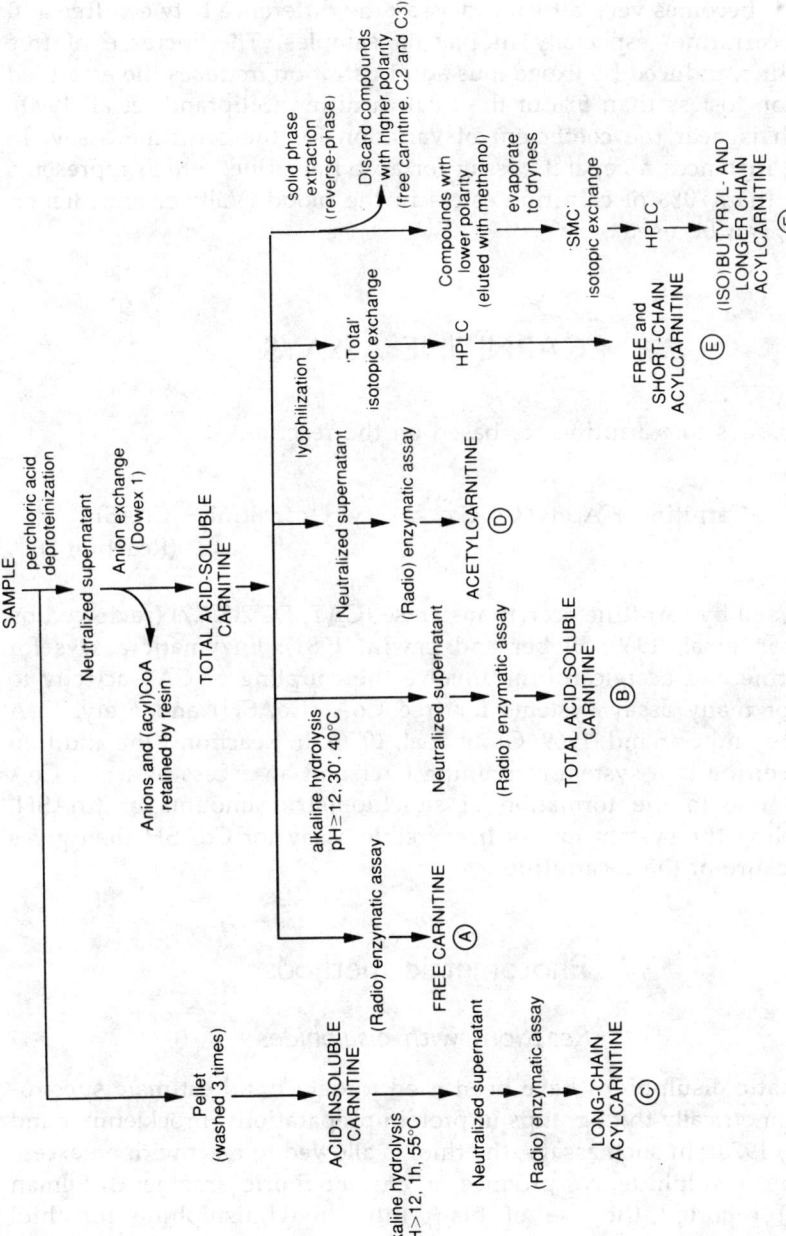

FIGURE 2. Sample work-up for the assays of the various carnitine fractions. SMC, short and medium chains. Mass spectrometry can be added for the identification of the chemical structure of individual acylcarnitines.

The need for a strategy to select the proper method for each situation is further stressed when exogenous carnitine is administered. In this case, it becomes very difficult to assay the difference between free and total carnitine, especially in plasma samples. The increase of free carnitine, induced by exogenous administration, reduces the esterified fraction to less than 5% of the total carnitine (Siliprandi et al, 1990), which is near the coefficient of variation for the carnitine assay. In some instances a separate assay for acetylcarnitine, which represents more than 70% of carnitine esters in the blood (Valkner and Bieber, 1982), can be used.

CARNITINE ASSAYS

The assays for carnitine are based on the reaction:

$$\text{L-Carnitine} + \text{Acetyl CoA} \overset{\text{CAT}}{\rightleftarrows} \text{Acetyl-L-carnitine} + \text{CoASH}$$
$$\text{(Reaction 1)}$$

catalysed by carnitine acetyltransferase (CAT, EC 2.3.1.7) (reviewed by Pearson et al, 1969; Bieber and Lewin, 1981). Enzymatic assays for carnitine and acetylcarnitine involve the coupling of CAT activity to one of many assay systems for free CoA (CoASH) and acetyl CoA (Tubbs and Garland, 1969; Groot et al, 1976). In Reaction 1 the addition of carnitine to a system containing CAT and an excess of acetyl CoA gives rise to the formation of stoichiometric amounts of CoASH. Coupling the system to any irreversible assay for CoASH then gives a measure of the L-carnitine.

Photometric methods

Reactions with disulphides

Aromatic disulphides have been used to detect and estimate spectro-photometrically thiol groups in protein preparations (Brocklehurst and Little, 1973). In such assays, the thiol is allowed to react with an excess of the disulphide to produce a chromophoric fragment. Ellman (1958) reported the use of bis-(p-nitrophenyl)disulphide for thiol determination and later (Ellman, 1959) enhanced its water-solubility by introduction of carboxyl groups into the benzene rings, resulting in the synthesis of 5,5′-dithiobis-(2-nitrobenzoic acid) (DTNB). The utilization of this compound for carnitine assay was introduced by Marquis and Fritz (1964) coupling CAT activity with the following reaction:

$$CoASH + DTNB \rightarrow CoA\text{-}S\text{-}S\text{-}NB + TNB^- + H^+ \qquad \text{(Reaction 2)}$$

The CoASH formed in Reaction 1 reacts with DTNB to form the yellow 5-thio-2-nitrobenzoate anion, TNB^- (absorption coefficient at 412 nm $(\epsilon_{412}) = 13\,600\ M^{-1}\,cm^{-1}$ at pH 8.0). This procedure is absolutely specific for L-carnitine (Marquis and Fritz, 1964). The increase in absorbancy is proportional to the amount of carnitine. Using microcuvettes (250 µl), the addition of 0.4 nmol of carnitine should result in an extinction increment of 0.02 Absorbance Units (AU). Such values are sufficient to detect the total carnitine concentration in the blood, but are not reliable for the estimation of normal plasma acylcarnitine which is usually below 10 nmol ml^{-1}.

This reaction (Reaction 2) is rapid, but shows a slow rate after 3–5 min. This slow rate is due to the reaction of the enzyme protein with DTNB. CAT is, in fact, slowly inactivated by DTNB. In addition, the pH has to be maintained close to 8.0 (Wieland et al, 1985). Values higher than 8.5 result in CAT inactivation, while at pH < 7 dissociation of TNB is incomplete (Jocelyn, 1962).

The major drawback to this method is represented by the interference of other thiol compounds that also react with DTNB. To avoid the interaction with tissue sulfhydryl groups, samples were heated at 90° C for 5 min at pH 8.5 (Marquis and Fritz, 1964). However, under these conditions acylcarnitines are not stable and so this procedure can be used only for total carnitine determination. More recently this problem has been solved by the oxidation of the sample with H_2O_2 which is removed with catalase prior to assaying (Wieland et al, 1985).

To circumvent some of the problems associated with DTNB, other thiol reagents able to produce chromophoric fragments have been used (Lilly et al, 1990). 4,4′-Dipyridyl disulphide (DTBP), reacting with sulfhydryl groups, produces 4-thiopyridone with an absorbance max at 324 nm (Grassetti and Murray, 1967). DTBP has some advantages over DTNB: (i) a higher extinction coefficient $(\epsilon_{324} = 19\,800\ M^{-1}\,cm^{-1})$; (ii) complete dissociation at pH > 5, making it more reliable at lower pHs. A lower degree of CAT inhibition (Ramsay and Tubbs, 1975) as well as a higher one (Parvin and Pande, 1977) have been reported for DTBP compared with DTNB.

Sorboyl CoA formation

CAT and the acyl CoA (ACS) synthetase can be coupled (Pearson et al, 1969) so that CoASH can be converted to sorboyl CoA (Wakil and Hübscher, 1960)

$$CoASH + Sorbate + ATP \xrightarrow{ACS} Sorboyl\ CoA + AMP + PP_i$$

(Reaction 3)

The reaction is completed in 6–15 min with extinction increments larger than those obtained with DTNB. This is due to the higher extinction coefficient of the thioester bond in sorboyl CoA ($\epsilon_{303} = 23\,500$ $M^{-1}\ cm^{-1}$). In fact, the double bonds of sorbate are responsible for both the increase and shift of absorbancy from the characteristic values of the thioester linkage of saturated fatty acids ($\epsilon_{232} = 4500\ M^{-1}\ cm^{-1}$). The sorboyl CoA formation is temperature-dependent; an increase in temperature lowers the pH of the TRIS buffer and the formation of more undissociated sorbic acid. Another limit of this procedure is the slowing down of the reaction as the sorbylation approaches completion (Pearson et al, 1969) due to the relatively high K_m for CoA (about 5 μM).

Fluorometric assay with BIPM

Fluorometry has also been employed in another modification of carnitine determination (Maehara et al, 1988). In this method, the release of CoASH catalysed by CAT is coupled to N-(p-(2-benzimidazolyl)-phenyl)-maleimide (BIPM). The sensitivity of the fluorometric assay is similar to the DTNB assay, but the background problems related to the presence of thiol groups in the sample are probably increased by the interference of unknown fluorescent substances. Interestingly, the authors reported a reduction of carnitine recovery induced by ascorbate which has not been described in other assays.

Coupled enzymatic methods

The term 'enzymatic' is used to distinguish the following reaction from the ones listed above and indicates that CAT activity is coupled to other enzymatic reactions.

α-Ketoglutarate dehydrogenase

CoA released from acetyl CoA in the CAT reaction can be converted to succinyl CoA in an irreversible reaction (Reaction 4) catalysed by α-ketoglutarate dehydrogenase (Pearson et al, 1969).

$$CoASH + NAD^+ + α\text{-Ketoglutarate}$$

$$\xrightarrow{αKGDH} \text{Succinyl CoA} + NADH(H^+) \quad \text{(Reaction 4)}$$

The reaction of $NADH(H^+)$ can be monitored by means of either a spectrophotometer or a fluorometer as described by Tubbs and Garland (1969) for CoASH assay. This method avoids some of the disadvantages of the DTNB assay, i.e. a gradual inactivation of CAT and reaction with thiol compounds other than CoASH. When the spectrophotometric procedure is followed, the lower absorption coefficient of $NADH(H^+)$ ($\epsilon_{340} = 6220$ M^{-1} cm^{-1}) reduces the sensitivity of this coupled method with respect to DTNB or DTBP. The use of a fluorometer increases the sensitivity at least tenfold so that 0.1–0.2 nmol of carnitine (or CoASH) can be measured. The complete irreversibility and the low K_m for CoASH (< 0.1 μM) of α-ketoglutarate dehydrogenase makes the coupling of this enzyme with CAT preferable to the sorboyl CoA method. The recent commercial availability of αKGDH has aroused new interest in this procedure (Schäfer and Reichmann, 1989).

Succinate thiokinase

Similar principles have been applied for the development of a more complex assay system (Williamson and Corkey, 1969).

$$CoASH + \text{Succinate} + ATP \xrightleftharpoons{ST} \text{Succinyl-CoA} + ADP + P_i \quad (5)$$

$$ADP + PEP \xrightarrow{PK} ATP + \text{Pyruvate} \quad (6)$$

$$\text{Pyruvate} + NADH(H^+) \xrightleftharpoons{LDH} \text{Lactate} + NAD^+ \quad (7)$$

CoASH released by CAT is converted into succinyl CoA by succinate thiokinase (ST) with concomitant hydrolysis of ATP to produce ADP. The resulting ADP is rephosphorylated to ATP at the expense of phosphoenolpyruvate (PEP). This irreversible reaction is catalysed by pyruvate kinase (PK) and yields pyruvate. In Reaction (7), the oxidation of NADH(H$^+$) by pyruvate decreases fluorescence (or light absorption) which is used as a quantitative indicator of carnitine concentrations.

Radioenzymatic assay

The sensitivity of the assays for carnitine was greatly augmented by the introduction of a radioisotopic assay (Cederblad and Linstedt, 1972). It depends on the incorporation of the acetyl moiety of [1-^{14}C]acetyl CoA into acetylcarnitine. The unreacted, negatively charged [1-^{14}C]acetyl CoA is then separated by means of anion exchange. Carnitine esters carrying the positive charge of the quaternary ammonium are not retained by the resin. A similar procedure was reported for assaying choline (Tencati and Rosenberg, 1973).

The Cederblad–Lindstedt assay (1972) has been modified because the presence of low molecular weight, short-chain acylcarnitines, such as acetylcarnitine can cause non-linear standard curves. In fact, in the original procedure the released CoASH was not trapped allowing the free reversibility of the CAT reaction. Under these conditions the endogenous acetylcarnitine causes an overestimation of free carnitine in relation to total carnitine. Another complication of the former Cederblad assay was the use of TRIS as a buffer which resulted in high blank values. TRIS can also be acetylated forming a radioactive compound that is not retained by anion exchange resin (Christiansen and Bremer, 1978), thus acetylated TRIS can be mistaken for carnitine. In a first attempt to improve the procedure, Reaction 1 was shifted to the right by (i) increasing acetyl-CoA/carnitine to 5 to 1 and (ii) adding DTNB to trap free CoA (Bohmer et al, 1974). Since, as mentioned previously, Ellman's reagent inhibits CAT, further improvements came from the substitution of DTNB with sodium tetrathionate (McGarry and Foster, 1976), and N-ethylmaleimide (NEM) (Parvin and Pande, 1977). NEM and sodium tetrathionate apparently do not inactivate CAT as rapidly as DTNB (Parvin and Pande, 1977; Bieber and Lewin, 1981) and so the displacement of the CAT equilibrium to the right is possible even in the presence of lower concentrations of acetyl CoA. The use of Hepes as a buffer, NEM as the thiol reagent and of Dowex 1 (-X8 or X-10, 200–400 mesh) as the anion exchange resin are now used (McGarry and Foster, 1985).

At present, the specific activities of commercial [1-^{14}C]acetyl-CoA range from 40 to 60 mCi mmol^{-1}. Thus theoretically it is possible to detect amounts of carnitine as low as 10 pmol, being equal to about 1000 d.p.m. In respect to the DTNB method, this represents an increase in sensitivity of more than 100 times. However, to minimize blank values (no carnitine present in the reaction tube) and reduce costs, [1-^{14}C]acetyl-CoA specific activity is usually diluted 1:3–5 with unlabelled acetyl CoA. Higher ratios can be employed for samples which contain considerable carnitine, such as urine.

The direct addition of the resin to the assay mixture is a convenient procedure (Pande and Parvin, 1980), but the classic 'passage-through-the-column' is preferred to minimize blank values and the coefficient of variation. A more expensive, but time-saving variation, is the utilization of small prepacked columns for solid-phase extraction (SAX Bond-Elut, Analytichem, USA or equivalent products from other companies) or the recently released ion exchange resins incorporated into membranes (AG 1-X8 Ion Exchange Membrane, Bio Rad Laboratories, USA). Low blank values can be obtained by washing the resin with bidistilled water just prior to the assay. It is important to note that when tissue free carnitine content is determined, the endogenous acetyl CoA can decrease the specific activity of [1-^{14}C]acetyl CoA, and it has to be eliminated by means of an anion-exchange resin (Kerner and Bieber, 1983).

For reproducible results in any method utilizing CAT, salts (ammonium sulphate) have to be removed from the commercial enzyme preparation either by centrifugation and resuspension in a low concentrated phosphate buffer (Pande, 1986) or by dialysis (Bieber and Kerner, 1986). Also, addition of EDTA to the assay mixture has been suggested (Pearson et al, 1969). Doubts have been raised concerning the optimal buffer to be used for the assay. Besides the problems deriving from the above mentioned TRIS acetylation, more recently Hepes and MOPS have been reported as competitive inhibitors for CAT (Tegelaers et al, 1989). These findings stress the necessity to correct sample data for a standard curve. Other 'unknowns' can impair this method, for instance, Sekas and Paul (1989) reported the inhibition of CAT by chenodeoxycolic acid, that could lead to artifactually low values of carnitine concentrations in bile.

Other methods

HPLC procedures, apart from being utilized for the separation and quantitation of the different acylcarnitine fractions (see below), have also been reported for carnitine assay (Takeyama et al, 1986; Minkler et al, 1987). In these methods, sample interference with CAT activity is avoided, but sensitivities are lower than those obtained with radioenzymatic assay.

ACETYLCARNITINE

Enzymatic method

When CAT activity is coupled to an acetyl CoA assay such as the one proposed by Ochoa et al (1951), NAD$^+$ reduction is proportional to the acetylcarnitine concentration in the sample (Fritz et al, 1963; Pearson and Tubbs, 1964). The reactions are as follows:

$$\text{Acetyl-L-carnitine} + \text{CoASH} \overset{\text{CAT}}{\rightleftharpoons} \text{L-Carnitine} + \text{Acetyl CoA}$$
(Reaction 1)

$$\text{Acetyl CoA} + \text{Oxaloacetate} \overset{\text{CS}}{\rightarrow} \text{Citrate} + \text{CoASH}$$
(Reaction 8)

$$\text{Malate} + \text{NAD}^+ \overset{\text{MDH}}{\rightleftharpoons} \text{Oxaloacetate} + \text{NADH(H}^+\text{)}$$
(Reaction 9)

In Reaction 1 CAT, by the reverse reaction, catalyses the transfer of the acetyl moiety from carnitine to CoA. Acetyl CoA, by condensation with oxaloacetate, catalysed by citrate synthase (CS), is irreversibly converted to citrate. The removal of oxaloacetate displaces the equilibrium of malate dehydrogenase (MDH); thus the presence of acetyl-L-carnitine in the system causes NAD reduction, which may be monitored spectrophotometrically or fluorometrically. If CAT is added last, the other reactions (Reactions 8 and 9) can be used to measure acetyl CoA.

NAD$^+$ reduction and citrate formation are stoichiometrically related only if oxaloacetate remains constant or its concentration is low with respect to that of NADH(H$^+$). When these prerequisites are not met, oxaloacetate can concomitantly become the substrate for citrate synthase and for MDH. The MDH reaction causes a simultaneous production and consumption of NADH(H$^+$). This results in an underestimation of both acetyl CoA and acetylcarnitine (Pearson, 1965). To overcome this problem, it has been suggested either (i) to add NADH(H$^+$) when MDH has reached its equilibrium prior to the execution of the citrate synthase and CAT catalysed reactions; or (ii) to calculate a correction factor (Pearson et al, 1969). As discussed for carnitine enzymatic assays, this method, especially in the case of spectrophotometric measurements, is not sufficient to detect acetylcarnitine in plasma or in small tissue samples, i.e. muscle biopsies. As will be discussed in the following section, radioenzymatic procedures are capable of detecting small quantities of acetylcarnitine (Pande, 1986).

Radioenzymatic method

Ochoa's procedure for measuring acetyl CoA became extremely sensitive with the introduction of a radioactive substrate, namely [U-^{14}C]oxaloacetate (Prinz et al, 1966). Mimicking Pearson's modification described for the enzymatic assay, the addition of CAT to this system results in a new sensitive procedure for assay of acetylcarnitine (Pande and Caramancion, 1981).

$$\text{Acetyl-L-carnitine} + \text{CoASH} \overset{\text{CAT}}{\rightleftarrows} \text{L-Carnitine} + \text{Acetyl CoA}$$
(Reaction 1)

$$\text{Acetyl CoA} + [^{14}\text{C}]\text{Oxaloacetate} \overset{\text{CS}}{\rightarrow} [^{14}\text{C}]\text{Citrate} + \text{CoASH}$$
(Reaction 8a)

$$[^{14}\text{C}]\text{Oxaloacetate} + \text{Glutamate} \overset{\text{GOT}}{\rightleftarrows} [^{14}\text{C}]\text{Aspartate} + \alpha\text{-Ketoglutarate}$$
(Reaction 10)

Reactions 1 and 8a were illustrated in the previous paragraph. The transamination of oxaloacetate to aspartate catalysed by glutamate–oxaloacetate transaminase (GOT) provides a means for separation of oxaloacetate from citrate. For the carnitine radioenzymatic assay, the anion exchange resin separates acetyl CoA from acetylcarnitine (Reaction 8a) but, both oxaloacetate and citrate are anions. Unreacted oxaloacetate can be removed by heating which increases the natural tendency of this α-ketoacid to spontaneously decarboxylate (Decker, 1985). In a more controlled fashion, Reaction 10 is utilized to convert the unreacted oxaloacetate to aspartate (Pande and Caramancion, 1981). Then, a cation exchange resin (i.e. Dowex 50-X8, H$^+$ form, 200–400 mesh) at a neutral pH allows the separation of citrate from aspartate. Citrate passes through the column and positively charged aspartate is retained. Since oxaloacetate, as already mentioned, is a very unstable compound, it has to be freshly prepared just prior to its utilization in the assay as shown in Figure 3. This is accomplished by reversing Reaction 10. When tissue samples are used, GOT has to be inactivated by perchloric acid precipitation in order to eliminate the possible isotopic dilution of the newly formed [U-^{14}C]oxaloacetate due to endogenous aspartate.

The high specific activity of [U-^{14}C]aspartate (> 200 Ci mol^{-1}) allows the estimation of > 10 pmol acetylcarnitine. Generally sample values are determined from a standard curve of acetylcarnitine ranging from 20–80 pmol. The assay is not affected by carnitine even when

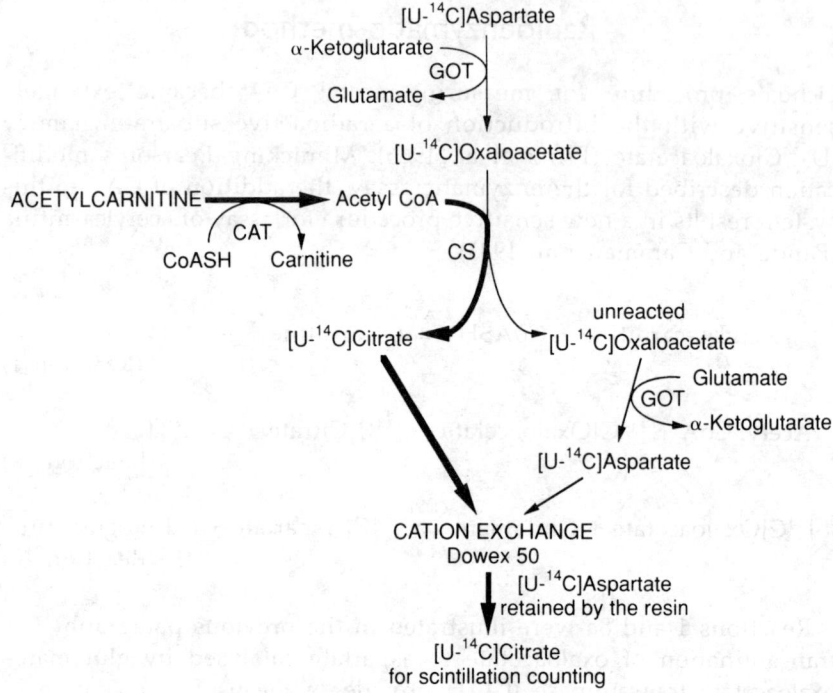

FIGURE 3. Radioenzymatic assay of acetylcarnitine. Bold arrows indicate the reactions directly involved in the formation of [^{14}C]citrate from acetylcarnitine. Ancillary reactions are indicated by lighter arrows.

carnitine/acetylcarnitine > 500. This is particularly useful for the estimation of acetylcarnitine in patients receiving L-carnitine. Propionyl CoA produced from propionyl-L-carnitine can react, although at a slower rate, with citrate synthase generating methylcitrate, which is indistinguishable from citrate under these assay conditions (Pande and Caramancion, 1981). This problem can be neglected in untreated samples since propionyl-L-carnitine is always a minor fraction of acetylcarnitine. However, it can be a serious source of error (overestimation) for patients with propionic acidaemia or when propionyl-L-carnitine is administered.

Attention must be paid to any condition leading to an accelerated rate of oxaloacetate decarboxylation (i.e. metals, alkalinization and heating). When this occurs, oxaloacetate can neither react with acetyl-CoA nor be converted back to aspartate. Since the degradation products are not retained by the cationic exchanger, an undesired increase of blank values results. The addition of EDTA to all steps minimizes this problem: this, combined with a passage through the resin column of the assay mixture, helps to maintain blank values below 1500 c.p.m. When tissues are analysed, pretreatment of the samples with an anion exchange resin removes interfering endogenous substances such as acetyl CoA, oxaloacetate, citrate and other anions. In order to eliminate citrate interference in blood samples, CoASH released by the CAT reaction can be oxidized. Thus, the reverse reaction of citrate synthase, giving acetyl CoA from endogenous citrate and CoASH, can be avoided (Cooper, 1986).

CARNITINE ESTERS: IDENTIFICATION AND QUANTITATION

It is relatively easy to separate the individual carnitine esters but much more difficult to detect them. A direct estimation of carnitine and of its esters can be based only on the light absorbance of the carboxyl group at 205–210 nm with a very low extinction coefficient ($\epsilon_{204} = 1780$ M^{-1} cm^{-1}). Thus, a chromatographic method based on a high-performance liquid chromatograph equipped with a reverse-phase column and a UV detector can be useful only for the recognition of impurities in concentrated standard solutions or in pharmaceutical formulations (Marzo et al, 1990).

Several procedures have been designed to improve the detection sensitivity following separation. In general, they can be divided into two main groups: indirect and direct methods. Only with the latter can the whole process, including sample treatment, separation and identification, be associated with the maintenance of the chemical integrity of carnitine esters. Otherwise, in the indirect procedures, mainly with gas chromatography (GC) or in some cases with high-performance liquid chromatography (HPLC), the assay only detects a fragment of the original molecule, namely the fatty acids released after alkaline hydrolysis. A special exception is represented by some applications of mass spectrometry (MS), i.e. fast-atom bombardment or thermospray, in which the molecules are fragmented and identified immediately upon their detection. Although, in principle, all these techniques could quantitatively assess the separated species, realistically a gold standard of acylcarnitine quantitation in biological samples has still to be achieved. This can be attributed to a series of factors:

1. the complex procedures for acylcarnitine extraction and purification, which in some cases show variable recoveries;
2. lack of appropriate standards (in some urine up to 20 different peaks can be revealed just in the region of carbon chains ranging from 5 to 10);
3. for some procedures, the low sensitivity permits the assay only after an extensive sample concentration;
4. HPLC methods utilizing a pretreatment of the sample with CAT (see above) are 'blind' for dicarboxylic (i.e. glutarylcarnitine) or other acylcarnitines (i.e. valproyl- or pivaloylcarnitine).

Gas chromatography

The detection and quantitation is performed on fatty acids obtained after saponification of the corresponding acylcarnitines (Choi and Bieber, 1977). Precautions and problems concern the separation of carnitine esters from interfering substances and especially from fatty acids. The necessary manoeuvres (up to 18) have been modified and reviewed by Bieber and colleagues (Bieber and Lewin, 1981; Bieber and Kerner, 1986). After the addition of the sample of valerylcarnitine as the internal standard, the essential steps to be performed on the neutralized perchloric acid supernatant are as follows:

1. Gel-chromatography (Bio-Gel P2) to remove materials with molecular weights less than 200 and greater than 400.
2. Elimination by means of anion-exchange (Dowex 1, carbonate form) of negatively charged molecules, i.e. free fatty acids, Krebs cycle intermediates and nucleotides.
3. Cation-exchange chromatography (Dowex 50, hydrogen form eluted with ammonium hydroxide-ethanol) for the separation of acylcarnitines from other acyl residues with a positive charge (mostly acetylcholine).
4. Saponification with KOH, evaporation to dryness, extraction with ether, conversion of the K^+ salts to the corresponding free fatty acids with HCl. Alternatively, following saponification and evaporation, the residue is dissolved in metaphosphoric acid for GC analysis.
5. The ether extract of the metaphosphoric acid solution is used in a GC system (Hewlett-Packard 5830 A gas chromatograph equipped with a 100–200 mesh Chromosorb WAW column,

Supelco, USA) which, with a temperature increment of $4°$ min^{-1} from $84°$ to $126°$, separates most of the mixtures.

For quantitation, the internal standard method is used. The detection limit of this method can be considered as low as 1 nmol for a specific acylcarnitine (Choi and Bieber, 1977).

Sources of error are represented by trace impurities present in organic solvents, especially in diethyl ether. The passage through both Dowex 1 and 50 can cause the retention of medium chain acylcarnitines due to hydrophobic interactions of relatively long carbon chains with the polystyrene matrix (Bieber and Kerner, 1986). In addition, after sample concentration, the solubility of longer acylcarnitines in acidic solutions is limited. It seems likely that the difficulties in recovery are due to the summation of small losses associated with each of the many steps employed.

HPLC and TLC

Many disadvantages encountered in the GC procedure can be overcome by HPLC providing that sensitive markers are incorporated into the (acyl)carnitines. So far the greatest sensitivity has been achieved by labelling the acylcarnitine with [³H] or [¹⁴C]L-carnitine (Kerner and Bieber, 1983). For this purpose radioactive carnitine, reacting with CAT in the presence of catalytic amounts of CoASH, is equilibrated into the (acyl)carnitines, which alternatively become substrates or products of the same reaction. This *isotopic exchange* is made possible by the reversibility of CAT; theoretically the distribution of radioactivity among the different carnitine fractions should reflect the relative amounts of each component in the sample if isotopic equilibration is attained and if the acylcarnitines are substrates for CAT. When equilibrium is attained, the alkylation of CoASH by NEM completely shifts the reaction to the right, that is towards [³H]acyl-L-carnitine formation (Figure 4).

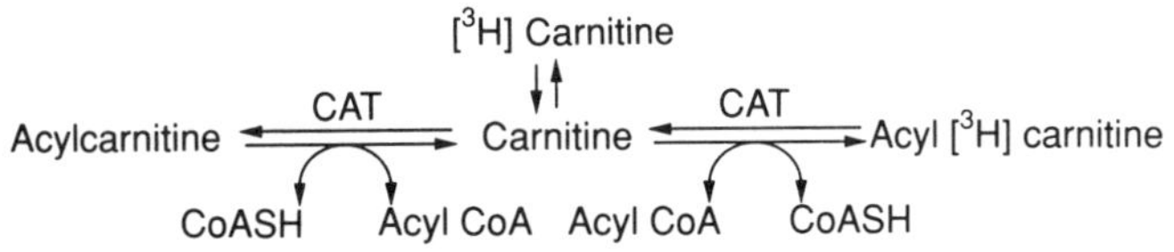

FIGURE 4. Isotopic exchange reaction which allows the incorporation of [³H]L-carnitine into the (acyl)carnitines.

This method is generally applied to acid-soluble carnitine. In principle any carnitine fraction can be exchanged, including the long-chain esters, but the commercial availability of only pigeon breast CAT set the practical limits of this method. However when peroxisomal carnitine octanoyl transferase (COT) was used, an improved exchange of medium-chain acylcarnitines was obtained (Bieber and Kerner, 1986).

The reaction time can be determined by using a very poor substrate for CAT such as isovalerylcarnitine. Although a 30-minute incubation appears to be adequate for a mixture of acylcarnitine standards (Kerner and Bieber, 1983), more time, i.e. up to 2 hours, was necessary for the complete exchange of acylcarnitines of biological samples, such as urine (Schmidt-Sommerfield et al, 1989). During prolonged incubation, temperature and pH become critical, since acylcarnitines are somewhat unstable at neutral pH. Furthermore, commercial CAT preparations can be contaminated with hydrolase activity, which subtracts acyl CoAs and/or acylcarnitines from the equilibrium. Therefore this contamination might be one of the explanations for the overestimation of free carnitine that often results when urinary acid-soluble carnitines are assayed with this method. This hydrolase activity can be a source of error for other HPLC methods. Dugan et al (1987) reported a disappearance of > 20% of acetyl CoA formed from acetylcarnitine after a 2 hour incubation.

Together with the isotopic exchange, Kerner and Bieber (1983) set up the procedures for the separation and the detection of the labelled acylcarnitines by means of thin-layer chromatography (TLC) and HPLC. For TLC, an aliquot of the incubation mixture is spotted onto a silica gel TLC plate with a mixture of free and standard acylcarnitines. The separation is obtained with the solvent system of Solberg and Bremer (1970) containing methanol:chloroform:water:concentrated ammonia:formic acid (55:50:10:7.5:2.5, v/v). Once separated, (acyl) carnitines are detected with iodine vapour, removed by scraping and counted.

The HPLC system was partly based on the separation of aromatic choline esters reported by Clausen et al (1983). The sample is applied to a reverse-phase column, usually with octadecylsilyl groups (ODS or C_{18}) and the column is developed using sodium butanesulfonate, pH 3.4 with acetic acid (solvent A), and 100% methanol (solvent B). The chromatogram shown in Figure 5 was obtained with a flow rate of 1 ml min^{-1} and the following gradient programme: 0–15 min from 0 to 21% solvent B; 15–25 min from 21 to 50%; 25–35 min from 50 to 70% solvent B. This latter condition is maintained for 15 min, followed by a decrease of solvent B to 0% in 10 min. The column is then equilibrated for 10 min in 100% solvent A. Although other solvent systems have been designed by changing pH or counterions in order to resolve isomers, particularly iso- from straight-chain of C-4 and C-5, a complete separation has not yet been achieved (Bieber et al, 1986).

The radioactivity in the column effluent can be monitored by means of fraction collection followed by scintillation counting or more conveniently using a radioactive flow detector (i.e. Flo-One, Radiomatic Packard, USA). In this case the eluate, mixed with a non-gelling scintillation cocktail (Pico-Fluor 40, Packard or similar products by other companies), is pumped through the detector cell intercalated between two photomultiplier tubes. Raw counts sampled from 10 to 30 times each minute are integrated by a specific software for the 'residence time', given by the ratio between the sum of HPLC and scintillation cocktail flows (F) and the volume of the cell (V). The same software also operates the background subtraction and the correction for the efficiency along the entire gradient with results expressed as DPM. At the end of each run the chromatogram and all the integrated parameters are printed. Data files can be stored and exported as ASCII

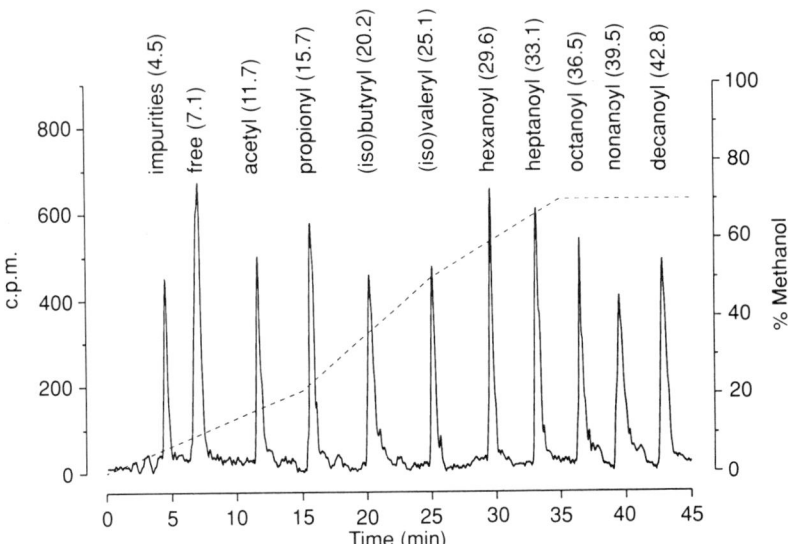

FIGURE 5. Radiochromatogram of acyl[^{3}H]carnitines. For each compound the acyl residue and the retention time between parentheses have been indicated. Dashed line represents the percentage of methanol in the solvent system.

files to the widespread spreadsheet, graphic or statistic software packages.

The selection of the cell volume and flow rate represents a compromise between sensitivity and selectivity (Reeve and Crozier, 1977). For instance, a 0.5 ml cell is ideal for the separation of many peaks, but, when c.p.m. are low (< 1000), there is an apparent decrease in sensitivity. This is due to the high multiplying factor applied by the software, which gives relatively high c.p.m. despite very low raw counts. On the other hand, with $F/V < 5$ the loss of resolution becomes noticeable.

The isotopic exchange coupled to the HPLC separation is very sensitive. In our experience reliable results were obtained with samples containing 50 pmol of total acid-soluble carnitine. Considering that 0.04 μCi of [^{3}H]L-carnitine is used for labelling, a 1000 c.p.m. area will be $\cong 1$ pmol. Furthermore, compared with the GC method, it allows the assay of relatively impure mixtures. The main disadvantage is the lack of CAT affinity for some acylcarnitines. Dicarboxylic acylcarnitines (i.e. glutarylcarnitine) and several 'unphysiological' esters (i.e. valproyl- or pivaloylcarnitine) are not detected. This can result in overestimation of free carnitine. Urine samples often contain considerable amounts of medium-chain acylcarnitines, other unknown carnitine esters or interfering compounds which decrease the recovery percentage of radioactivity in the esterified fractions. Several procedures have been used to overcome this problem. Pretreatment of the sample by molecular sieving (Bio-Gel P2) gives satisfactory results (Schmidt-Sommerfield et al, 1989). More recently we used solid-phase extraction (Sep-Pak C_{18}, Waters, USA) to rid the sample of carnitine and acetylcarnitine (which can be determined separately), and to concentrate the C4-C10 acylcarnitine fraction (see Figure 2). Besides improvement in recovery, this procedure permits the detection of medium-chain acylcarnitines in plasma or when exogenous carnitine is administered. In both cases, since the ratio between free carnitine and all carnitine esters except acetylcarnitine is too high, the free carnitine in the sample dilutes the radioactivity making the other compounds undetectable.

This particular HPLC system can also be used to investigate carnitine-dependent reactions in isolated mitochondria (Lysiak et al, 1988) or perfused hearts (Di Lisa et al, 1989). However, the need for special equipment and the high cost for processing each sample limits the use of radioisotopic exchange in routine clinical testing.

Other HPLC methods have been developed and are employed taking advantage of common laboratory resources, such as UV detectors. By reversing the CAT reaction (Reaction 1), carnitine esters can be enzymatically converted to the corresponding acyl CoAs (Dugan et al, 1987). These esters are then separated with a reverse-phase column and a mobile phase containing 0.025 M tetraethylammonium phosphate in a linear gradient of 1 to 50% methanol. The spectrophotometric detection ($\lambda = 254$ nm for detectors equipped with a fixed wavelength, or 259 nm when a variable wavelength is available) is based on the adenine portion of coenzyme A ($\epsilon_{259} = 14\,600$ M^{-1} cm^{-1}). The disadvantages of this method are represented by (i) critical reaction conditions analogous to those described for the isotopic exchange; (ii) sensitivity sufficient only for urine samples; (iii) lack of detection for (iso)butyrylcarnitine and acylcarnitines longer than six carbons, which are normal constituents of human urine. This latter problem could probably be ameliorated by changing reaction conditions and/or the HPLC gradient.

Others have approached the problem by attempting to 'label' the carboxylic group of carnitine. The assay system is based on the carboxyl-O-alkylation with bromophenacyl compounds ($\epsilon_{240-260} = 38\,000-45\,000$ M^{-1} cm^{-1}), thus resulting in a severalfold increase of the detection limit (Grushka et al, 1975; Ingalls et al, 1984). After a series of improvements to their first report (Minkler et al, 1984), Minkler et al (1990) reported a procedure of derivatization with 4'-bromophenacyl trifluoromethanesulfonate which allows at 254 nm the detection of carnitine and its esters from C2 (acetylcarnitine) to C18 (stearoyl-carnitine) in the nanomolar range. This method appears to be easier and cheaper than the isotopic exchange, but its detection limit does not seem to be adequate for plasma or tissues. The other limitation is that all other carboxyl containing compounds in the sample can also be labelled. However, Bhuiyan and Bartlett (1988) used a similar procedure (Tracey et al, 1986) for the analysis of carnitine esters, not only in urine, but also in plasma. The analysis of their results is not clear. The concentration of the added internal standard was 50–200-fold higher than the concentration of the compound tested. Alternatively Hoppel et al (1986) suggested the use of HPLC for carnitine ester separation. Subsequently, fractions are collected at predetermined times and, after alkaline hydrolysis, carnitine is assayed by conventional methods. A similar procedure has been applied for the separation and quantitation of γ-butyrobetaine (Sandor et al, 1988).

Mass spectrometry

MS has been used for the unequivocal identification of the various acylcarnitines. For an indirect analysis, GC can be coupled to an instream mass spectrometer resulting in on-line acquisition of the mass spectra (Chalmers and Lawson, 1982; Roe et al, 1985; Bieber and Kerner, 1986). Acyl groups liberated by milk alkaline hydrolysis, extracted into ether have been successfully analysed as either methyl or trimethylsilyl ester derivatives (Roe et al, 1985). Extensive sample purification and concentration are needed since the method appears to be reliable for levels approaching 100 nmol ml^{-1}. For the MS of authentic acylcarnitines (direct analysis) two different approaches have been used: (i) fast-atom bombardment (FAB)-MS applied either to raw samples (Millington et al, 1984) or to compounds purified by previous chromatographic steps (Kerner and Bieber, 1985); (ii) use of MS-detecting devices, such as thermospray ionization, directly connected to the outlet of an HPLC system (Yergey et al, 1984; Millington et al, 1989).

For FAB-MS, samples are applied to a stainless steel target coated with glycerol and p-toluenesulphonic acid (glycerol matrix) and spectra are generated by bombardment of the target with xenon atoms (Kerner and Bieber, 1985). The interference of alkali metals and urea with the matrix was initially overcome by using isotope dilution. For this purpose, [^{2}H$_3$]acetylcarnitine was added as the internal standard and both a qualitative and quantitative estimate was made possible (Millington et al, 1984). Subsequent improvements were obtained first by treating urine samples with cation exchange chromatography (Roe et al, 1984) and then by methylating (Millington and Maltby, 1985). Methyl esters of acylcarnitines increase the sensitivity tenfold. Since mass spectra of acylcarnitine methyl esters show a common fragment at m/z 99, a scan of the precursors of this fragment has been recently used to generate very clean acylcarnitine profiles of biological extracts (Millington et al, 1989). With this background correction, the sensitivity of the assay has been increased to detect concentrations as low as 1.0 nmol ml^{-1}. A relative lack of specificity is the major drawback of methylation, since a given methyl ester is mass spectrometrically indistinguishable from the free acid of the next higher homolog. A useful improvement is the analysis of [^{2}H$_3$-Me]methyl acylcarnitines made with perdeuteromethanol in the place of the unlabelled methyl esters (Montgomery and Mamer, 1989). The increment of 17 Da to the molecular mass results in the formation of derivatives that are distinct in mass from the other homologues.

When structural information is required, more sophisticated equipment is necessary. FAB-MS is associated to tandem mass spectrometry (MS/MS) providing high-energy collisional activation of the molecular ions (Millington, 1986). With this procedure isomers (Millington, 1986), as well as the occurrence of double bonds and branched chains (Kerner and Bieber, 1985), can be characterized.

An interesting application of MS has been shown by Millington et al (1989). After intravenous injection of [^{2}H$_3$-*methyl*]L-carnitine in a patient with medium-chain acyl-CoA dehydrogenase (MCAD) deficiency, plasma samples analysed with MS/MS showed isotope incorporation into the acylcarnitines. In the future, this safe procedure could represent a very rapid device for the screening and diagnosis of secondary carnitine deficiencies.

The major shortcomings of MS techniques are the complexity and the cost of the equipment. Furthermore the sensitivity, except in the most sophisticated applications, is generally low so that samples have to undergo purification and concentration procedures. This disadvantage is of little concern when the identification of a specific carnitine ester and its structure represents the goal.

REFERENCES

Beinert H, Green DE, Hele P et al (1953) *J. Biol. Chem.* 203: 35–45.

Bhuiyan AKMJ & Bartlett K (1988) *Biochem. Soc. Trans.* 16: 796–797.

Bieber LL & Kerner J (1986) *Methods Enzymol.* 123: 264–276.

Bieber LL & Lewin LM (1981) *Methods Enzymol.* 72: 276–287.

Bieber LL, Lysiak W & Kerner J (1986) In Borum PR (ed.) *Clinical Aspects of Human Carnitine Deficiency* pp 66–74. New York: Pergamon Press.

Bohmer T, Rydning A & Solberg HE (1974) *Clin. Chim. Acta* 57: 55–61.

Bremer J (1983) *Physiol. Rev.* 63: 1420–1480.

Brocklehurst K & Little G (1973) *Biochem. J.* 133: 67–80.

Carter HE, Bhattacharyya PK, Weidman KR & Fraenkel G (1952) *Arch. Biochem. Biophys.* 38: 405–416.

Cederblad G & Lindstedt S (1972) *Clin. Chim. Acta* 37: 235–243.

Cederblad G, Larsson H, Nordstrom H & Schildt B (1980) *Burns* 8: 102–108.

Cederblad G, Harper P & Lindgren K (1986) *Clin. Chem.* 32: 342–346.

Chalmers RA & Lawson AM (1982) *Organic Acids in Man.* London: Chapman and Hall.

Chase JFA, Pearson DJ & Tubbs PK (1965) *Biochim. Biophys. Acta* 96: 162–165.

Choi YR & Bieber LL (1977) *Anal. Biochem.* 79: 413–418.

Christianson DD, Wall JS, Cavins JF & Dimler RJ (1963) *J. Chromatogr.* 10: 432–438.

Christiansen RZ & Bremer J (1978) *FEBS Lett.* 86: 99–102.

Clausen S, Olsen O & Sorensen H (1983) *J. Chromatogr.* 260: 193–199.

Cooper MB, Forte CA & Jones DA (1986) *Clin. Chim. Acta* 159: 291–299.

Decker K (1985) In Bergmeyer HU (ed.) *Methods of Enzymatic Analysis*, vol. 7, pp 193–200. Weinheim: VCH Verlags-Gesellschaft.

Di Lisa F, Menabò R & Siliprandi N (1989) *J. Mol. Cell. Cardiol.* 21 (supplement 2): S30.

Dugan RE, Schmidt MJ, Hoganson GE et al (1987) *Anal. Biochem.* 160: 275–280.

Ellman GL (1958) *Arch. Biochem. Biophys.* 74: 443–450.

Ellman GL (1959) *Arch. Biochem. Biophys.* 82: 70–77.

Fishlock RC, Bieber LL & Snoswell AM (1984) *Clin. Chem.* 30: 316–318.

Friedman S (1958) *Arch. Biochem. Biophys.* 75: 24–30.

Friedman S & Fraenkel G (1955) *Arch. Biochem. Biophys.* 59: 491–501.

Friedman S, McFarlane JE, Bhattacharyya PK and Fraenkel G (1955) *Arch. Biochem. Biophys.* 59: 484–490.

Fritz IB (1955) *Acta Physiol. Scand.* 34: 367–385.

Fritz IB, Schultz SK & Srere PA (1963) *J. Biol. Chem.* 236: 2509–2517.

Grassetti DR & Murray JF (1967) *Arch. Biochem. Biophys.* 119: 41–49.

Groot PHE, Scholte HR & Hülsmann WC (1976) *Adv. Lipid Res.* 14: 75–126.

Grushka E, Durst HD & Kikta EJ (1975) *J. Chromatogr.* 112: 673–680.

Hestrin S (1949) *J. Biol. Chem.* 180: 249–261.

Hoppel CL, Brass EP, Gibbons AP & Turkaly JS (1986) *Anal. Biochem.* 156: 111–117.

Ingalls ST, Minkler PE, Hoppel CL & Nordlander JE (1984) *J. Chromatogr.* 299: 365–376.

Jocelyn PC (1962) *Biochem. J.* 85: 480–495.

Kerner J & Bieber LL (1983) *Anal. Biochem.* 134: 459–466.

Kerner J & Bieber LL (1985) *Prep. Biochem.* 15: 237–257.

Lilly K, Bugaisky GE, Umeda PK & Bieber LL (1990) *Arch. Biochem. Biophys.* 280: 167–174.

Lysiak W, Lilly K, Di Lisa F et al (1988) *J. Biol Chem.* 263: 1151–1156.

McGarry JD & Foster DW (1976) *J. Lipid Res.* 17: 277–281.

McGarry JD & Foster DW (1985) In Bergmeyer HU (ed.) *Methods of Enzymatic Analysis*, vol. 8, pp 474–481. Weinheim: VCH Verlags-Gesellschaft.

Maehara M, Kinoshita S & Watanabe K (1988) *Clin. Chim. Acta* 171: 311–316.

Marquis NR & Fritz IB (1964) *J. Lipid Res.* 5: 184–187.

Marzo A, Cardace G, Monti N et al (1990) *J. Chromatogr.* 527: 247–258.

Melegh B, Kerner J & Bieber LL (1987) *Biochem. Pharmacol.* 36: 3405–3409.

Millington DS (1986) In Gaskell SJ (ed.) *Mass Spectrometry in Biomedical Research* pp 97–114. New York: Wiley.

Millington DS, Roe CR & Maltby DA (1984) *Biomed. Mass Spectrom.* 11: 236–241.

Millington DS, Bohan TP, Roe CR et al (1985) *Clin. Chim. Acta* 145: 69–76.

Millington DS, Norwood DL, Kodo N et al (1989) *Anal. Biochem.* 180: 331–339.

Minkler PE, Ingalls ST, Kormos DE et al (1984) *J. Chromatogr.* 336: 271–283.

Minkler PE, Ingalls ST & Hoppel CL (1987) *J. Chromatogr.* 420: 385–393.

Minkler PE, Ingalls ST & Hoppel CL (1990) *Anal. Biochem.* 185: 29–35.

Montgomery JA & Mamer OA (1989) *Anal. Biochem.* 176: 85–95.

Naftalin L & Mitchell R (1958) *Clin. Chim. Acta* 3: 197–199.

Ochoa S, Stern JR & Schneider J (1951) *J. Biol. Chem.* 193: 691–702.

Pande SV (1986) *Methods Enzymol.* 123: 259–263.

Pande SV & Caramancion N (1981) *Anal. Biochem.* 112: 30–38.

Pande SV & Parvin R (1980) *J. Biol. Chem.* 255: 2994–3001.

Parvin R & Pande SV (1977) *Anal. Biochem.* 79: 190–201.

Pearson DJ (1965) *Biochem. J.* 95: 23c–24c.

Pearson DJ & Tubbs PK (1964) *Nature* 202: 91.

Pearson DJ, Chase JFA & Tubbs PK (1969) *Methods Enzymol.* 13: 612–622.

Prinz W, Schoner W, Haag U & Seubert W (1966) *Biochem. Z.* 346: 206–211.

Ramsay RR & Tubbs PK (1975) *FEBS Lett.* 54: 21–25.

Reeve DD & Crozier A (1977) *J. Chromatogr.* 137: 271–282.

Roe CR, Millington DS, Maltby DA et al (1984) *J. Clin. Invest.* 74: 2290–2295.

Roe CR, Millington DS, Maltby DA et al (1985) *Ped. Res.* 19: 459–466.

Roe CR, Millington DS & Maltby DA (1986) in Borum PR (ed.) *Clinical Aspects of Human Carnitine Deficiency* pp 97–107. New York: Pergamon Press.

Sandor A, Minkler PE, Ingalls ST & Hoppel CL (1988) *Clin. Chim. Acta* 176: 17–28.

Schäfer J & Reichmann H (1989) *Clin. Chim. Acta* 182: 87–94.

Schmidt-Sommerfeld E, Penn D, Kerner J & Bieber LL (1989) *Clin. Chim. Acta* 181: 231–238.

Seccombe DW, Dodek P, Frohlich J et al (1976) *Clin. Chem.* 22: 1589–1592.

Sekas G & Paul HS (1989) *Anal. Biochem.* 179: 262–267.

Siliprandi N, Sartorelli L, Ciman M & Di Lisa F (1989) *Clin. Chim. Acta* 183: 3–12.

Siliprandi N, Di Lisa F, Pieralisi G et al (1990) *Biochim. Biophys. Acta* 1034: 17–21.

Solberg HE & Bremer J (1970) *Biochim. Biophys. Acta* 222: 372–380.

Takeyama N, Takagi D, Adachi K & Tanaka T (1986) *Anal. Biochem.* 158: 346–354.

Tegelaers FPW, Margery MG & Seelen PJ (1989) *J. Clin. Chem. Clin. Biochem.* 27: 967–972.

Tencati JR & Rosenberg RN (1973) *Biochim. Biophys. Acta* 293: 542–551.

Tracey BM, Chalmers RA, Rosankiewicz JR et al (1986) *Biochem. Soc. Trans.* 14: 700–701.

Tubbs PK & Garland PB (1969) *Methods Enzymol.* 13: 535–551.

Valkner KJ & Bieber LL (1982) *Biochem. Medicine* 28: 197–203.

Vickers S, Duncan CAH, White SD et al (1985) *Xenobiotica* 15: 453–458.

Wakil SJ & Hübscher G (1960) *J. Biol. Chem.* 235: 1554–1558.

Wieland OH, Deufel T & Paetzke-Brunner I (1985) In Bergmeyer HU (ed.) *Methods of Enzymatic Analysis,* vol. 8, pp 481–488. Weinheim: VCH Verlags-Gesellschaft.

Williamson JR & Corkey BE (1969) *Methods Enzymol.* 13: 434–513.

Yergey AL, Liberato DL & Millington DS (1984) *Anal. Biochem.* 139: 278–283.

4

PHARMACOKINETICS OF L-CARNITINE IN HUMAN SUBJECTS

V. Rizza, R. Lorefice, N. Rizza and V. Calabrese

L-Carnitine (L-β-hydroxy-4-N-trimethylaminobutyric acid) is an essential nutrient in animals, including humans (Boots et al, 1980; Paulson and Shug, 1981). It was discovered approximately 80 years ago and chemically characterized as a small, highly polar, water soluble compound having a molecular weight of 162. Its biological importance did not emerge until the 1960s when Fritz and colleagues (Fritz and Schultz, 1965) showed its essential requirement in mitochondrial β-oxidation of long-chain fatty acids. Since then several roles for L-carnitine in mammalian metabolism have been proposed involving conjugation of acyl residues to the β-hydroxyl group on the carnitine molecule, with subsequent translocation from one cellular compartment to another. The process affects both availability of activated acyl residues and availability of coenzyme A (CoA). A number of reports on cellular intermediary metabolism have shown that in the presence of L-carnitine, a large amount of specific acylcarnitines are generated within the mitochondria. The production and efflux of acylcarnitines from mitochondria is tissue- and substrate-specific and dependent on L-carnitine concentration (Kysiak et al, 1986). The acetylated form of L-carnitine, acetyl-L-

63

L-Carnitine and Its Role in Medicine:
From Function to Therapy. ISBN 0–12–253940–0

carnitine, is the major acylcarnitine found in animal tissues (Bieber et al, 1982). Hence, free L-carnitine and, to a much lesser extent, acetyl-L-carnitine can be considered respectively as the major and minor shuttling forms of L-carnitine found in both intracellular and extracellular fluids.

All animals and man are able to synthesize L-carnitine, even though an exogenous supply of L-carnitine is necessary to balance the daily requirements. The principal sources are red meat and dairy products. Over 90% of body L-carnitine is present in skeletal and cardiac muscles, and the remainder is found in liver, kidney and other tissues. Extracellular fluids, including plasma, contain approximately 0.6% of the body's carnitine. Tissue concentrations of L-carnitine exceed the plasma concentration ($0.04-0.06$ μmoles ml^{-1}) by one or two orders of magnitude indicating the need for an energy-dependent active transport mechanism to maintain this membrane gradient (De Vivo and Tein, 1990).

The discovery of various human carnitine deficiency syndromes (Engel and Angelini, 1973) has suggested that the causes of this potentially fatal disorder might involve defects in the biosynthesis and catabolism of carnitine, as well as abnormalities in the renal handling and transport mechanism affecting uptake and/or release of carnitine. To better understand the development of a carnitine deficiency in humans, and to investigate its therapeutic potential, knowledge of the pharmacokinetics of the drug is necessary.

This chapter describes the pharmacokinetics of L-carnitine in healthy subjects following intravenous and oral administration of the drug, and ascertains various pharmacokinetic parameters derived by using techniques of compartmental analysis.

MATERIALS AND METHODS

Six volunteers, between the ages of 28 and 33 (34 ± 2.3, mean $\pm$ SD) were entered in this study. The mean weight $\pm$ SD was 71.3 kg $\pm$ 1.9 kg (range 64–77 kg). The weight of each subject did not deviate more than 30% above or below the 50th percentile for people in that age group. All volunteers were judged healthy according to medical history and preliminary clinical and laboratory examinations. The subjects were informed of the purpose of the study and the drug they would receive. All volunteers gave written consent to participate in the study. The study was carried out at Medical Semiotics Department, University of Rome (La Sapienza), Rome, Italy in collaboration with the Clinical Research Department of the Sigma Tau S.p.A. The hospital's ethical committee approved the protocol.

Drugs and reagents

L-Carnitine (Lot No. 316) was kindly supplied by the Sigma Tau S.p.A., Pomezia, Italy. Ampules (1 g) and tablets (500 mg) were supplied for intravenous injection and oral use respectively. Biochemicals used in the study included: Carnitine acetyltransferase, acetyl CoA (CoASH), 2-oxoglutarate, 2-oxoglutarate dehydrogenase and NAD, and were purchased from the Sigma Chemical Co. All chemicals and reagents used were the purest grade available commercially.

Study design

The pharmacokinetics of L-carnitine was studied at two dosage levels of 30 mg kg^{-1} and 100 mg kg^{-1}, administered by two routes, namely intravenous and oral. The dosage and route of administration was described in the experimental protocol. Each subject in the group was monitored for carnitine urinary excretion and blood carnitine levels over a period of 24 h before the experimental trial. On the day of the experimental trial, starting at 8:00 a.m., all subjects were asked to fast overnight and to report to the study site at least 1 h prior to the start of the experiment. Pre-dose urine and blood samples were taken before intravenous injection or ingestion of L-carnitine. Blood samples were taken through a short catheter inserted percutaneously into a forearm vein.

Each subject received an intravenous bolus dose of L-carnitine (30 mg kg^{-1}) in the contralateral forearm vein within a period of 5 min. A washout period of 1 week was allowed before the experiment was repeated at a dosage level of 100 mg kg^{-1} L-carnitine.

Samples of blood (3 ml) were routinely collected in heparinized (10 U ml^{-1}) test tubes at the following time intervals: −5, 0.08, 0.16, 0.33, 0.5, 1, 2, 3, 4, 5, 6, 8, 10, 12, 24 h. Blood samples were centrifuged at 1000 r.p.m. for 10 min and 1 ml aliquots of plasma was removed and stored at −20° C. Urine samples were collected at 0–4, 4–8, 8–12, 12–24 and 24–48 hours. The total volume of urine was recorded and aliquots of each urine sample was stored at −20° C until ready for analysis of L-carnitine concentration.

The protocol for the oral administration of L-carnitine was essentially as described for the intravenous dosage. The dosage levels were 30 mg kg^{-1} and 100 mg kg^{-1} respectively. Carnitine was ingested with approximately 300–400 ml water. Blood and urine samples were collected from each individual at increasing time intervals as described for intravenous dosing, and samples were stored frozen until analysed.

Multiple oral dosing of L-carnitine. Five volunteers were asked to ingest 2 g of L-carnitine every 12 h for a period of 6 days. Each subject was asked to report at least three times each day to the study centre for blood sampling and for returning urine specimens collected over the interval of 24 hours. The subjects in this study were maintained on an isocaloric diet, low in carnitine, so as to minimize carnitine intake from dietary sources.

Assay procedure for free L-carnitine

A spectrophotometric procedure described by Schafer and Reichmann (1989) with minor modifications was used to measure L-carnitine concentration in blood and urine. Essentially, the assay is based on a coupled reaction as illustrated below:

$$\text{L-Carnitine} + \text{Acetyl CoA} \overset{\text{CAT}}{\rightleftharpoons} \text{Acetyl-L-carnitine} + \text{CoASH}$$
(Reaction 1)

$$\text{NAD} + \text{CoASH} + \text{2-Oxoglutarate} \overset{\text{OGDH}}{\rightleftharpoons} \text{Succinyl CoA} + \text{NADH}$$
(Reaction 2)

Extinction measurements of NADH ($\epsilon = 6.22 \times 10^{E3}$) at 340 nm were used to calculate L-carnitine concentration in biological fluids. Plasma and urine samples were deproteinized by passage through amicon membranes (MPS 1) and aliquots of the sample were assayed in triplicate for each time point. In plasma samples containing known added concentrations of L-carnitine (20 μmol l^{-1} and 50 μmol l^{-1}), the concentration found averaged 17.7 and 48.1 μmol l^{-1}, respectively, and the accuracy was 88.5% for the lower concentration and 96.2% for the higher concentration. The precision of the assay at the 95 percentile confidence level established by replicate analyses of samples generally did not vary by more than 8%.

Data analysis

The concentration of L-carnitine in plasma and urine was analysed by a coupled enzyme reaction (Schafer and Reichman, 1989). The disposition of L-carnitine in the body after intravenous dosing has often been described by a biexponential disposition model (Gibladi and Perrier, 1982). This approach has proved very useful, especially for predicting plasma concentration of L-carnitine in the first 6 h post-dosing. However, for longer time periods, a triexponential model better describes drug disposition. The following triexponential equations were fitted to plasma and urine concentration obtained from each volunteer.

$$C = \sum_{i=1}^{3} C_i \, e^{-\beta_i t}$$

$$U_e = \sum_{i=1}^{3} Cl_r C_i \, (1 - e^{-\beta_i t/\beta_i})$$

where C is the plasma concentration at any time, C_i and β_i are the disposition rate constants of the ith exponential term which may be expressed in terms of the individual intercompartmental transfer rate constants and elimination rate constants. U_e is the cumulative amount of L-carnitine excreted in urine. This approach was chosen after showing that the incremental renal clearance Cl_r did not change with time. Fitting was made by non-linear regression analysis using the ordinary least squares algorithm. Estimates of Cl_r were obtained by the following relationship: $Cl_r = U_e \, (0\text{-}t_x)/\text{AUC} \, (0\text{-}t_x)$, in which t_x is the time of last measurable plasma concentration. The values of Cl_r, C_i and α were estimated by curve-fitting techniques in the standard manner. AUC is the area under the curve. The data sets of all six volunteers were modelled independently and the model chosen proved suitable for each of them. The area under the plasma concentration–time curve (AUC, 0–24 h), total clearance (Cl), non-renal clearance (Cl_{nr}) and volume of distribution at steady state (V_{ss}) were obtained using the following expressions:

$$\text{AUC} = \sum_{i=1}^{3} C_i/\beta_i$$

$$Cl = D/\text{AUC}$$

$$Cl_{nr} = Cl - Cl_r$$

$$V_{ss} = Cl \text{MRT}$$

in which D is the dose of L-carnitine administered and MRT is the mean residence time calculated as the ratio of the area under the first moment curve (AUMC) and the AUC. The amount excreted in the urine in infinite time, U (0–) was calculated by:

$$U(0-) = U(0-48 \text{ h}) + dU/dt/\beta 3$$

where dU/dt is the rate of excretion of L-carnitine in urine in the last interval, and $\beta 3$ is the terminal exponential coefficient estimated from the semilogarithmic plot of the rate of excretion vs. the midpoint time of the collection interval.

The maximum and minimum plasma concentration at steady state $C_{ss,max}$ and $C_{ss,min}$ and the accumulation ratio (R) during multiple dosing were calculated using the following relationship:

$$C_n(t) = C_1(t) + \frac{Be^{-\lambda_n \tau} [1 - e^{-(n-1)\lambda_n \tau}] e^{-\lambda_n \tau}}{1 - e^{-\lambda_n \tau}}$$

The accumulation ratio (R) of L-carnitine was quantified by determining the ratio of the $C_{ss,max}/C_{1,max}$, or as the ratio of $C_{ss,min}/C_{1,min}$, where $C_{1,max}$ and $C_{1,min}$ represent the maximum and minimum drug concentration, respectively, after the first dose. Time intervals of 6 and 12 h were considered for developing the steady-state model for oral administration of L-carnitine (30 mg kg^{-1}). Student's t test was used for statistical comparison of groups. Differences were considered to be significant at $p < 0.05$.

RESULTS

The basal level of urinary excretion of L-carnitine in all six subjects was 205 μmol per 24 h $\pm$ SD. During the course of the experimental period lasting approximately 1 month, with four intermittent wash out periods lasting 1 week, the subjects were encouraged to maintain a low carnitine diet and were instructed on the use of reference charts to record the carnitine content ingested per 100 g of food item.

Intravenous administration

The concentration of L-carnitine at different time intervals post-dosing is illustrated in Table 1. The data compares the mean plasma values ± SD determined for all subjects in the study group after intravenous bolus dose of 30 mg kg^{-1} and 100 mg kg^{-1} L-carnitine. A plot of the plasma concentration–time points measured for each subject showed that the curves exhibited multiexponential decline which were best fitted to a triexponential model especially when considering longer time intervals of L-carnitine concentration in plasma. Figure 1a (30 mg kg^{-1}) and Figure 1b (100 mg kg^{-1}) illustrate the best-fit curve of the mean plasma values listed in Table 1. The triexponential equation derived by non-linear least squares analysis, and shown in the figures, gave a good estimate of the plasma concentration of L-carnitine at different time intervals post intravenous dosing.

Other pharmacokinetic parameters are shown in Table 2: the values of the zero time intercepts, C_1, C_2, and C_3, as well as the area under the curve (AUC) were proportional to the dose administered, being higher at the larger dose. The half-life ($t_{\frac{1}{2}}$) of the drug in the distribution phase was significantly lower for the larger dose, as evidenced by the

TABLE 1.

Mean plasma concentration minus endogenous values after administration of 30 mg kg^{-1} and 100 mg kg^{-1} L-carnitine intravenously

Time (h)	30 mg kg^{-1} μmol l^{-1} ± SD	100 mg kg^{-1} μmol l^{-1} ± SD
0.00	37.2 ± 6.1	37.2 ± 6.1
0.08	1444.8 ± 157.9	2913.9 ± 320.4
0.16	1177.8 ± 129.8	2635.7 ± 237.5
0.33	1083.2 ± 157.6	2398.4 ± 239.1
0.50	718.3 ± 72.7	2210.3 ± 265.2
1.00	222.5 ± 29.0	1482.3 ± 133.3
2.00	163.3 ± 18.1	819.9 ± 81.9
3.00	114.1 ± 13.8	627.2 ± 56.4
4.00	57.7 ± 9.4	380.7 ± 49.4
6.00	33.9 ± 5.2	225.1 ± 24.7
8.00	13.1 ± 4.5	237.5 ± 23.7
10.00	17.2 ± 2.0	42.4 ± 5.5
12.00	12.6 ± 1.9	40.3 ± 8.8
24.00	3.9 ± 0.4	110.1 ± 14.3
Body weight mean ± SS	71.3 ± 2.3	71.3 ± 2.3

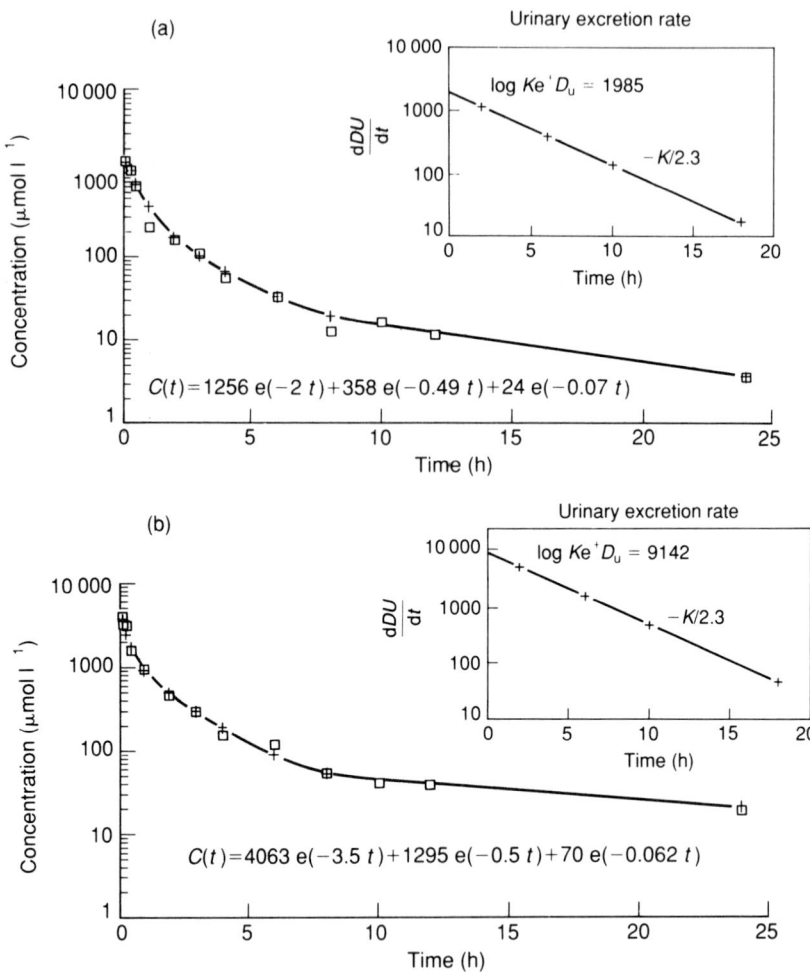

FIGURE I. Plasma concentration–time profile minus endogenous values after intravenous administration of (a) 30 mg kg^{-1} L-carnitine and (b) 100 mg kg^{-1} L-carnitine.

higher value of the fast disposition slope (β_1). The differences seen in the overall elimination rate β_2, even though lower at the higher dose, were not statistically significant for the two dosage levels. The terminal phase of the distribution slope (β_3) gave a significantly longer half-life for the higher dose, hence, suggesting a dose dependency on the mean residence time (MRT) of the drug in the body. Total clearance (Cl), renal clearance (Cl$_r$) and non-renal clearance (Cl$_{nr}$) were significantly higher for the larger dose. For the two dosage levels, the Cl$_r$

TABLE 2.
Pharmacokinetic parameters of L-carnitine calculated for 30 mg kg^{-1} and 100 mg kg^{-1} doses administered intravenously

Parameters	Dose	
	30 mg kg^{-1}	100 mg kg^{-1}
C_1 (μmol l^{-1})	1256.4 ± 356.1	4063.4 ± 509.6
C_2 (μmol l^{-1})	358.1 ± 75.2	1295.4 ± 430.7
C_3 (μmol l^{-1})	24.0 ± 4.5	70.3 ± 18.2
β_1 (l h^{-1})	2.00 ± 0.4	3.5 ± 0.63
β_2 (l h^{-1})	0.49 ± 0.1	0.5 ± 0.14
β_3 (l h^{-1})	0.07 ± 0.01	0.062 ± 0.013
$t_{\frac{1}{2}}\beta_1$ (h)	0.34 ± 0.07	0.19 ± 0.032
$t_{\frac{1}{2}}\beta_2$ (h)	1.41 ± 0.31	1.38 ± 0.35
$t_{\frac{1}{2}}\beta_3$ (h)	9.24 ± 2.21	11.55 ± 2.42
Cl_t (l h^{-1})	8.03 ± 0.54	9.89 ± 2.76
Cl_r (l h^{-1})	6.97 ± 0.83	7.89 ± 1.57
Cl_{nr} (l h^{-1})	1.06 ± 0.16	2.05 ± 0.38
V_d (l)	36.95 ± 7.75	34.09 ± 7.49
MRT (h)	4.21 ± 0.79	5.60 ± 1.12
AUC(0–24) (μmol h l^{-1})	1377.15 ± 335.38	4013.12 ± 1003.25
AUC(0–∞) (μmol h l^{-1})	1648.31 ± 428.20	4445.11 ± 800.10
AUMC(0–∞) (μmol h l^{-1})	5618.00 ± 1179.20	24892.00 ± 6471.92
K_e (l h^{-1})	0.14 ± 0.035	0.19 ± 0.04

TABLE 3.
Urinary excretion of L-carnitine at different time intervals after administration of 30 mg kg^{-1} and 100 mg kg^{-1} intravenously

Time (h)	basal (μmol ± SD)	30 mg kg^{-1} (μmol ± SD)	100 mg kg^{-1} (μmol ± SD)
0–4	38.98 ± 5.42	9619 ± 193	30618 ± 3368
4–8	38.01 ± 6.94	1055 ± 96	3993 ± 319
8–12	38.34 ± 11.04	410 ± 85	1093 ± 66
12–24	68.93 ± 17.19	414 ± 98	665 ± 40
Recovery % Dose		86	82

was less than the renal blood flow, indicating a low extraction ratio
of the drug. The volume of distribution of the drug did not show
statistically significant differences at the two dosage levels. The volume
of distribution was in the range typical for drugs distribution within
the intracellular fluid. The cumulative excretion data, calculated at
different time intervals over a period of 24 h, are listed in Table 3. A
plot of log excretion rate (dU_e/dt), versus midpoint time of urinary
collection period is shown in the insert to Figure 1a. The elimination
rate constant determined from the zero time intercept in the graph
was $0.14 \, h^{-1}$. The recovery of L-carnitine found in the 24-h urine,
expressed as percentage of the administered dose, did not differ
significantly for the two different doses. It should be mentioned,
however, that non-renal clearance increased with the higher dosage
level, conceivably involving greater biliary recycling of the drug.

Oral administration

The mean plasma concentration values ± SD following oral administration of L-carnitine are shown in Table 4. The zero time point in the

TABLE 4.

Mean plasma concentration minus endogenous values after oral administration of
$30 \, mg \, kg^{-1}$ and $100 \, mg \, kg^{-1}$ L-carnitine

Time (h)	30 mg kg^{-1} (Mean ± SD)	100 mg kg^{-1} (Mean ± SD)
0	60.42 ± 6.07	60.42 ± 6.07
0.5	5.11 ± 1.98	5.40 ± 1.18
1	6.20 ± 2.41	14.92 ± 2.98
2	23.69 ± 6.62	65.09 ± 12.36
3	27.10 ± 8.11	90.74 ± 22.68
4	25.72 ± 7.31	88.32 ± 20.31
5	23.00 ± 7.12	72.37 ± 13.75
6	18.50 ± 5.68	50.43 ± 5.54
8	9.30 ± 2.82	35.79 ± 6.44
10	7.20 ± 2.95	32.21 ± 5.79
12	4.50 ± 1.46	17.43 ± 2.61
14	4.00 ± 1.18	15.37 ± 3.38
18	2.60 ± 1.55	9.65 ± 2.21
24	0.20 ± 0.52	4.09 ± 0.44

table represents the endogenous carnitine values. Figures 2a and 2b show a profile of the plasma concentration–time points illustrated in Table 1. The shaded region of the curve represents the distribution of the data points for the time interval. The mean pharmacokinetic parameters listed in Table 5 show that the maximum plasma concentration, as well as the AUC, were proportional to the administered dose. The time to reach maximum blood concentration (t_{max}) was slightly longer for the higher dose. No statistically significant differences

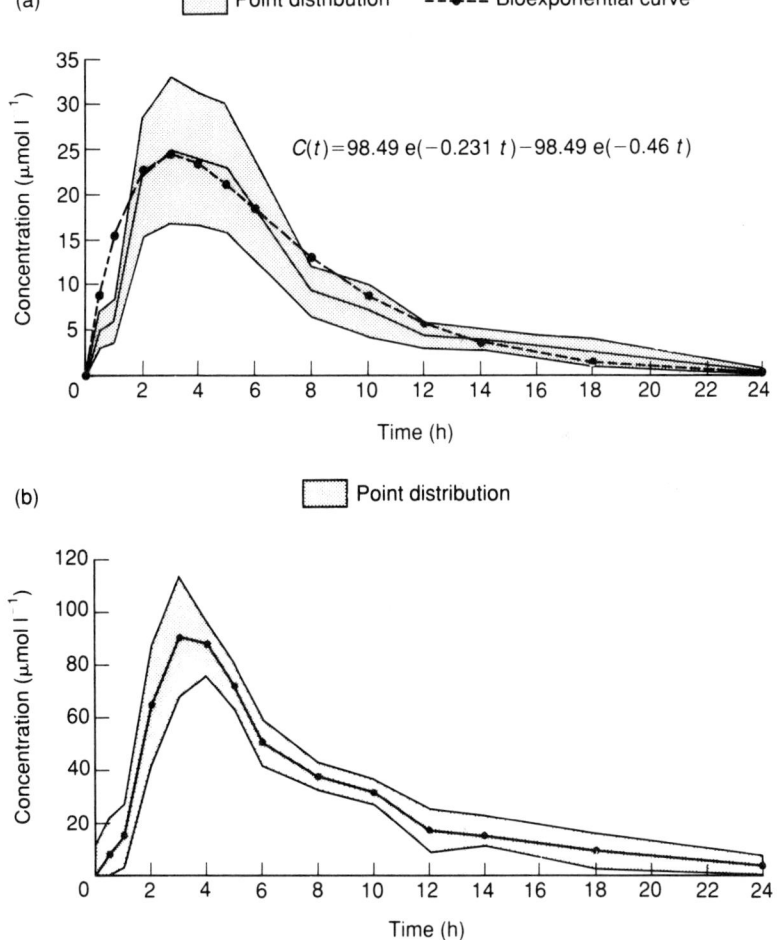

FIGURE 2. Plasma concentration–time profile minus endogenous values after oral administration of (a) 30 mg kg^{-1} and (b) 100 mg kg^{-1} L-carnitine.

TABLE 5.

Pharmacokinetic parameters of L-carnitine calculated for 30 mg kg^{-1} and 100 mg kg^{-1} oral dose

Parameters	Dose	
	30 mg kg^{-1}	100 mg kg^{-1}
C_{max} (μmol/l)	24.62 ± 3.93	90.81 ± 19.07
T_{max} (hrs)	2.98 ± 0.58	3.52 ± 0.56
$T_{\frac{1}{2}}$ (hrs)	3.02 ± 0.75	4.07 ± 0.44
Cl_t (l/h)	8.69 ± 2.08	9.70 ± 2.23
V_d (l)	37.62 ± 7.78	36.58 ± 8.41
AUC(0–24) (μmol h l^{-1})	197.25 ± 43.34	727.12 ± 116.33
AUC(0–∞) (μmol h l^{-1})	213.18 ± 38.34	945.11 ± 141.75
F (%)	0.16 ± 0.03	0.14 ± 0.02

were observed for the volume of distribution (V_d) or total body clearance (C_t). The half-life of the drug calculated from the elimination phase of the curve showed that the overall differences between the two dosage levels were relatively small; the higher dose having a slightly larger value. Since the urine concentrations at different time intervals were not available, further attempts to define the disposition of the drug in the body were not made. However, on the basis of the 24-h urine collected from each volunteer, a total recovery of unchanged drug was found to be approximately 4–7%. Estimation of the bioavailability of the drug showed that 13% and 21% of the drug dose was absorbed, respectively, at each dosage level. The range of bioavailability is in keeping with other reports in the literature (Welling et al, 1979; Gudjonsson et al, 1985).

Multiple dosing regimen

Studies on multiple dosing regimens with L-carnitine at 30 mg kg^{-1} showed that administration of the drug at time intervals four times longer than the elimination half-life, had no significant accumulation ratio and a considerably larger fluctuation between the $C_{ss,max}$ and the $C_{ss,min}$. However, repeated doses of drug at time intervals of 6 h (approximately two half-lives) showed that the accumulation ratio between the $C_{ss,min}/C_{1,min}$ and the $C_{ss,max}/C_{1,max}$ was approximately 1.27–1.44. Where $C_{ss,min}$ and $C_{ss,max}$ are the minimum and maximum blood levels, respectively, at the plateau, $C_{1,min}$ and $C_{1,max}$ are the minimum and maximum blood concentrations after the first dose. A computer-simulated, multiple-dosing plasma concentration–time profile is shown in Figure 3. The curve was derived from best-fit parameters calculated from single oral dose of 30 mg kg^{-1}, at different time intervals, after repeated dosage. Carnitine concentration in the blood samples during multiple dosing was assayed primarily to evaluate the accumulation of drug. A comparison between the calculated values, and the values actually found, showed that the simulated curve at dosing intervals of 6 h, gave an overestimation of the experimental data points of approximately 14–18%. This error is inherent in the techniques used for back-extrapolation, the monoexponential line from the graphically determined C_0, which generally lies below the monoexponential slope.

DISCUSSION

We studied the pharmacokinetics of L-carnitine at two dosage levels in healthy volunteers following intravenous and oral administration. Significant correlations were found between a triexponential model and plasma concentration–time data, suggesting that kinetic features of L-carnitine disposition may be interpreted and predicted over a period of 24 h post-dosing. It should be mentioned, however, that

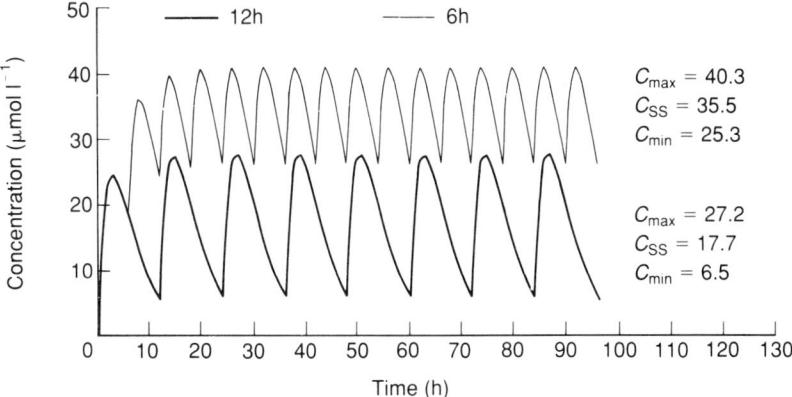

FIGURE 3. Concentration–time profile after multiple oral administration of 30 mg kg^{-1} L-carnitine.

some methodological problems were encountered in determining L-carnitine concentrations at the longer time periods post-dosing. The variance associated to the estimated mean plasma values at 24 h, for the six individuals, is high and conceivably might overestimate the pharmacokinetic parameters associated with the terminal distribution phase, as well as mean residence time of the drug in the body. This feature was more pronounced especially at the higher dosage levels. As the dosage level of drug increased, the total Cl as well as the renal and non-renal clearance of the drug increased. The half-life of the drug calculated from the elimination phase of the triexponential function did not show a statistically significant difference. In contrast, the distribution and terminal elimination half-life were significantly different at the two dosage levels. The estimates of the pharmacokinetic parameters after intravenous dosage, as well as bioavailability of the drug were in agreement with those reported by Harper et al (1988). Plasma protein binding of the drug did not appear as a significant factor in determining L-carnitine content in the blood. However, binding to red blood cells appears to be a more significant phenomenon in determining blood levels of the drug. In vitro incubation of L-carnitine with whole blood from volunteers in the study group, showed that incubation of red blood cells at 37° C, for 30 min, sequestered approximately 20–30% of the initial L-carnitine concentration added. The binding of L-carnitine to red cells may be important in the disposition of L-carnitine in the body. Conceivably, the uptake and release of L-carnitine by red blood cells may have important consequences not only on the blood concentration–time profile of the drug, but also on the disposition of the drug in the body.

The accumulation ratio of L-carnitine during multiple oral dosing regimen of 30 mg kg^{-1} L-carnitine was calculated from the experimental data points. The calculated curve assuming linear first-order kinetics, gave an overestimated prediction of the experimental points of approximately 14–18%. These results would suggest that there is some binding of the drug to red blood cells as well as to cellular macromolecules within the body.

REFERENCES

Bieber LL, Emaus R, Valkner K & Farrel S (1982) Fed. Proc. 41: 2858–2862.
Boots MR, Wolfe ML, Boots SG & Bobbitt JI (1980) J. Pharm. Sci. 69: 202–204.
De Vivo D & Tein I (1990) Int. Pediatr. 5(2): 134–141.

Engel AG & Angelini C (1973) *Science* 173: 899–902.

Fritz IB & Schultz SR (1965) *J. Biol. Chem.* 240: 2188–2192.

Gibladi M & Perrier D (eds) (1982) *Pharmacokinetics*, 2nd edn. New York: Marcel Dekker.

Gudjonsson H, Li BUK, Shug AL & Olsen WA (1985) *Gastroenterology* 88: 1880–1887.

Harper P, Elwin CE & Cederblad G (1988) *Eur. J. Clin. Pharmacol.* 35: 555–562.

Kysiak W, Toth PP, Suelter CH & Bieber LL (1986) *J. Biol. Chem.* 261, 29: 13698–13701.

Paulson DJ & Shug AL (1981) *Life Sci.* 28: 2931–2938.

Schafer J & Reichmann (1989) *Clin. Chim. Acta* 182: 87–94.

Welling PG, Thomsen JH, Shug AL & Tse FLS (1979) *Int. J. Clin. Pharmacol. Biopharm* 70: 56–60.

Part Ib

Applications to therapy

5

CLINICAL AND BIOMEDICAL PHENOTYPES OF CARNITINE DEFICIENCIES

S. DiDonato, B. Garavaglia, M. Rimoldi, and F. Carrara

FUNCTION

Carnitine, β-hydroxy-γ-N-trimethylamino-butyrate, performs a crucial role in energy supply by controlling the influx of long-chain fatty acids into mitochondria. L-Carnitine, two carnitine palmitoyltransferases, CPT I and II, located respectively in the outer and inner mitochondrial membrane, and a carnitine–acylcarnitine translocase embedded in the inner mitochondrial membrane, are required in mammalian tissues to transfer long-chain acyl CoAs across the inner membrane for β-oxidation in the matrix (Bremer, 1983). Furthermore, intramitochondrial carnitine and the matrix enzyme carnitine acetyltransferase (CAT) can react with short- and medium-chain acyl CoAs to produce acylcarnitines, which can be shuttled out of mitochondria (Bieber et al, 1982). Through this mechanism, carnitine is able to modulate the intracellular concentrations of free CoA and acetyl CoA via reversible formation of acetylcarnitine (Bloisi et al, 1990). Therefore, besides

L-Carnitine and Its Role in Medicine:
From Function to Therapy. ISBN 0–12–253940–0

shuttling long-chain fatty acids into mitochondria, carnitine facilitates the oxidation of pyruvate (Uziel et al, 1988) and branched-chain ketoacids (Bieber et al, 1982) and, by preventing their accumulation, it contributes to the protection of cells from the potentially membrane-destabilizing acyl CoAs (Bremer, 1983).

The relevance of carnitine in intermediary metabolism has been stressed by the important work of McGarry et al (1989), who reported elevated levels of carnitine in rats that had been starved, made diabetic or treated with glucagon: these animals showed concomitantly increased long-chain fatty acid oxidation and ketogenesis. These authors showed also that malonyl CoA, the first intermediate of fatty acid biosynthesis, is a potent inhibitor of CPT I, the acyltransferase located in the outer membrane in mitochondria, therefore suggesting a reciprocal control of hepatic fatty acid biosynthesis and oxidation by malonyl CoA and carnitine in normal and ketotic states (McGarry and Foster, 1979). With a carbohydrate diet, when the plasma ratio of glucagon to insulin is low, the malonyl CoA concentration arises with concomitantly enhanced fatty acid synthesis and suppression of fatty acid oxidation. Conversely, in the fasting state or uncontrolled diabetes, where the plasma glucagon:insulin ratio is high, the malonyl CoA levels fall and the carnitine levels increase in the liver: fatty acid synthesis is diminished and CPT becomes depressed, favouring fatty acid oxidation and ketogenesis (McGarry et al, 1989).

Although there is general agreement on this scheme of metabolic regulation proposed by McGarry et al (1989), some doubts have been raised about the existence of a CPT I enzyme with malonyl CoA-binding properties. Indeed, there is some evidence from the literature that a malonyl CoA-binding protein (MCBP) is present at the outer mitochondrial membrane, but this protein seems to lack CPT activity (Lund and Woldegiorgis, 1986). The recent molecular cloning of a cDNA encoding the entire sequence of human CPT should help in addressing these ambiguities (Finocchiaro et al, 1990). Another possible physiological role for carnitine comes from the work of Bieber et al (1982), who demonstrated high levels of branched-chain acylcarnitines in beef liver suggesting that carnitine might help in the oxidation of branched-chain amino acids. Finally, carnitine may also shuttle acyl moieties, shortened by the peroxisomal β-oxidation system, from peroxisomes to mitochondria for further oxidation (Engel, 1986).

Metabolism

Approximately 75% of the carnitine source for the body stores comes from the diet: red meat in adults and human milk in infants are the principal sources. In man the liver and the kidney synthesize the remaining 25% from the immediate precursor γ-butyrobetaine: protein-bound lysine and methionine are required for carnitine biosynthesis (Engel, 1986; Scholte and de Jonge, 1987). Carnitine is present in tissues and biological fluids in free and esterified forms. In humans, acylcarnitine esters account for about 25% of total carnitine in serum and for about 15% of total carnitine in liver and skeletal muscle. Total carnitine concentration in human tissues is higher in the heart and skeletal muscle (3.5–6.0 and 2.0–4.6 μmol g^{-1}, respectively) than in the liver and the brain (1.0–1.9 and 0.5–1.0 μmol g^{-1}, respectively): these values reflect the higher rates of fatty acid oxidative metabolism in the former tissues. Due to the bulk of skeletal muscle, and its high carnitine concentration, 95% of the total body carnitine (approximately 100 mmol in a 70 kg adult) is stored in muscle. The remaining body carnitine is in heart, liver and kidney, with less than 1% in biological fluids. Carnitine in blood is 20–60 times less concentrated (30–60 nmol ml^{-1}) than in tissues (Engel, 1986; Scholte and DeJonge, 1987; DeVivo and Tein, 1990).

Therefore carnitine, either introduced in the diet, or synthesized de novo in the liver and kidney, must be actively concentrated from the blood into fatty acid-metabolizing organs, such as skeletal muscle. Cell receptors with high affinity for carnitine have been identified in muscle (Rebouche, 1977), heart cells (Bohmer et al, 1977) and cultured fibroblasts (Rebouche and Engel, 1982). The liver (Christensen and Bremer, 1976) and the brain (Huth et al, 1981) have low-affinity receptors for carnitine, while the intestinal epithelial cells (Shaw et al, 1983) and the renal tubular cells (Rebouche and Mack, 1984) have intermediate-affinity receptors for carnitine. The kidney, in addition to its contribution in carnitine biosynthesis, is crucial in regulating the plasma and tissue levels of carnitine: the renal threshold for free carnitine is approximately 40 μmol l^{-1}, a value close to that in plasma, and the proximal tubule actively transports carnitine across its membrane thus minimizing the loss of carnitine from the body (Engel, 1986).

Thus, a complex metabolic equilibrium exists between the various carnitine fractions in the different body compartments, and between the carnitine pool of tissues and blood, as well as the fraction excreted in the urine (Bremer, 1983).

HUMAN DISORDERS

Since fatty acid oxidation is essential for ketone body synthesis in the liver and for energy production in the muscle, and carnitine is crucial for long-chain fatty acid oxidation, disorders associated with carnitine deficiency would be expected to impair liver and muscle function. Carnitine deficiency was recognized as a cause of human myopathy by Engel and Angelini (1973) and of hepatic encephalomyopathy by Karpati et al (1975). Since then, and as the means to measure the concentrations of carnitine have become more available, it became clear that carnitine deficiency was a relatively common finding in patients with a number of inherited metabolic and acquired diseases: both *primary carnitine deficiencies* (Treem et al, 1988) and *secondary carnitine deficiencies* were identified (DiDonato, 1987; Stanley, 1987). The association of human diseases with critically low tissue carnitine suggested a therapeutic role for L-carnitine (the active physiological isomer) (Editorial, 1990).

Three forms of primary carnitine deficiency (CD) have been described: myopathic, systemic, and progressive cardiomyopathy with systemic CD. However, the definition of 'primary' CD for most cases reported in the literature was based on negative criteria (i.e. lack of evidence for an associated genetic or acquired disorder able to lower tissue carnitine stores) and many of the earlier cases have undergone reassessment during the past decade in light of new information (DeVivo and Tein, 1990). Indeed, the pathogenesis of these earlier cases of CD is obscure, although different possible mechanisms have been suggested. Lack of receptors for carnitine in skeletal muscle in muscle CD, and defective carnitine biosynthesis or generalized absence of carnitine receptors in systemic CD have been proposed, but never proven (Engel, 1986). The reports in the literature have been contradictory: in many patients the mechanisms able to cause CD have been re-examined and many cases have been reclassified (DiDonato, 1987; DeVivo and Tein, 1990). In spite of these ambiguities in the classification of patients in the literature, primary CD is now recognized as a true nosological entity characterized by progressive cardiomyopathy, low carnitine in plasma, heart, muscle, and liver, lipid accumulation in skeletal muscle and other organs, and a defect in carnitine transport which can be demonstrated in cultured fibroblasts (Treem et al, 1988; Erikssonn et al, 1988; Tein et al, 1990).

Secondary CDs include numerous genetic and acquired conditions which are associated to a depletion of tissue carnitine stores. Among the genetic causes of secondary CD, the most frequently reported are the organic acidurias (such as propionic, methylmalonic and isovaleric acidurias) (Chalmers et al, 1984; DiDonato et al, 1984a), and the genetic defects of β-oxidation, such as short-chain acyl CoA dehydrogenase (SCAD), medium-chain acyl CoA dehydrogenase (MCAD), and long-chain acyl CoA dehydrogenase (LCAD) deficiencies and glutaric aciduria type II (DiDonato, 1987; Stanley, 1987). Table 1 summarizes the main forms of primary and secondary CD recognized in man.

PRIMARY CARNITINE DEFICIENCIES

Myopathic carnitine deficiency

Carnitine deficiency was recognized as a cause of human myopathy in 1973 (Engel and Angelini, 1973). Since then several patients with progressive muscular weakness and wasting, accumulation of lipid droplets in type I muscle fibres, and low carnitine in skeletal muscle but not in plasma, liver or heart, have been described (Cornelio and DiDonato, 1985; Scholte and de Jonge, 1987). Carnitine esters are

TABLE I.
Carnitine deficiencies in man

Type of deficiency	Reference
Primary CD (clinically identified)	
Muscle CD	Engel and Angelini (1973)
Systemic CD	Karpati et al (1975)
Familial cardiomyopathy	Tripp et al (1981)
Primary CD (biochemically identified)	
Defective carnitine transport	Treem et al (1988)
Secondary CD (genetically determined)	
Organic acidurias	Chalmers et al (1984)
Defects of β-oxidation	Stanley (1987)
Respiratory chain defects	Sengers et al (1987)
Secondary CD (acquired)	
Haemodialysis	Bohmer et al (1978)
Pivampicillin	Holme et al (1989)
Valproate	Editorial (1990)

normal, and there is no abnormal excretion of organic acids in the urines. Treatment with oral L-carnitine (2–6 g day^{-1}) improves patients' clinical status, but is unable to modify the low carnitine content in muscle (Engel, 1986).

Since the description of secondary CDs, the existence of a true form of primary CD affecting only skeletal muscle has been questioned. First, it is difficult to differentiate myopathic and systemic CD because, often, extramuscular tissues, such as liver or heart, are not available to be tested (Scholte and de Jonge, 1987). Furthermore, genetic defects of β-oxidation can mimic muscle CD, but have been rarely explored in the patients described in the literature (Stanley, 1987) (see below). However, the first patient with muscle CD described by Engel and Angelini had the following features: the carnitine content was low in muscle and normal in plasma; the oxidation of palmitate, defective in muscle homogenates, was normalized by carnitine; the patient improved under carnitine supplementation; carnitine uptake was specifically impaired in skeletal muscle (Engel, 1986). It is reasonable to think that this patient might have suffered from primary muscle CD.

Systemic carnitine deficiency

The first patient with this disorder, described by Karpati et al in 1975, had weakness, wasting and generalized lipid storage in muscle and liver, established after he had suffered from several episodes of Reye's-like hepatic encephalopathy associated with dicarboxylic aciduria. This patient was treated with carnitine and fully recovered. Many infants suffering from hepatic encephalopathy, reduced plasma and tissue carnitine and lipid storage were described later under the heading of systemic CD: in most patients the overt myopathy was absent and muscle signs were restricted to mild weakness and hypotonia (Cornelio and DiDonato, 1985). Total carnitine was found low in plasma, muscle, liver, and heart; carnitine esters, however, could be higher than normal in plasma and tissues (Engel, 1986; Scholte and de Jonge, 1987). Since carnitine content in the liver is low, ketone body production with fasting may be impaired (DiDonato et al, 1980). Increased urinary excretion of carnitine, especially in the esterified form, has been reported in some patients: abnormal renal handling of carnitine was suggested to contribute to the pathogenesis of the disorder (Engel et al, 1981). Several cases of systemic CD have been treated with oral L-carnitine: under treatment the metabolic attacks disappeared, muscle strength improved, and carnitine content increased in the tissues of some of the patients reported (Chapoy et al, 1980; DiDonato et al, 1984b).

Although there was no cardiac involvement in most patients with systemic CD, it was a main symptom in the infant reported by Chapoy et al (1980). This patient however, was probably affected by the cardiomyopathic form of systemic CD, described later by Tripp et al (1981), and Waber et al (1982) (see below).

Several considerations question the existence of this type of primary CD. First, the disease was thought to be genetic and inherited as an autosomal recessive trait, on the basis of intermediate values of tissue and plasma carnitine found in obligate heterozygotes of a family with two affected twin siblings (DiDonato et al, 1984c); this family, however, was further investigated and the two sisters were shown to be affected by glutaric aciduria type II (DiDonato, unpublished data). Second, the first patient with systemic CD described in the literature excreted dicarboxylic acids in his urine (Karpati et al, 1975), similarly to patients with MCAD and LCAD deficiencies (Stanley, 1987), but at difference with patients with the cardiomyopathic form of primary CD (Treem et al, 1988). Finally, biochemical studies in subjects with systemic CD, proved recently that some of these patients had a deficiency of the β-oxidation enzyme medium-chain acyl CoA dehydrogenase (Zierz et al, 1988), while other patients had defects of the flavoproteins linking the primary dehydrogenases to the respiratory chain (DiDonato et al, 1986a). Therefore, many of the cases reported in the literature with systemic CD, similarly to those with muscle CD, may have suffered from other disorders, namely primary defects of β-oxidation enzymes (Stanley, 1987).

Progressive cardiomyopathy and systemic CD

Among the patients with systemic CD, a subgroup is characterized by the peculiar phenotype of progressive dilatative cardiomyopathy which, untreated, leads to death. Carnitine content is low in the patients' muscle, heart, liver and plasma. The disease is described in familial form, suggesting autosomal recessive inheritance (Chapoy et al, 1980; Tripp et al, 1981; Waber et al, 1982). Although the patients have a generalized deficiency of carnitine in tissues, signs of liver and muscle dysfunction are generally limited to hypoglycaemia and hypotonia, and the pathology is confined to progressive, dilatative, life-threatening, cardiomyopathy. Clinical response to carnitine supplementation is dramatic. Treated patients soon recover a normal heart function and can perform a normal life, whilst untreated patients die of cardiac insufficiency at an early age (Tripp et al, 1981). Excellent therapeutic results with carnitine supplementation have been reported in American (Tein et al, 1990), European (Taillard et al, 1988), and Japanese families (Matsuishi et al, 1985) with this disorder. Although some degree of clinical heterogeneity was suggested by the description of infants (Treem et al, 1988) with hypoketotic hypoglycaemia and marked hypotonia, but absence of cardiac involvement, a recent overview shows that most patients have either cardiomyopathy or hypoglycaemia, or both (Tein et al, 1990).

Interestingly, in some patients both the intestinal uptake and the renal readsorption of carnitine are impaired (Waber et al, 1982; Rodriguez–Pereira et al, 1988) suggesting that the signs and symptoms might be due to a reduced availability of carnitine, which in turn is secondary to a defect in membrane transport involving the gut, the kidney and other organs. A defect of carnitine transport across the cell membranes was subsequently demonstrated in cultured fibroblasts from several patients (Treem et al, 1988; Eriksson et al, 1989; Tein et al, 1990).

As a whole, these data suggest that a common transport system with high affinity for carnitine might exist in human fibroblasts, muscle, kidney and, possibly, intestinal mucosa, and may be impaired in patients with this disease. This conclusion however, is somewhat hampered by the current notion that although the heart, skeletal muscle and fibroblasts have similar K_m values for carnitine uptake (in the order of 2–6 μM), the kidney and intestinal mucosa show higher K_m for carnitine transport (in the order of 100–200 μM) (Scholte and de Jonge, 1987; DeVivo and Tein, 1990).

Family studies have shown that obligate heterozygotes for this disease show intermediate values of carnitine in plasma and muscle (Tein et al, 1990). Moreover, transport in cultured cells from heterozygotes shows normal K_m for carnitine, but the V_{max} are approximately 50% of those of controls, suggesting that: (i) the disease is autosomal recessive; (ii) it is due to absence of high affinity receptors for carnitine in homozygotes; and (iii) the heterozygotes have about half the normal number of receptors in their cells (Garavaglia et al, 1991).

Patients with this disease, due to a genetically determined defect in carnitine transport, appear to have 'true primary' CD.

SECONDARY CARNITINE DEFICIENCIES

As previously discussed, the pathogenesis of primary CD is not clearly understood in many patients described under the heading of muscular and systemic CD. Conversely, in patients with secondary CD of genetic origin, the pathogenesis of CD has been studied in depth, especially in subjects with organic acidurias and primary β-oxidation defects (Chalmers et al, 1984; Stanley, 1987). Indeed, detailed studies have shown that in these patients with mitochondrial diseases the acyl CoAs, which accumulate in mitochondria because of specific blocks in metabolism, can react with matrix carnitine to form acylcarnitines. These esters can leave the mitochondrion in virtue of the inner membrane carnitine–acylcarnitine translocase and, in contrast to their corresponding acyl CoAs, are eventually lost from the cell and excreted in the urine (Chalmers et al, 1984; DiDonato et al, 1984a). The presence of an intramitochondrial carnitine acetyltransferase, an enzyme with broad specificity for short-chain acyl CoAs, ensures the formation of the corresponding acylcarnitines in these disorders (Bremer, 1983). The initial loss of intracellular carnitine, in the form of acylcarnitines, would be buffered by free carnitine in plasma, which is synthesized in kidney and liver, or ingested with food. However, owing to continuous formation of acyl CoAs, when chronic acylcarnitine excretion exceeds the amounts of dietary and endogenous carnitine, the carnitine balance in the body would become negative, with a depletion of tissue carnitine stores (DiDonato et al, 1984a). Since data from several laboratories suggest that there is a renal threshold for free carnitine but not for carnitine esters in man, the type of distribution of carnitines in the plasma of patients with secondary CD (i.e. low free carnitine and increased short-chain carnitines) should enhance the loss of carnitine from the body (Rebouche and Engel, 1983). Another hypothetic mechanism for carnitine depletion is based on the possibility that increased acylcarnitine levels might impair carnitine transport in the tubular cells. Both mechanisms may contribute to the renal carnitine loss observed in secondary CD (Engel, 1986).

Since the driving force for carnitine depletion in these disorders is the continuous synthesis of acylcarnitines due to a block in acyl CoA metabolism, we expect to find in the patients' urine specific patterns of urinary acylcarnitines matching the corresponding acyl CoAs. Moreover, specific patterns of acylcarnitines in urine can be a useful tool for the diagnosis of the primary genetic defect (DiDonato, 1987).

Organic acidurias

The organic acidurias are genetic disorders of mitochondrial metabolism, which lead to the accumulation in tissues and biological fluids of organic acids, which cannot be further catabolized. They include defects in the catabolism of straight-chain fatty acids, the catabolism of the branched-chain amino acids and the numerous forms of infantile lactic acidosis (Saudubray et al, 1984). Accumulated acids are excreted in urines in free or esterified form: the gas chromatographic and mass spectrometric analysis of these acid compounds allows the diagnosis of the genetic disorder underlying the acidotic syndrome (Chalmers et al, 1984). Indeed, most organic acidurias are poorly characterized clinically. Patients are infants with poor growth, acidosis, metabolic attacks, and early death. Sometimes a peculiar odour can orientate the diagnosis (Saudubray et al, 1984). Among the more common organic acidurias, secondary CD has been described in propionic acidaemia and methylmalonic aciduria (Chalmers et al, 1984; DiDonato et al, 1984a), isovaleric aciduria (Roe et al, 1984), 3-methylglucagonic aciduria (Roe et al, 1986) and glutaric aciduria type I (Seccombe et al, 1986). Although mitochondrial defects of β-oxidation go along with increased excretion of organic acids in urines (i.e. the dicarboxylic acidurias and glutaric aciduria type II), these disorders are generally treated as separate entities from the previously described organic acidurias.

Defects of β-oxidation

The acyl CoA dehydrogenation deficiencies of straight-chain acyl CoAs comprise a group of inborn defects in the enzyme system that catalyses the oxidation of fatty acids. These disorders appear to be relatively common and, in some instances, can mimic primary CD (DiDonato, 1987; Stanley, 1987).

LCAD deficiency

The systemic study of young patients with fasting intolerance and defects in fatty acid metabolism, led Hale et al (1985) to identify three children, from unrelated families, with non-ketotic hypoglycaemia and LCAD deficiency. All patients had failure to thrive, hepatomegaly, cardiomegaly, hypotonia, encephalopathic metabolic crises and dicarboxylic aciduria. Total and free carnitine were lowered in patients' plasma, liver and muscle, but long-chain carnitine esters were increased.

Although the patients were weak and hypotonic, they were not primarily myopathic. LCAD activity was less than 10% of control values in patients' fibroblasts, leukocytes and liver, while the activities of MCAD, SCAD and isovaleryl CoA dehydrogenase were in the normal range. In agreement with these findings CO_2 production from cultured fibroblasts of the patients was impaired with long-chain fatty acids, but normal with medium- and short-chain substrates. Carnitine treatment improved the cardiac hypertrophy and prevented metabolic attacks, but failed to affect hypotonia and weakness (Hale et al, 1985).

MCAD deficiency

Episodes of metabolic encephalopathy, hypoglycaemia, defective synthesis of ketones, hepatomegaly with fatty degeneration of the liver are characteristic of Reye's syndrome, one of the major causes of sudden infant death (Howat et al, 1985). Some of these infants were shown to have dicarboxylic aciduria, with adipic, suberic, and sebacic acids in their urines (Rhead et al, 1983). Total carnitine content was markedly low in their tissues (Stanley et al, 1983). Genetic deficiency of MCAD was proven in the patients' cultured fibroblasts, lymphocytes and liver (Kolvraa et al, 1982; Rhead et al, 1983; Stanley et al, 1983). Accordingly, cultured cells from patients did not oxidize medium-chain fatty acids, but normally oxidized long- and short-chain substrates. More recently, immunoprecipitation assays with anti-MCAD antibodies and northern blot analysis of cellular mRNA, have shown either reduced synthesis of a normal-sized MCAD precursor and mature protein, or the synthesis of a MCAD enzyme of abnormal size in the cells from different affected individuals. The data suggest that both point mutations and aberrant splicing of primary transcription products may cause MCAD deficiency in man (Strauss et al, 1990).

MCAD deficiency has been recognized to be one of the most frequent genetic metabolic diseases, with more than 50 patients recognized up to now (Rinaldo et al, 1988). The diagnosis is greatly facilitated by recent FAB–MS (fast atom bombardment–mass spectroscopy) data showing that increased urinary levels of the more common dicarboxylic acids are associated in this disease with the excretion of hexanoylglycine, suberylglycine and phenylpropionylglycine: these metabolites have been considered pathognomonic of the disease (Rinaldo et al, 1988). In partial contrast with these findings, other FAB–MS studies revealed a unique profile in urinary organic acids of MCAD patients: octanoylcarnitine, associated with other medium-chain acylcarnitines, was described as the major metabolite in this disease, being present, and diagnostic, even between metabolic attacks (Roe et al, 1985).

Carnitine therapy in two MCAD patients improved urinary organic acid profile, reduced hepatomegaly and prevented metabolic attacks: however, in other patients' carnitine was unable to influence the clinical course and failed to restore to normal muscle carnitine content (Treem et al, 1989).

SCAD deficiency

This disease has been documented in a few patients. Two were infants with failure to thrive and non-ketotic hypoglycaemia (Amendt et al, 1987); one infant had vomiting, myopathy and low muscle carnitine (Coates et al, 1988); one was an adult with a lipid storage myopathy (Turnbull et al, 1984); another adult, described in abstract form (DiDonato et al, 1986b), also had progressive myopathy. All patients excreted increased amounts of ethylmalonic and methylsuccinic acids, two metabolites expected to accumulate in case of SCAD deficiency.

The myopathic patient, a 53-year-old woman, had weakness and wasting at the proximal muscle of the limbs, low carnitine in skeletal muscle and lipid storage. She normally oxidized ketones in liver, as deduced by normal ketogenesis with fasting. In muscle the oxidation of short-chain fatty acids was impaired, while the oxidation of octanoate and palmitate was similar to controls. SCAD activity was only partially reduced in her muscle mitochondria (Turnbull et al, 1984). This observation, together with the notion of absence of tissue specific isoenzymes for SCAD, has raised some doubts about the existence of a myopathic form of SCAD (DiDonato and Gellera, 1990) since both riboflavin deficiency and systemic SCAD deficiency may cause myopathic phenotypes (DiDonato et al, 1989).

Defects in the electron-transferring flavoproteins

Glutaric aciduria type II (GA II) is a human genetic disorder characterized by the excretion in urines of numerous organic acids, which derive from at least six different acyl CoA substrates. Consequently, the disorder has been classified as multiple acyl CoA dehydrogenase (MAD) deficiency (Gregersen, 1985; Rhead et al, 1987). Detailed biochemical and molecular studies have shown that the disease is biochemically heterogeneous since it can be associated to a deficiency of either electron-transfer flavoprotein or its dehydrogenase (Frerman and Goodman, 1985). A third type of glutaric aciduria type II with no identified aetiology and treatable with riboflavin (i.e. riboflavin-responsive multiple acyl CoA dehydrogenase deficiency) has been reported (Gregersen et al, 1982).

ETF and ETF-dehydrogenase deficiencies

Typical patients with GA II present neonatal acidosis and urinary excretion of glutaric, ethylmalonic, isovaleric, isobutyric, 2-methyl-butyric, and saturated and unsaturated dicarboxylic acids and sarcosine. In cultured cells from the patients, there is defective oxidation of several metabolites that are oxidized through different and specific acyl CoA dehydrogenases, (i.e. SCAD, MCAD and LCAD, isovaleryl CoA dehydrogenase, 2-methyl branched-chain acyl CoA dehydrogenase, glutaryl CoA dehydrogenase, and sarcosine dehydrogenase) (Gregersen, 1985). These primary flavoprotein dehydrogenases transfer electrons to the common FAD-containing electron-transfer flavoprotein (ETF) that, in turn, reduces the iron–sulphur-flavoprotein ETF-dehydrogenase (ETF-DH). This latter enzyme is thought to reduce coenzyme Q at the respiratory chain level. Frerman and Goodman (1985), and Christensen et al (1984) have independently shown that ETF is deficient in some of the patients with GA II, while in others the defect is localized at the level of ETF-DH. Most of GA II patients described in the literature have the acute infantile form of the disease, which may be life-threatening and is associated with generalized carnitine deficiency. Some GA II patients have a late-onset and milder disease, frequently presenting with hypotonia, lipid myopathy and low carnitine content in plasma, muscle and liver (Rhead et al, 1987; DiDonato et al, 1986a). A detailed study of a patient with GA II of late-onset, showed deficiency of carnitine in plasma, muscle, liver, kidney and heart: interestingly, an excess of butyryl-, isovaleryl-, isobutyryl-, and hexanoylcarnitines were found in the patient's urine, as expected in case of ETF-DH deficiency (DiDonato et al, 1986a). In some instances the patients with mild forms of MAD, excrete in their urines only ethylmalonic and adipic acids (ethylmalonic–adipic aciduria, EMA) (Mantagos et al, 1979). However, there is no evidence that these patients can be distinguished on a biochemical–genetic basis from patients with GA II (Stanley, 1987).

Riboflavin-responsive glutaric aciduria type II

This disorder has been described both in infants with acute metabolic attacks (Gregersen et al, 1982), and in adult patients with progressive myopathy and lipid storage (DeVisser et al, 1986). The patients have a urinary pattern of organic acids compatible with either GA II or EMA. Carnitine content in plasma and tissues is variably reduced. The clinical and biochemical responses to oral riboflavin supplementation are dramatic: the patients improve and organic aciduria normalizes (Harpey et al, 1983; DeVisser et al, 1986; DiDonato et al, 1989). Multiple defects of the acyl CoA dehydrogenases have been shown in muscle mitochondria isolated from these patients. Recent studies show that the enzyme deficiency involves all the primary dehydrogenases but is more marked at the level of SCAD and MCAD (DiDonato and Gellera, 1990). Interestingly, riboflavin was able to restore to normal the activity of the deficient dehydrogenases in some patients (DiDonato et al, 1989).

Other secondary carnitine deficiencies

Respiratory chain defects

A few patients with defects of the respiratory chain complexes, namely complex I, or NADH–coenzyme Q reductase (Clarke et al, 1984), complex II plus III, or succinate–cytochrome c reductase (Sengers et al, 1987), complex IV, or cytochrome c oxidase (Rimoldi et al, 1982), and complex V or ATP synthetase (Engel et al, 1986), have been reported to have lowered carnitine content either in plasma or muscle, or in both. The significance of these observations is unclear, since most patients with respiratory chain defects have normal carnitine content in their tissues and body fluids (Engel, 1986). Moreover, levels of plasma carnitine are known to fluctuate, especially in infants with generalized metabolic diseases (Saudubray et al, 1984).

Methylenetetrahydrofolate reductase deficiency

An infant with profound methylenetetrahydrofolate reductase deficiency, leukoencephalopathy, tetraparesis, lipid storage myopathy, low methionine in serum, and low carnitine in plasma and muscle, responded dramatically to folate, methionine and carnitine supplementation. The authors suggested that, since S-adenosylmethionine is necessary for carnitine biosynthesis, the disease could be an example of CD due to reduced endogenous synthesis of carnitine (Allen et al, 1980).

Renal Fanconi syndrome and haemodialysis

Any cause of renal Fanconi syndrome leads to systemic carnitine deficiency, which can be severe enough to cause liver dysfunction, lipid storage and weakness and wasting in muscle (Editorial, 1990). Furthermore, abnormalities of carnitine metabolism have been reported by several authors in haemodialysed patients (Bohmer et al, 1978): the plasma free carnitine/acylcarnitine ratio is lowered in plasma and muscle carnitine content may be reduced (Engel, 1986). Whether this relative CD is due to reduced carnitine synthesis or excessive loss into dialysate is uncertain, but many authors suggest that moderate amounts of carnitine in the exchange fluid may help the patients (Editorial, 1990).

Valproate therapy

Some patients treated with sodium valproate excrete valproylcarnitine and have low concentrations of free carnitine in plasma with an increased acyl/free carnitine ratio (Editorial, 1990). Valproic acid is a branched-chain acid (2-propyl-pentenoic acid) which gives rise to valproyl CoA in mitochondria. Although the metabolism of valproyl CoA is not fully understood, it has been suggested that it could be metabolized by the 2-methyl branched-chain acyl CoA dehydrogenase, the mitochondrial enzyme active on isobutyryl- and 2-methylbutyryl CoA (i.e. the two intermediates of valine and isoleucine metabolism, respectively) (Ito et al, 1990). Indeed, valproyl CoA has strong structural relationships with the latter substrates, since it is branched at the 2-carbon position. Moreover, 2-propyl-pentenoyl CoA, the desaturation product of valproyl CoA has been identified after incubation of valproyl CoA and purified rat liver 2-methyl branched-chain acyl CoA dehydrogenase. It has been suggested therefore that the enzymatic basis for valproate toxicity observed in some patients might reside in mutations of the 2-methyl branched-chain dehydrogenase, making these subjects intolerant to high doses of this compound (Ito et al, 1990).

Pivampicillin therapy

Another drug, pivampicillin, has been shown to cause CD in treated patients. In these subjects carnitine depletion has been observed both in plasma and muscle. Similarly to patients under valproate therapy, or those with genetic organic acidurias, the mechanism for carnitine loss is thought to be the excessive excretion of carnitine in the form of acyl ester, i.e. pivaloylcarnitine (Holme et al, 1989).

THERAPEUTIC ROLE OF CARNITINE IN SECONDARY CARNITINE DEFICIENCIES

In organic acidurias and in defects of β-oxidation, L-carnitine was shown to have positive metabolic effects, probably because exogenously administered carnitine was able 'to buffer' the excess of acyl CoAs, which accumulates in mitochondria as a consequence of specific metabolic blocks (Chalmers et al, 1984; DiDonato et al, 1984a; Stanley, 1987). Whether this metabolic effect of carnitine is associated to measurable clinical benefits is uncertain. Improvement of the general conditions and muscle tone, and reduction of recurrent metabolic attacks have been reported in some patients with organic acidurias (Roe and Bohen, 1982), but not in others (Seccombe et al, 1982), who continued to suffer acute metabolic attacks in spite of treatment. Probably these patients need an accurate and meticulous dietary treatment in addition to oral carnitine supplementation (Saudubray et al, 1984; Treem et al, 1989).

Acknowledgements

This work has been supported in part by a grant of the Associazione Italiana per la promozione delle Ricerche Neurologiche (ARIN), Milano. The authors are gratefully indebted to Barbara Bertagnolio and Cinzia Gellera, Dept Biochemistry & Genetics, Istituto Nazionale Neurologico, Milano, for critical reading of the manuscript.

REFERENCES

Allen RJ, Wong P, Rothenberg SP et al (1980) *Ann. Neurol.* 8: 211.
Amendt BA, Green C, Sweetman L et al (1987) *J. Clin. Invest.* 79: 1303–1309.
Bieber LL, Emans R, Valkeur K & Farrel S (1982) *Fed. Proc.* 41: 2858–2862.
Bloisi W, Colombo I, Garavaglia B et al (1990) *Eur. J. Biochem.* 189: 539–546.
Bohmer T, Eiklid K & Jonsen J (1977) *Biochim. Biophys. Acta* 465: 627–634.
Bohmer T, Bergrem H & Eiklid K (1978) *Lancet* i: 126–128.
Bremer J (1983) *Physiol. Rev.* 63: 1420–1480.

Broquist HR (1982) *Fed. Proc.* 41: 2840–2842.
Chalmers RA, Roe RC, Stacey CE & Hoppel CL (1984) *Pediatr. Res.* 18: 1325–1328.
Chapoy PR, Angelini C, Brown WJ et al (1980) *New Engl. J. Med.* 303: 1389–1394.
Christensen RZ & Bremer J (1976) *Biochim. Biophys. Acta* 448: 562–568.
Christensen N, Kolvraa S & Gregersen N (1984) *Pediatr. Res.* 18: 663–667.
Clark JB, Hayes DJ, Morgan-Hughes JA & Byrne E (1984) *J. Inher. Metab.* 7 (supplement 1): 62–74.
Coates PM, Hale DE, Finocchiaro G et al (1988) *J. Clin. Invest.* 81: 171–175.
Cornelio F & DiDonato S (1985) *J. Neurol.* 232: 329–340.
DeVisser M, Scholte HR, Schutgens RBH et al (1986) *Neurology* 36: 367–372.
DeVivo DC & Tein I (1990) *Int. Pediat.* 5: 134–140.
DiDonato S (1987) In Gitzelman R, Baerlocher K & Steinmann B (eds) *Carnitine in der Medizine* pp 91–100. Stuttgart; New York: Schattauer.
DiDonato S & Gellera C (1990) In Tanaka K & Coates P (eds) *Fatty Acid Oxidation: Clinical, Biochemical and Molecular Aspects* pp. 325–332. New York: Alan R. Liss.
DiDonato S, Peluchetti D, Rimoldi M et al (1980) *Clin. Chim. Acta* 100: 209–214.
DiDonato S, Rimoldi M, Garavaglia B et al (1984a) *Clin. Chim. Acta* 139: 13–20.
DiDonato S, Peluchetti D, Rimoldi M et al (1984b) *Neurology* 34: 157–162.
DiDonato S, Peluchetti D, Cornelio F et al (1984c) *Ann. Neurol.* 11: 190–192.
DiDonato S, Frerman FE, Rimoldi M et al (1986a) *Neurology* 36: 957–963.
DiDonato S, Cornelio F, Gellera C et al (1986b) *Muscle and Nerve* 9: 178.
DiDonato S, Gellera C, Peluchetti D et al (1989) *Ann. Neurol.* 25: 479–484.
Editorial (1990) *Lancet* i: 631–633.
Engel AG (1986) In Engel AG & Banker BQ (eds), *Myology, Basic and Clinical*, 5 pp. 1663–1696. New York: McCraw-Hill.
Engel AG & Angelini C (1973) *Science* 179: 899–902.
Engel AG, Rebouche CJ, Wilson MD et al (1981) *Neurology* 31: 819–825.
Eriksson BO, Lindstedt S & Nordin I (1988) *Eur. J. Pediatr.* 147: 662–663.
Eriksson BO, Gustafson B, Lindstedt S & Nordin I (1989) *J. Inher. Metab. Dis.* 12: 108–111.
Finocchiaro G, Taroni F, Rocchi M et al (1991) *Proc. Natl Acad. Sci. USA* 188: 661–665.
Frerman FE & Goodman SI (1985) *Proc. Natl Acad. Sci. USA* 82: 4517–4520.
Garavaglie B, Vziel GL, Dvorzak F et al (1991) *Neurology* (in press).
Gregersen N (1985) *Scand. J. Clin. Lab. Invest.* 45 (supplement 174): 11–60.
Gregersen N, Wintzensen H, Kolvraa S et al (1982) *Pediatr. Res.* 16: 861–868.
Hale DE, Batshaw ML, Coates PM et al (1985) *Pediatr. Res.* 19: 666–671.
Harpey JP, Charpentier C, Goodman SI et al (1983) *J. Pediatr.* 103: 394–398.
Holme E, Greter J, Jacobson CE et al (1989) *Lancet* i: 469–472.
Howat AJ, Bennet MJ, Variend S et al (1985) *Br. Med. J.* 290: 1771–1773.
Huth PJ, Schmidt MJ, Hall PV et al (1981) *J. Neurochem.* 36: 715–723.
Ito M, Ikeda Y, Arnez GJ et al (1990) *Biochim. Biophys. Acta* 1034: 213–218.
Karpati G, Carpenter S, Engel AG et al (1975) *Neurology* 25: 16–24.
Kolvraa S, Gregersen N, Christensen E et al (1982) *Clin. Chim. Acta* 126: 53–67.
Lund H & Woldegiorgis G (1986) *Biochim. Biophys. Acta* 878: 243–249.
Mantagos S, Genel M & Tanaka K (1979) *J. Clin. Invest.* 64: 1580–1589.
Matsuishi T, Hirata K, Terasawa K et al (1985) *Neuropediatrics* 16: 6–12.
McGarry JD & Foster DW (1979). *J. Biol. Chem.* 254: 8163–8168.

McGarry JD, Woeltje KF, Kuwajima M & Foster DW (1989) *Diabetes/Metabolism Reviews* 5: 271–284.
Rebouche CJ (1977) *Biochim. Biophys. Acta* 471: 145–155.
Rebouche CJ & Engel AG (1982) *In Vitro* 18: 495–502.
Rebouche CL & Engel AG (1983) *Mayo Clin. Proc.* 58: 832–841.
Rebouche CJ & Mack DL (1984) *Arch. Biochem. Biophys.* 235: 393–401.
Rhead WJ, Amendt BA, Fritchman KS et al (1983) *Science* 221: 73–75.
Rhead WJ, Wolff JA, Lipson M et al (1987) *Pediatr. Res.* 21: 371–376.
Rimoldi M, Bottacchi E, Rossi L et al (1982) *J. Neurol.* 227: 201–207.
Rinaldo P, O'Shea JJ, Coates PM et al (1988) *New Engl. J. Med.* 319: 1308–1313.
Rodriguez-Pereira R, Scholte HR, Luyt-Houven IEM & Vaandrager-Verduin MHM (1988) *Eur. J. Pediatr.* 148: 193–197.
Roe RC & Bohen TP (1982) *Lancet* i: 1401.
Roe CR, Millington DS, Maltby DA et al (1984) *J. Clin. Invest.* 74: 2290–2295.
Roe CR, Millington DAM, Bohan TP et al (1985) *Pediatr. Res.* 19: 459–466.
Roe CR, Millington DS & Maltby DA (1986) *J. Clin. Invest.* 77: 1391–1394.
Saudubray JM, Ogier H, Charpentier C et al (1984) *J. Inher. Metab. Dis.* 7 (supplement 1): 2–9.
Scholte HR & de Jonge PC (1987) In Gitzelman R, Baerlocker K & Steinmann B (eds) *Carnitine in der Medizine* pp. 22–59. Stuttgart: Schattauer.
Shaw RD, Li BUK, Hamilton JW et al (1983) *Am. J. Physiol.* 245: 4376–4381.
Seccombe DW, Snyder P & Parsons HG (1982) *Lancet* ii: 1401.
Seccombe DW, James L & Booth F (1986) *Neurology* 36: 264–267.
Sengers RCA, Fisher JC, Trijbels JMF et al (1987) *Eur. J. Pediatr.* 140: 332–337.
Stanley CA (1987) *Adv. Pediatr.* 34: 59–88.
Stanley CA, Hale DE, Coates PM et al (1983) *Pediatr. Res.* 17: 877–884.
Strauss AW, Duran M, Zhang Z et al (1990) In Tanaka K & Coates P (eds) *Fatty Acid Oxidation: Clinical, Biochemical and Molecular Aspects* pp. 609–623. New York: Alan R. Liss.
Taillard F, Mundler O, Tillous-Borde I et al (1988) *Eur. Heart J.* 9: 811–818.
Tein I, DeVivo DC, Bierman F et al (1990) *Pediatr. Res.* 28: 247–255.
Treem WR, Stanley CA, Finegold DN et al (1988) *New Engl. J. Med.* 319: 1331–1336.
Treem WR, Stanley CA & Goodman SI (1989) *J. Inher. Metab. Dis.* 12: 112–119.
Tripp ME, Katcher ML, Peters HA et al (1981) *New Engl. J. Med.* 305: 385–390.
Turnbull DM, Bartlett K, Stevens DL et al (1984) *New Engl. J. Med.* 311: 1232–1236.
Uziel G, Garavaglia B & DiDonato S (1988) *Muscle and Nerve* 11: 720–724.
Waber LJ, Valle D, Neill C et al (1982) *J. Pediatr.* 101: 700–705.
Zierz S, Engel AG & Romshe CA (1988) In DiDonato S, DiMauro S, Mamoli A & Rowland PL (eds) *Advances in Neurology*, 48: pp 231–237. New York: Raven Press.

PART II

PAEDIATRIC MEDICINE

Carnitine and paediatrics: an
overview
G. Sherwood

During the 1960s, the condition called 'familial steatosis' was reported
in many children who invariably died with massive lipid accumulation
in liver, skeletal muscle and/or cardiac muscle. The basic cause
remained unclear. During the 1970s, these cases were assigned to the
diagnostic category of 'systemic carnitine deficiency'. A primary
disorder in the intake, synthesis, tissue uptake and/or renal excretion
of carnitine was suspected. Carnitine treatment was expected to be
completely curative. This proved to be so only in some cases. During
the 1980s, it was discovered that primary disorders of carnitine
metabolism were the culprits in only a small proportion of cases. In
most cases, free carnitine became deficient/insufficient because it was
being sequestered away in the form of acylcarnitine esters as a
consequence of the accumulation of various acyl compounds. In other
words, the primary defect involved disorders of fatty acid metabolism
with carnitine deficiency/insufficiency being a secondary phenomenon.

Thus, from the clinical viewpoint, it has taken 25 years or so to
begin to construct the correct questions to ask about the role of

L-Carnitine and Its Role in Medicine
From Function to Therapy. ISBN 0–12–253940–0

endogenous carnitine in the pathogenesis of various paediatric disorders and the role of exogenous carnitine in the therapy of those conditions.

This section contains individual chapters that discuss selected paediatric topics. Drs Novak and Schmidt-Sommerfeld address issues pertaining to the role of carnitine in the perinatal period when fatty acids are so essential as an energy source. Drs Angelini and Tein relate the current understanding of primary defects in the tissue uptake of carnitine. Dr Bennett provides a review of the known disorders of fatty acid oxidation and how they result in secondary problems with carnitine metabolism. Finally, Drs Winter and Dionisi-Vici share their clinical experiences with a variety of common paediatric conditions in which low carnitine levels have been found.

Missing in this section are chapters relating to conditions in which acyl compounds not directly related to fatty acid oxidation accumulate. Carnitine deficiency/insufficiency also occurs in the classical organic acidopathies such as methylmalonic and propionic acidaemia as well as with the administration of sodium valproate, the widely used, branched-chain fatty acid anticonvulsant. The release of new important information in regard to the role of carnitine in these conditions is imminent. The situation is similar for matters pertaining to the enzymes that transport long-chain fatty acids across the mitochondrial membranes, i.e. the carnitine palmitoyl transferase and carnitine translocase systems. It was deemed more appropriate that discussion of these topics not be presented until additional data clarifies this very confused area.

Part IIa

Perinatology

6

CARNITINE IN PERINATAL METABOLISM OF LIPIDS

M. Novak

In fetal tissues of mammals the metabolic energy is obtained mainly from the oxidative metabolism of carbohydrates. Birth represents a sudden increase in energy requirements. In addition to ongoing needs for growth and differentiation, there are new requirements to generate metabolic energy for breathing, movement and maintenance of body temperature. Considerable data is now available concerning the effects of varying feeding practices and composition of nutrients on lipid metabolism after birth.

After delivery, the normal neonate adapts to fatty acids as a major source of calories. Within hours, accelerated lipolysis elevates free fatty acid concentrations and fatty acids are supplied by a high fat diet of milk.

When fatty acids are used for energy production they are processed mainly in the mitochondria by β-oxidation. L-Carnitine is a naturally

L-Carnitine and Its Role in Medicine:
From Function to Therapy. ISBN 0–12–253940–0

occurring compound found in humans and other mammals. It acts as a cofactor in the mechanism by which fatty acids are transported into the mitochondria for β-oxidation (Fritz and Marquis, 1965) and regeneration of free coenzyme A (CoA) from acyl CoA intermediates (Bremer, 1983). It is reasonable to assume that the need for carnitine in tissues is increased when the rate of fatty acid oxidation is high.

This chapter discusses research into the sources and functions of carnitine in physiological processes vital for the newborn infant. Data obtained from experimental animals are mentioned to help clarify the mechanism postulated from results obtained in human studies.

PRENATAL SOURCES OF CARNITINE

In humans and other mammals, carnitine is normally available via diet and de novo synthesis from dietary precursors (Mitchell, 1978; Broquist and Borum, 1982; Rebouche, 1982). The transplacental transport of carnitine or precursors from the maternal plasma appears important for the formation of carnitine depots in fetal tissues.

Plasma carnitine concentration decreases during pregnancy with lowest concentrations being found at term (Hahn et al, 1977; Scholte et al, 1978). Lowest levels of amniotic fluid acylcarnitines are found in late pregnancy (Novak et al, 1979). The postulation that maternal blood and fetal urine may be a source of carnitine and acylcarnitines of the amniotic fluid is supported by several observations. Various alterations influencing maternal and fetal metabolism affect the concentration of free carnitine or acylcarnitines in plasma and amniotic fluid. Elevated concentrations of acylcarnitines were found in amniotic fluid obtained from pregnancies complicated by toxaemia and/or insulin-dependent diabetes mellitus (Schmidt-Sommerfeld et al, 1981). High proportions of acylcarnitines were detected in amniotic fluid, cord blood plasma and urine before birth and at birth in an infant with propionic acidaemia (Benke et al, 1986). In cord blood obtained from newborns with cystic fibrosis, acylcarnitines were low (Lloyd-Still et al, 1990). These and other observations may explain the inconsistent results obtained by the comparison of free and esterified carnitine levels in the umbilical artery and vein.

There is a positive correlation between maternal venous and umbilical venous blood concentrations of free carnitine and acylcarnitines in newborns of various gestational ages (Shenai et al, 1983; Cederblad et al, 1985; Sachan et al, 1989). These data suggest a transplacental transfer of carnitine from the maternal blood to the fetus.

The transfer and metabolism of carnitine and acylcarnitines in the human term placenta have been studied by Schmidt-Sommerfeld et al (1985a) using an in vitro perfusion method. In term placenta, the calculated maximal carnitine transfer is far in excess of the estimated fetal carnitine requirements. However in humans there is no information on whether carnitine biosynthesis in the fetus is a significant contributor to its carnitine status. Perfusion studies indicate that transplacental transport may ensure sufficient amounts of carnitine even in the absence of carnitine biosynthesis in fetal tissues.

It is possible to increase the carnitine supply to the fetus. Some attention has been given to the effects of antepartum administration of L-carnitine on the metabolism of the human placenta (Gengler et al, 1988) or fetus (Salzer et al, 1983). Stronger efforts have been made to elucidate the role of carnitine after birth and to establish the value of carnitine therapy in infants.

RESERVES OF METABOLIC ENERGY AND THE TRANSITION TO AN INCREASED FAT CATABOLISM AFTER BIRTH

After delivery, the neonate is faced with marked metabolic challenges. Many vital functions are assumed by the mother during prenatal life. With the interruption of the continuous supply of placentally transported nutrients the neonate depends on the utilization of metabolic fuels derived from endogenous sources. The length of this period depends on varying feeding practices.

The release of energy-yielding substrates from depots accumulated prenatally is initiated by hormonal changes at birth (Girard and Ferre, 1982). Glycogen from muscle, liver and other tissues represents a minor source of metabolic fuel for the newborn (Shelley, 1961; Hahn and Koldovsky, 1966). Glycogen depots are exhausted within hours after birth. Although fat constitutes about 15% of the body weight, the proportion may vary in newborn infants after altered gestation.

The rapid increase of free glycerol and free fatty acids (FFA) in plasma of newborn infants (Novak et al, 1964; Van Duyne, 1965) gave first evidence of an accelerated release of these substrates from adipose tissue. However, the interpretation of plasma concentrations is

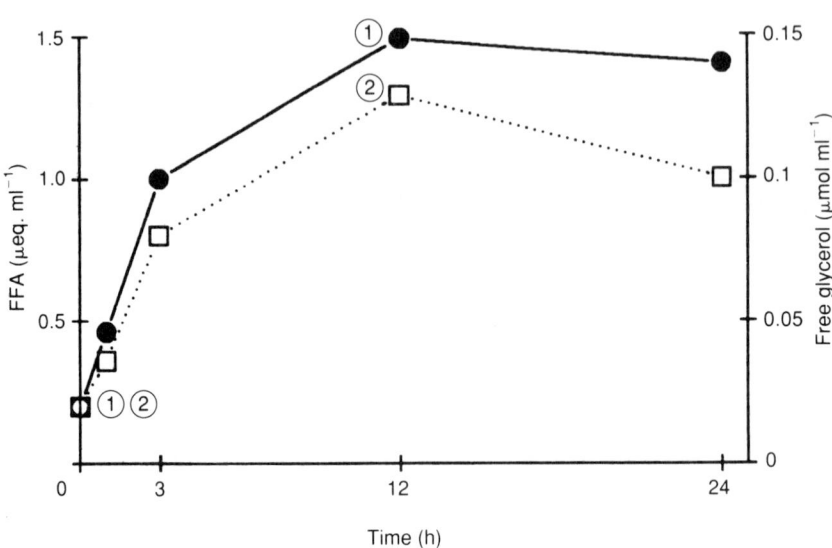

FIGURE I. Increase of FFA (●) and free glycerol (□) in plasma of full-term infants, $p < 0.0001$; $p < 0.0005$.

complicated; they may be elevated because of increased release or decreased uptake by tissues. Further studies on subcutaneous white adipose tissue of newborn infants revealed that these units of metabolic energy (glycerol, FFA) were in fact released by adipose tissue and exported to other tissues for utilization (Novak et al, 1965a, 1965b; Novak et al, 1973).

THE ROLE OF CARNITINE IN ADIPOSE TISSUE AFTER BIRTH

Adipose tissue has been shown to be influenced by the adaptive mechanisms necessary for the neonate to cope with the extrauterine environment as documented above. Considerable work has been done on morphological, functional and metabolic characteristics of white and brown adipose tissue (Jeanrenaud and Hepp, 1970; Lindberg, 1970). Developmental aspects have been reviewed (Hahn and Novak, 1975). The metabolic development of white adipose tissue of human newborns has been studied in samples obtained by subcutaneous biopsy (Novak et al, 1971).

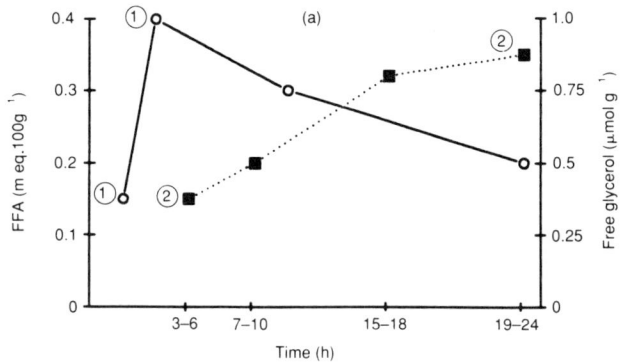

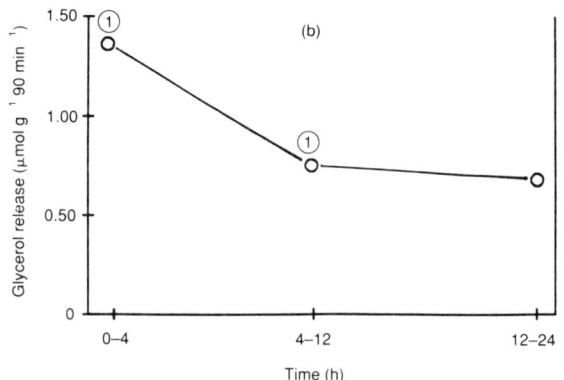

FIGURE 2. (a) Increase of free glycerol (○) and FFA (■) content of white adipose tissue after birth. $p < 0.001$; $p < 0.01$. (b) Glycerol release from white adipose tissue. $p < 0.01$.

Numerous results have confirmed that β-oxidation of long-chain fatty acids becomes increasingly important for energy production in adipocytes cells after birth. In vitro studies of both brown and white adipose tissue revealed that the accumulation of FFA occurs when the glycogen stores become depleted. This hormone-stimulated lipolysis is tightly regulated by ATP and cyclic AMP (Skala et al, 1972). The decline of ATP, adenyl cyclase, cyclic AMP and of the activity of cyclic AMP-dependent protein kinase in white adipose tissue of newborn infants (Novak et al, 1973) and brown adipose tissue of neonatal rats parallels the decrease in glycogen content and glycolysis. In vitro glycerol release from the subcutaneous white adipose tissue of newborn infants was enhanced by L-carnitine (Novak et al, 1975), suggesting that the elevation of carnitine-dependent fatty acid oxidation is related to energy requirement. Simultaneously, an abundance of FFA or acyl CoA may act in a variety of hormone-mediated regulatory processes in adipose tissue.

Although the exact mechanism of this inhibition is not known, the availability of carnitine may affect the regulatory processes by which adipose tissue provides metabolic fuels for other tissues. The activity of carnitine palmitoyl transferase (CPT), β-hydroxyacyl CoA dehydrogenase and carnitine content increase after birth in brown adipose tissue of newborn rat (Hahn and Novak, 1975) and white adipose tissue of newborn infants (Schmidt-Sommerfeld et al, 1978). These changes coincide with carnitine intake from the diet.

THE ROLE OF CARNITINE IN THE REGULATION OF HEPATIC METABOLISM OF FATTY ACIDS AFTER BIRTH

Liver glycogen stores accumulate during late fetal life in all mammals but are rapidly mobilized at birth to provide glucose for tissues and cells that are entirely dependent upon glucose to maintain their function. The supply of FFA to the liver depends on the amount of adipose tissue depots and fatty acid release. Several regulatory mechanisms operate for the control of hepatic fatty acid oxidation. Immediately after birth, there is a transient hypoglycaemia (Wilkinson, 1969), increase in plasma glucagon and catecholamines (Girard and Ferrè, 1982) and fall in plasma insulin (Girard, 1990). Studies in experimental animals have shown that carnitine has an important role in these changes. The production of ketone bodies in the liver is accompanied by an increase in carnitine content (McGarry et al, 1975) and appears to be regulated by carnitine palmitoyl transferase 1 (CPT-1). This enzyme controls the rate of entry of activated fatty acids into mitochondria (McGarry and Foster, 1980). Further studies on hepatocytes and isolated mitochondria revealed that the increase in the capacity for long-chain fatty acid oxidation and ketogenesis resulted from a decrease in lipogenesis and malonyl CoA concentration (Ferrè et al, 1983; Herbin et al, 1987). Thus, this mechanism may ensure a sensitive response to decreased availability of carbohydrates and provide control of ketone body production as alternative fuels in times of fasting.

With the severance of the umbilical cord at birth, the fetoplacental transfer of carnitine is interrupted. Before the onset of feeding the neonate fully depends on fetal carnitine deposits and on endogenous carnitine biosynthesis. Some experimental data provided evidence that early postnatal ketogenesis is stimulated by carnitine from milk (Hahn et al, 1979). Injection of the radio-isotopically labelled carnitine (Hahn and Skala, 1975) or γ-butyrobetaine (Robles-Valdes et al, 1976) into nursing rats resulted in the appearance of labelled carnitine in the milk with subsequent accumulation in the liver of suckling pups. Autopsy studies suggested that neonatal total parenteral nutrition (TPN) decreased carnitine stores in the liver (Penn et al, 1985) and may interfere with normal development of carnitine reserves in various tissues (Nakano et al, 1989).

Fatty acid oxidation in the liver provides cofactors (acetyl CoA, NADH and ATP) for gluconeogenesis as well as ketogenesis. Early neonatal hypoglycaemia may result in part from reduced gluconeogenesis and may relate to lower capacity to oxidize long-chain fatty acids (Girard, 1986). Hypoglycaemia, increased levels of FFA and defective ketogenesis are potential consequences of certain hereditary disorders of fatty acid β-oxidation (Bachman et al, 1988; Roe and Coates, 1989; Pollit, 1990).

After birth, there is a period when long-chain fatty acids accumulate in tissues to an extent, resulting in an oversaturation of mitochondrial β-oxidation. Under such conditions, long-chain fatty acids may be increasingly metabolized in peroxisomes where their carbon chains are shortened (Brofman et al, 1979; Lazarov, 1982). These shortened fatty acids are converted to acylcarnitines (Bieber et al, 1982) and may be transferred into mitochondria for further oxidation. When the mitochondrial β-oxidation is overloaded or impaired there is increased ω-oxidation of fatty acids in microsomes (Mortensen, 1984). The resulting elevation of dicarboxylic acids in the urine has been often interpreted as indicative of these conditions (Karpati et al, 1975; Nyhan, 1988; Olson et al, 1989).

CARNITINE AND CORRELATES OF NEONATAL LIPID METABOLISM IN PLASMA AND URINE

The relative changes in the concentration of glucose, free glycerol, FFA, acetoacetate and β-hydroxybutyrate reflect the transition to an increased fat catabolism after birth. It has been evident for some time that glycerol and FFA levels are increasing faster than ketone bodies (Hahn and Novak, 1985). Ketone bodies are formed in the liver when the supply of FFA exceeds the mitochondrial capacity to oxidize them completely to H_2O and CO_2. There is also a substantial increase of acylcarnitines in plasma (Novak et al, 1979) and acylcarnitines represent a predominant fraction of total carnitine in the urine before the onset of feeding (Cederblad et al, 1982). The negative correlation between free carnitine and β-hydroxybutyrate and the positive correlation of acetylcarnitine with β-hydroxybutyrate suggested an increased hepatic formation of acetyl CoA, exceeding the capacity for its oxidation via the Krebs cycle. These data suggest that carnitine serves as an acceptor for the excessively formed acetyl groups and thus prevents the depletion of free coenzyme A. High concentrations of carnitine may decrease ketogenesis by reducing the acetyl CoA pool under some conditions (Yeh, 1981).

It should be noted, however, that plasma and particularly urine of newborn infants may contain a wide spectrum of acylcarnitines in addition to acetylcarnitine (Schmidt-Sommerfeld et al, 1989; Schmidt-Sommerfeld and Penn, 1990). Some of these acylcarnitines may derive from breakdown of amino acids or other precursors. Their formation is important for the maintenance of a free CoA pool as described in a variety of metabolic processes.

INVESTIGATIONS ON CARNITINE AND LIPID METABOLISM IN NEWBORN INFANTS RECEIVING TOTAL PARENTERAL NUTRITION (TPN)

In contrast to the mixture of fat and glucose obtained by infants on standard oral feeding, newborns treated by customary TPN receive glucose as a predominant source of calories. Considerable evidence has documented an accelerated insulin-stimulated glucose utilization under these conditions and indices reflecting lipid catabolism (free glycerol, FFA and ketone bodies) have been markedly reduced (Hahn and Koldovsky, 1966; Girard and Ferre, 1982). Initial plasma levels of acylcarnitines fell rapidly and were significantly decreased at 12–24 h of age in premature infants who had received 10% glucose as the only source of calories in the first hours of life (Chung et al, 1981). Free carnitine was significantly decreased at 2–4 days of age. Plasma lipoprotein profile showed an increase in the very low density lipoprotein (VLDL) fraction. An abnormal elevation of triglycerides, in the absence of milk feeding or supplemental lipid emulsion, suggested an accelerated hepatic re-esterification of FFA.

From these results it appears that the majority of FFA released from adipose tissue in response to an accelerated hormonally-stimulated lipolysis was re-esterified in the liver and transported for deposition. The effect of exogenous carnitine on plasma indices of lipid catabolism in infants receiving continuous TPN and carnitine supplements can be detected only following reduction of glucose or fasting challenge (Orzali et al, 1983; Schmidt-Sommerfeld et al, 1985b; Helms et al, 1986, 1990). However, irrespective of variables such as gestational age or nutritional treatment, carnitine supplementation always elevated acylcarnitines in plasma or urine. Undoubtedly, some other metabolic pathways were affected that were not related to the oxidative metabolism of fatty acids. Carnitine may promote some other effects such as metabolism of nitrogen compounds (Melegh, 1990) or stimulation of growth (Helms et al, 1990) in parenterally alimented premature

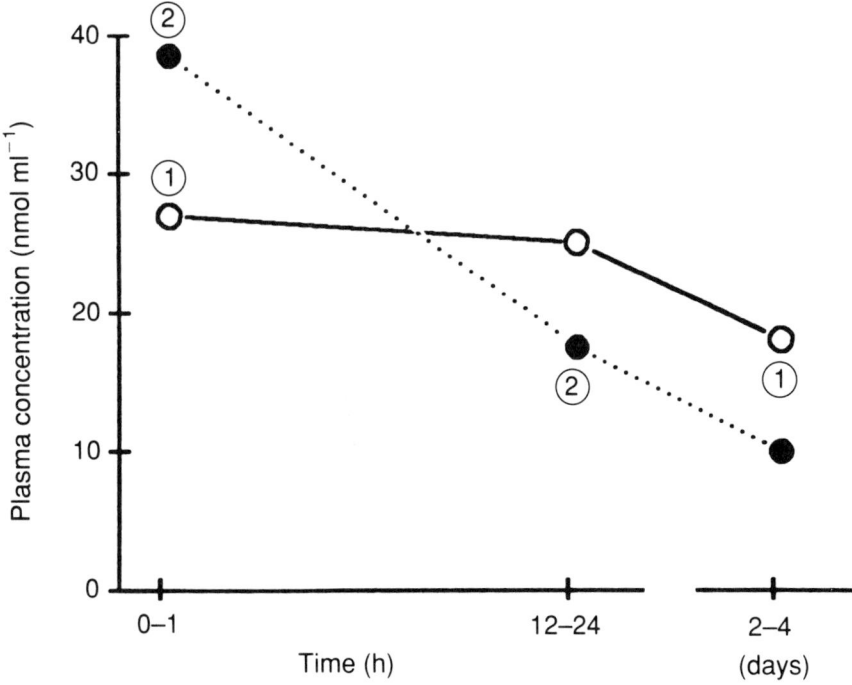

FIGURE 3. Decrease of plasma free carnitine ($\bigcirc$) and acylcarnitines ($\bullet$) in premature infants in response to 10% i.v. glucose. $p < 0.002$; $p < 0.025$.

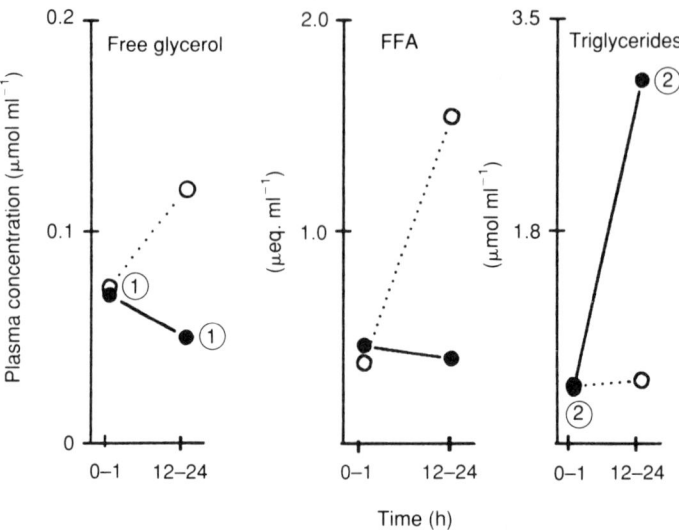

FIGURE 4. Plasma concentrations of free glycerol, FFA and triglycerides in premature infants in response to 10% i.v. glucose (●) (O, initial concentrations in orally-fed infants) 1 $p < 0.05$; 2 $p < 0.001$.

infants. These findings may not fall beyond the scope of perinatal lipid metabolism and are discussed in more detail elsewhere.

THEORETICAL CONSIDERATIONS EVALUATING THE IMPORTANCE OF EXOGENOUS CARNITINE IN INFANTS

Plasma concentrations of carnitine significantly decreased in premature infants receiving TPN and increased again with the institution of oral feeding (Schiff et al, 1979). Comparison of plasma levels in infants given carnitine-free soy-based formulas and in infants fed carnitine-containing formulas or human milk has shown that dietary intake is a main determinant of carnitine levels after birth (Novak, 1990). In agreement with this observation, investigations on the development of biosynthesis of carnitine in humans had shown that the activity of the hepatic γ-butyrobetaine hydroxylase was low in infants (Rebouche and Engel, 1980). Carnitine precursors added to carnitine-free soy-based formula caused plasma and urine concentrations of carnitine to

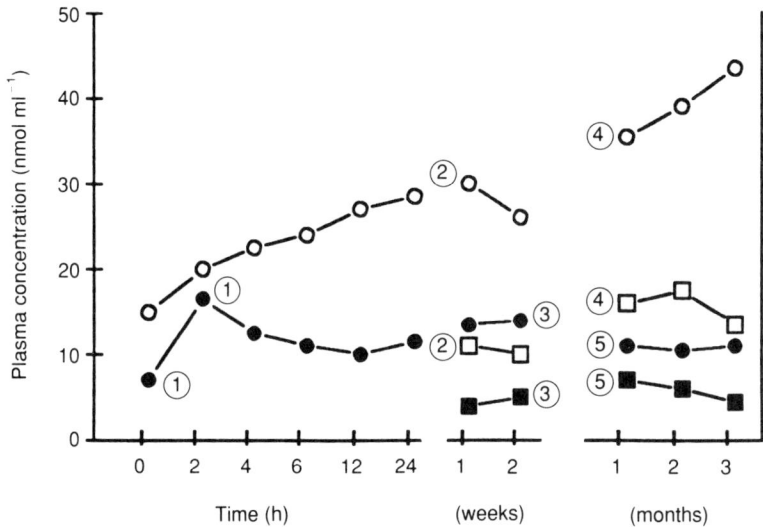

FIGURE 5. Plasma concentrations of free carnitine (○, □) and acylcarnitines (●, ■) during first hours, weeks and months (○, ●, Breast milk or carnitine-containing formulas; □, ■, carnitine-free, soy-based formulas). 1 $p < 0.005$; 2 $p < 0.001$; 3 $p < 0.001$; 4 $p < 0.01$; 5 $p < 0.01$.

rise. Olson and Rebouche (1987) provided evidence that the conversion of γ-butyrobetaine to carnitine was not a rate-limiting step of carnitine biosynthesis in human infants. The different response to γ-butyrobetaine compared with ε-N-trimethyl-L-lysine has shown the potential contribution of two enzymatic steps. However, whether these enzyme systems alone hold the key to understanding the low plasma carnitine levels in newborn infants remains unanswered.

The greater excretion of short-chain acylcarnitines than of free carnitine observed in infants has been attributed to active renal tubular reabsorption of free carnitine and preferential elimination of acylcarnitines (Valkner and Bieber, 1982). The relative proportion of acylcarnitines in plasma of newborn infants is higher than in adults. The different renal handling of carnitine or high excretion rate of acylcarnitines in infants compared with adults has been considered as a possible determinant of lower carnitine levels in infants (Novak et al, 1978). However, no evidence of a developmental regulation in the renal handling of carnitine was found by Olson and Rebouche (1989). The low carnitine plasma levels of infants deprived of exogenous carnitine were explained by rapid incorporation of carnitine into growing tissues combined with relatively low rate of carnitine biosynthesis (Olson and Rebouche, 1987, 1989). Some supportive evidence for this hypothesis may be the persistence of rapidly growing cells after birth, characterized morphologically by a relatively larger cytoplasmic compartment and by abundant mitochondria whose number depends on the requirement for metabolic energy.

The question of whether carnitine should be considered an essential nutrient for the human infant has been the topic of several reviews (Borum, 1981, 1985; Rebouche, 1986). Data from studies in healthy full-term infants given soy-based formulas with or without added carnitine have suggested differences in lipid metabolism. However, lack of exogenous carnitine alone did not induce clinical syndromes of carnitine deficiency. On the other hand, there is a number of highly heterogeneous metabolic disorders in which the accumulation of acyl CoA thioesters occurs at the expense of free CoA and free carnitine. Such a situation is common in a large number of genetic or other metabolic diseases.

It is important to consider that metabolism undergoes very rapid changes immediately after birth which may be characterized chiefly by accelerated catabolism. Under these circumstances the metabolic errors affecting carnitine, lipid metabolism and energy homeostasis are difficult to recognize by using only routine laboratory methods. Acute events capable of causing metabolic decompensation under stressful catabolic conditions (infection, prolonged fast) were more often identified later during infancy. Here, carnitine treatment resulted in a successful normalization of metabolism and an improvement of the clinical status.

REFERENCES

Bachmann C, Catzeflis C, Hale DE et al (1988) *International Symposium on Clinical Biochemical and Molecular Aspect of Fatty Acid Oxidation, Philadelphia, November 6–9.*
Benke PJ, Novak M & Goldberg F (1986) In Borum PR (ed.) *Clinical Aspects of Human Carnitine Deficiency* p. 141. New York: Pergamon Press.
Bieber LL, Valkner KJ & Farell S (1982) *Ann. NY Acad. Sci.* 386: 395–396.
Borum PR (1981) *Nutr. Rev.* 39: 385–390.
Borum PR (1985) *Can. J. Physiol. Pharmacol.* 63: 571–576.
Bremer J (1983) *Physiol. Rev.* 63: 1420–1480.
Brofman M, Inestrosa NC & Leighton F (1979) *Biochem. Biophys. Res. Commun.* 88: 1030–1036.
Broquist HP & Borum PR (1982) *Adv. Nutr. Res.* 4: 181–204.
Cederblad G, Finnstrom O & Marthensson J (1982) *Biochem. Med.* 27: 260–267.

Cederblad G, Niklasson A, Ridgren B et al (1985) *Acta Paediatr. Scand.* 74: 500–504.

Chung D, Novak M, Monkus EF & Buch M (1981) *XVI International Congress of Pediatrics*, Barcelona, Spain, p. 17 (Abstract).

Ferrè P, Satabin P, Decaux JF et al (1983) *Biochem. J.* 214: 937–942.

Fritz IR & Marquis NR (1965) *Proc. Natl Acad. Sci. USA* 54: 1226–1233.

Gengler H, Enzelsberger H & Salzer H (1988) *Z. Geburtshilfe Perinatol.* 192(4): 155–157.

Girard J (1986) *Biol. Neonate* 50: 237–258.

Girard J (1990) *Biol. Neonate* 58 (supplement 1): 3–15.

Girard J & Ferrè P (1982) In Jones CT (ed.) *The Biochemical Development of the Fetus and Neonate* pp. 517–551. Amsterdam: Elsevier Biomedical.

Hahn P & Koldovsky O (eds) (1966) *Utilization of Nutrients During Postnatal Development*. Oxford: Pergamon Press.

Hahn P & Novak M (1975) *J. Lipid Res.* 16: 79–91.

Hahn P & Novak M (1985) *Fed. Proc.* 44: 2369–2372.

Hahn P & Skala J (1975) *Comp. Biochem. Physiol.* 51B: 507–515.

Hahn P, Skala JP, Secombe DW et al (1977) *Pediatr. Res.* 11: 878–880.

Hahn P, Secombe DW & Towell ME (1979) *S. Z. Levine Conf. 1st Intl. Meeting 187*, Paris.

Helms RA, Whitington PF, Mauer EC et al (1986) *J. Pediatr.* 109: 984–988.

Helms RA, Mauer EC, Hay WW et al (1990) *J. Pediatr. Gastroenterol. Nutr.* 14: 448–453.

Herbin C, Pegorier JP, Duee PH et al (1987) *Eur. J. Biochem.* 165: 201–207.

Jeanrenaud B & Hepp D (eds) *Adipose Tissue. Regulation and Metabolic Functions*, Stuttgart: Georg Thième Verlag; New York, London: Academic Press.

Karpati G, Carpenter S, Engel AG et al (1975) *Neurology* 25: 16–24.

Lazarov PB (1982) In Sies H (ed.) *Metabolic Compartmentation* pp. 317–329. New York: Academic Press.

Lindberg O (ed.) (1970) *Brown Adipose Tissue*. New York, London, Amsterdam: Elsevier Publishing.

Lloyd-Still JD, Bohan T, Hughes S & Wessel HU (1990) *Acta Paediatr. Scand.* 79(4): 427–430.

McGarry JD & Foster DW (1980) *Annu. Rev. Biochem.* 49: 395–420.

McGarry JD, Robles-Valdes C & Foster DW (1975) *Proc. Natl Acad. Sci. USA* 72: 4385–4388.

Melegh B (1990) *Biol. Neonate* 58 (supplement 1): 93–106.

Mitchell ME (1978) *Am. J. Clin. Nutr.* 31: 293.

Mortensen PB (1984) *Dan. Med. Bull.* 31: 121–145.

Nakano C, Takashima S & Takeshita K (1989) *Early Hum. Dev.* 19: 21–27.

Novak M (1990) *Biol. Neonate* 58 (supplement 1): 89–92.

Novak M, Hahn P & Melichar V (1964) *Biol. Neonate* 7: 179–184.

Novak M, Melichar V & Hahn P (1965a) *J. Lipid Res.* 6: 91–95.

Novak M, Melichar V & Hahn P (1965b) *Biol. Neonate* 8: 253–257.

Novak M, Monkus E & Pardo V (1971) *Biol. Neonate* 19: 306–321.

Novak M, Monkus E & Wolf H (1973) *Pediatr. Res.* 9: 769–777.

Novak M, Penn-Walker D, Hahn P & Monkus EF (1975) *Biol. Neonate* 25: 85–94.

Novak M, Monkus EF, Buch M et al (1978) *J. Pediatr. Gastroenterol. Nutr.* 7: 222–224.

Novak M, Wieser PB, Buch M & Hahn P (1979) *Pediatr. Res.* 13: 10–15.

Nyhan WL (1988) N. Engl. J. Med. 17: 1344–1346.

Olson AL & Rebouche CJ (1987) J. Nutr. 117: 1024–1031.

Olson AL & Rebouche CJ (1989) Early Hum. Dev. 19: 29–38.

Olson AL, Nelson SE & Rebouche CJ (1989) Am. J. Clin. Nutr. 49: 624–628.

Orzali A, Donzelli F, Enzi G & Rubaltelli F (1983) Biol. Neonate 43: 186–190.

Penn D, Ludwigs B, Schmidt-Sommerfeld E & Pascu F (1985) Biol. Neonate 47: 130–135.

Persson B & Gentz J (1966) Acta Paediatr. Scand. 55: 353–362.

Pollit RJ (1990) In Tanaka K & Coates PJM (eds) Fatty Acid Oxidation, Clinical, Biochemical and Molecular Aspects pp. 495–502. New York: Alan R Liss.

Rebouche CJ (1982) Fed. Proc. 41: 2848–2852.

Rebouche CJ (1986) J. Nutr. 116: 704–706.

Rebouche CJ & Engel AG (1980) Biochim. Biophys. Acta 630: 22–29.

Robles-Valdes C, McGarry JD & Foster DW (1976) J. Biol. Chem. 251: 6007–6012.

Roe CR & Coates PN (1989) In Scriver CR, Beaudet AL & Sly WS et al (eds) The Metabolic Basis of Inherited Disease pp. 889–914. New York: McGraw-Hill.

Sachan DS, Smith RB, Plattsmier J & Lorch V (1989) Am. J. Perinatol. 6(1): 14–17.

Salzer H, Husslein P, Löhninger A et al (1983) Wien. Klin. Wochenschr. 95(20): 724–728.

Schiff D, Chan G, Secombe D & Hahn P (1979) J. Pediatr. 95: 1034–1046.

Schmidt-Sommerfeld E & Penn D (1990) Biol. Neonate 58 (supplement): 81–88.

Schmidt-Sommerfeld E, Novak M, Penn D et al (1978) Pediatr. Res. 12: 660–664.

Schmidt-Sommerfeld E, Penn D & Wolf H (1981) Early Hum. Dev. 5: 233–242.

Schmidt-Sommerfeld E, Penn D, Sodha RJ et al (1985a) Pediatr. Res. 19: 700–706.

Schmidt-Sommerfeld E, Penn D & Wolf H (1985b) J. Pediatr. Gastroenterol. Nutr. 4: 795–798.

Schmidt-Sommerfeld E, Penn D, Kerner J & Bieber LL (1989) Clin. Chim. Acta 181: 231–238.

Scholte HR, Stinis JT & Jennekens FGI (1978) N. Engl. J. Med. 229: 1079.

Shelley H (1961) Br. Med. Bull. 17: 137–143.

Shenai J, Borum PR, Mohan P & Donlery SD (1983) Pediatr. Res. 17: 579–583.

Skala J, Novak E, Hahn P & Drumond J (1972) Int. J. Biochem. 3: 229–242.

Valkner KJ & Bieber LL (1982) Biochem. Med. 28: 197–203.

Van Duyne CM (1965) Biol. Neonate 66(9): 115–123.

Wilkinson AW (1969) Proc. Nutr. Soc. 28: 61–66.

Yeh YY (1981) J. Nutr. III: 831–840.

7

ROLE OF CARNITINE IN CHILDREN RECEIVING TOTAL PARENTERAL NUTRITION

Eberhard Schmidt-Sommerfeld and D. Penn

Total parenteral nutrition (TPN) has become a widely accepted means of nutritional support for children and adults who do not tolerate enteral feedings or in whom circumvention of the gastrointestinal tract is desirable. However, our knowledge about macro- and micronutrient requirements in parenteral nutrition is still incomplete. The young child is especially vulnerable to a parenteral feeding regimen since the immaturity of many metabolic pathways early in life affects not only the tolerance for proteins, fats and carbohydrates, but also the availability of cofactors which may be inadequately synthesized.

Carnitine, an essential cofactor for the transport of acyl groups across the mitochondrial membrane is supplied by dietary intake, primarily in meat and milk products, and endogenous biosynthesis. The latter is believed to be sufficient in the adult organism so that adequate blood and tissue levels of carnitine can be maintained over extended periods of time without carnitine intake (Rebouche and Paulson, 1986). However, this may not be the case in the young child.

L-Carnitine and Its Role in Medicine:
From Function to Therapy. ISBN 0–12–253940–0

CARNITINE BIOSYNTHESIS AND STATUS DURING HUMAN DEVELOPMENT

During human pregnancy, there is a decrease of maternal plasma concentrations of carnitine which are lowest at term (Hahn et al, 1977; Scholte and Stinis, 1978). Immediately after delivery, there is a positive correlation between maternal venous and umbilical venous blood concentrations of both free and esterified carnitine suggesting placental transfer (Schmidt-Sommerfeld et al, 1981; Cederblad et al, 1985). Reports of maternal/fetal plasma concentration gradients of free and esterified carnitine are inconsistent (Hahn et al, 1977; Bargen-Lockner et al, 1981; Novak et al, 1981; Schmidt-Sommerfeld et al, 1981). Such gradients may be dependent upon acute changes in maternal and/or fetal fat metabolism at the time of birth. Investigation of carnitine transfer across the in vitro perfused human placenta at term demonstrated that, in contrast to most amino acids, L-carnitine is not transported against a concentration gradient from the maternal to the fetal circulation (Figure 1). Nonetheless, the calculated maximal carnitine transfer from the maternal to the fetal side greatly exceeded the estimated fetal carnitine requirement (Schmidt-Sommerfeld et al, 1985). This does not exclude the possibility that the human fetus is capable of synthesizing substantial amounts of carnitine. In fact, it has recently been shown that the rat fetus contributes up to 50% of its own carnitine stores by endogenous biosynthesis (Davis, 1989). Equivalent data in the human are not available.

Although carnitine plasma concentrations at birth are higher in premature than in full-term infants (Novak et al, 1979), probably due to higher maternal plasma levels earlier in gestation, carnitine stores in human muscle are positively correlated with gestational age (Figure 2; Penn et al, 1985; Nakano et al, 1989). From measurements in autopsy material, the skeletal muscle carnitine pool of the term neonate was calculated to be about four times smaller and that of the very premature infant 10 times smaller than that of the adult on a per kg body-weight basis (Penn et al, 1985). This indicates that the newborn infant, especially the premature, is born with limited carnitine reserves.

The rate-limiting step of carnitine biosynthesis in the human is still unknown (for review see Rebouche and Paulson, 1986). Likewise, it is not known how carnitine biosynthesis is regulated developmentally. Research in this area has focused on γ-butyrobetaine hydroxylase, the last enzyme in the carnitine biosynthetic pathway converting γ-butyrobetaine to carnitine. In the human, this enzyme is present only

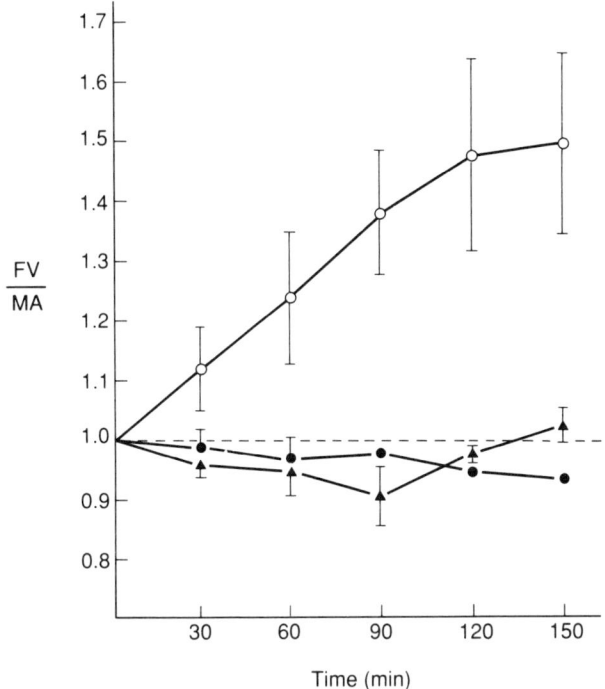

Time (min)

FIGURE 1. Dual perfusion of an isolated human placental lobe: Maternal and fetal perfusates contained equal concentrations of ^{3}H-L-lysine and L-carnitine or L-acetylcarnitine. At time 0 the fetal circulation was closed and the maternal circulation remained open. While an increasing fetal/maternal (FV/MA) concentration gradient was demonstrated for ^{3}H-L-lysine (○), no such gradient developed for L-carnitine (●) or L-acetylcarnitine (▲). From Schmidt-Sommerfeld et al (1985).

in the liver, kidney and brain but not in muscle and heart where most of the body's carnitine is stored. The activity of γ-butyrobetaine hydroxylase was found to be low in liver, but normal in the kidney of infants (Olson and Rebouche, 1987). Moreover, the same authors provided evidence, by feeding infants ε-N-trimethyllysine or γ-butyrobetaine and measuring carnitine excretion, that the rate-limiting step in carnitine biosynthesis is prior to the conversion of γ-butyrobetaine to carnitine. Similar data were obtained in adults and the authors speculated that the rate-limiting step is either at the level of one of the enzymes involved in the conversion of free trimethyllysine to γ-butyrobetaine or at the level of trimethyllysine uptake into cells (Rebouche et al, 1989). The step of the carnitine biosynthetic pathway where developmental regulation takes place remains to be determined.

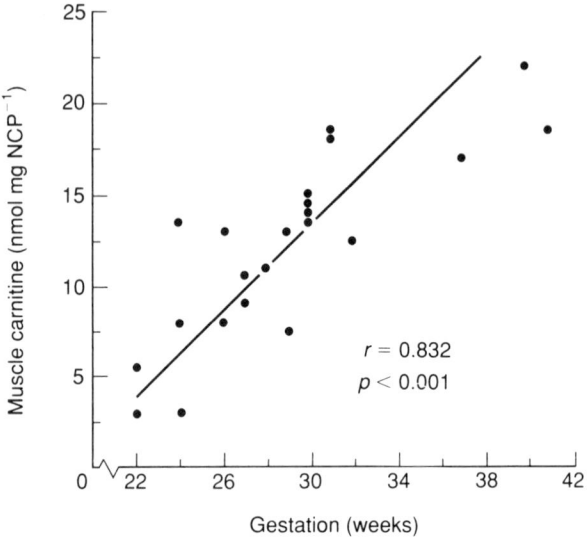

FIGURE 2. Positive correlation between muscle total carnitine concentrations in infants <24 h old and gestational age. From Shenai and Borum (1984).

In conclusion, although the rate-limiting step of carnitine biosynthesis in the human fetus and newborn is still unknown, there is evidence that carnitine stores are low in the fetus early in gestation and increase towards term. This may put the premature infant at a special risk to develop carnitine deficiency if exogenous carnitine is not provided through nutrition.

CARNITINE STATUS OF CHILDREN DURING TPN

Although parenteral nutrition solutions provide sufficient lysine and methionine as precursors of carnitine biosynthesis, they currently do not contain carnitine.

Schiff et al (1979) were the first to report carnitine plasma concentrations in infants receiving TPN (Figure 3). The gestational age of their infants ranged from 26 to 40 weeks. Mean plasma carnitine determined during a period of TPN was about 50% of that measured during a period of oral feedings. Postnatal ages, duration of TPN and the amounts of carnitine containing feedings were not given. We studied 12 premature infants receiving TPN for the first 5 days of life

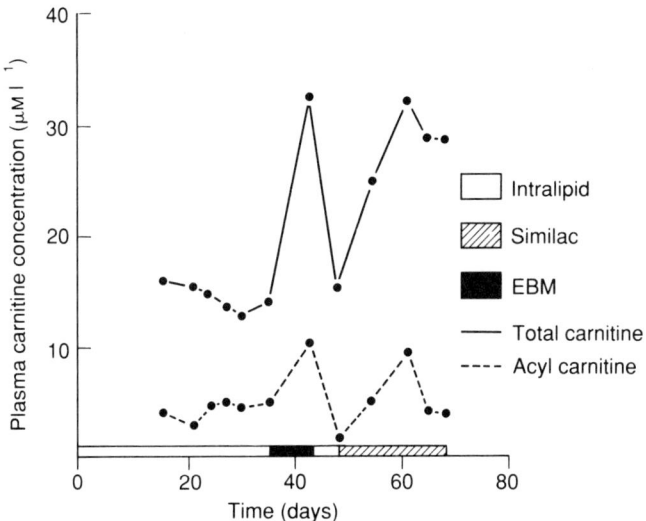

FIGURE 3. First report of plasma carnitine concentrations in a premature infant receiving TPN with Intralipid. Carnitine concentrations fell during carnitine-free TPN (Travasol and Intralipid) and rose during carnitine-containing oral feedings (Similac or expressed breast-milk, EBM). From Schiff et al (1979).

and compared them with eight control infants who were orally fed with a carnitine-containing formula starting on the second day of life (Penn et al, 1980). Gestational age (mean 34 weeks) and birth-weight were comparable in the two groups. There was a decrease in plasma carnitine concentrations to 50% of the values obtained on the first day of life after only 5 days of TPN and a subsequent increase with the onset of oral feedings. The control infants maintained their initial carnitine plasma levels.

A later study (Helms et al, 1986) showed that if the duration of carnitine-free TPN was extended to over 1 month, carnitine plasma concentrations became even lower in premature as well as in term infants (average <30% of normal). Short-term TPN in a population of mostly term infants caused only a moderate depression of carnitine plasma concentrations (Orzali et al, 1984). Smith et al (1988) measured plasma carnitine concentrations in 36 premature infants receiving TPN with supplemental oral feedings. Lowest values (mean total carnitine 8.2 μmol/l[1]) were found in the lowest birth-weight group (<1000g), but this group also received TPN over the longest period of time (mean 35 days). Positive correlations between plasma total carnitine and the calculated carnitine intake were found in all gestational age groups. The accumulated data suggest that postnatal age and/or duration of carnitine-free TPN as well as gestational age are important factors determining the carnitine status.

Urinary excretion of carnitine in premature infants is greatly reduced during TPN (Penn et al, 1980; Helms et al, 1986; Larsson et al, 1990) suggesting an intact renal conservation mechanism.

Little information is available about the effect of TPN on carnitine tissue concentrations in neonates. In autopsy specimens, carnitine concentrations in muscle, heart and liver of premature infants receiving at least 10 days of carnitine-free TPN were lower than those of a comparable infant population receiving carnitine-containing oral feedings (Figure 4).

The carnitine status of children beyond infancy receiving TPN has only recently been studied. Carnitine plasma concentrations and urinary carnitine excretion were measured in 25 children and adolescents with gastrointestinal disease receiving TPN for longer than 1 month (Schmidt-Sommerfeld et al, 1990). The patients were divided into two groups on the basis of their carnitine status. Those who had subnormal carnitine plasma concentrations (<50% of normal mean for age) were less than 12 years old, whereas those who were generally able to maintain their carnitine plasma concentrations within 2 SD of normal

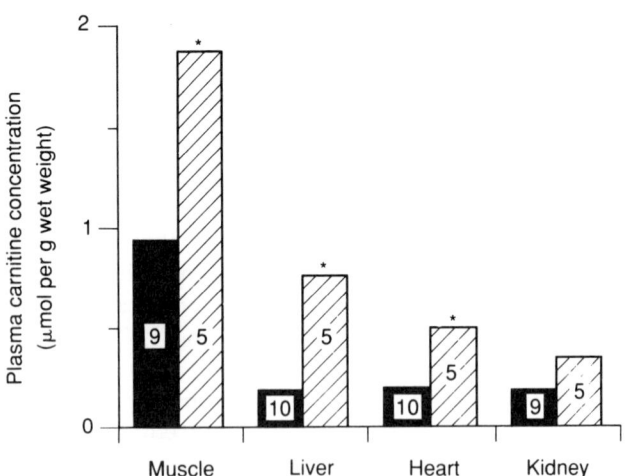

FIGURE 4. Carnitine tissue concentrations at autopsy in premature infants >10 days old receiving carnitine-free TPN (■) compared with a group receiving >7.5 μmol L-carnitine kg^{-1} per day through oral feedings (▨). Asterisk indicates significant differences. Redrawn after data from Penn et al (1985).

controls were older than 12 years. Age was the only variable to correlate significantly with plasma carnitine concentrations during TPN (Figure 5) suggesting that the ability to synthesize carnitine may be age-dependent. However, the type of disease was also different between the two patient groups: whereas the older patients had inflammatory bowel disease with limited involvement of the small intestine, the younger patients had extensive small bowel disease with impaired intestinal absorption. The latter may have led to decreased carnitine reserves due to carnitine malabsorption even before the onset of TPN. Longitudinal observations revealed that after an initial decrease to subnormal levels, carnitine plasma concentrations stabilized at a new, lower steady state during continuing carnitine-free TPN.

Urinary carnitine and carnitine ester excretion in these patients was studied in detail (Schmidt-Sommerfeld et al, 1990). Children with low carnitine plasma concentrations and intact renal tubular function excreted very low amounts of free carnitine and short-chain carnitine esters, but the excretion of complex medium-chain acylcarnitines was

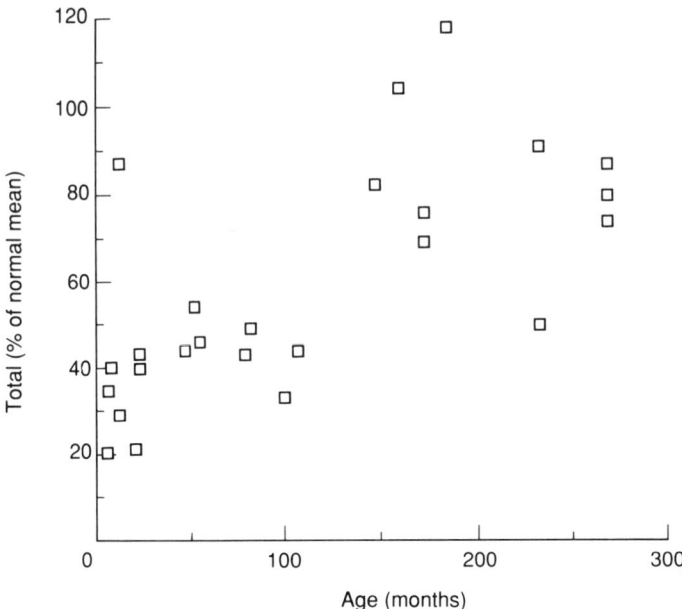

FIGURE 5. Relationship between total carnitine plasma concentrations (expressed as % of the normal mean for age) and age of children and adolescents with gastrointestinal disease receiving TPN for >1 month. $r = 0.68$, $p < 0.001$. From Schmidt-Sommerfeld et al (1990).

relatively preserved. The origin of such carnitine esters is unknown, but may be renal. It was speculated that carnitine has a role in the removal of presumably slowly metabolized acyl moieties from the body. This metabolic pathway may proceed despite hypocarnitinaemia during TPN, thus contributing to the risk of carnitine deficiency in younger children.

In contrast to young children, adults may be able to maintain normal carnitine plasma concentrations during TPN over a longer period of time (Hahn et al, 1982). However, Bowyer et al (1986) reported decreased carnitine plasma concentrations in 35% of their adult patients with gastrointestinal disease receiving long-term home parenteral nutrition. In their patient population, the mean decrease (65% of control values) was less pronounced than that reported for infants on long-term TPN. One patient with low plasma carnitine also had decreased liver carnitine content. In a later study, the same authors found decreased liver carnitine concentrations in all four patients with low carnitine plasma levels who underwent a liver biopsy for abnormal liver enzymes (Bowyer et al, 1988). Other investigators (Berner et al, 1990) found plasma carnitine concentrations in adult patients receiving prolonged TPN to be very similar to those reported by Bowyer et al (1986). In this study, decreased plasma concentrations of lysine were found despite sufficient lysine intake. The question was raised whether decreased plasma carnitine concentrations might be caused by inadequate availability of the precursor lysine. This appears to be an unlikely explanation in view of the fact that lysine feeding has very little effect on carnitine biosynthesis in the human (Rebouche et al, 1989). Furthermore, in the rat, a lysine-deficient diet did not influence the rate of biosynthesis of peptide-bound trimethyllysine, the methylated precursor of carnitine (Davis, 1990). In a population of neurological patients receiving combined parenteral nutrition and enteral tube feeding, total carnitine concentrations in plasma decreased to 60% of the initial value after a period of 8 weeks (Schäfer and Reichmann, 1990).

As is the case in children, carnitine excretion in adult patients receiving long-term TPN may be reduced (Worthley et al, 1984). However, it has been shown to be increased during periods of stress-induced catabolism, e.g. in the immediate post-operative period (Pichard et al, 1989), with multiple injury (Cederblad et al, 1983; Iapichino et al, 1988), during sepsis and after burns (Nanni et al, 1985). In such situations, carnitine plasma concentrations do not reflect carnitine tissue stores and may mask carnitine tissue depletion.

In conclusion, premature infants on short-term TPN and full-term infants on long-term TPN develop a decrease in plasma carnitine concentrations to levels considerably lower than those found in adult patients on long-term TPN. Postnatal age and/or duration of TPN as well as gestational age determine the carnitine status. In children beyond infancy, age and type of disease seem to play a role in the development of low carnitine plasma concentrations. Urinary carnitine excretion is reduced during TPN except in catabolic situations. Carnitine tissue concentrations are decreased in premature infants receiving TPN.

METABOLIC AND CLINICAL CONSEQUENCES OF NUTRITIONAL CARNITINE DEFICIENCY

Data pertaining to the question whether low carnitine plasma and tissue concentrations have an adverse effect on metabolic pathways in children is still accumulating. In our first study addressing this question, we found that premature infants receiving enteral and/or parenteral alimentation had total carnitine plasma concentrations that correlated positively with the amount of carnitine taken in and with plasma levels of β-OH-butyrate (BOB), but negatively with plasma levels of free fatty acids (FFA) after a 4-h infusion of fat (Intralipid 1 g kg^{-1}) without glucose (Schmidt-Sommerfeld et al, 1982). This provided evidence that the capacity of the premature infant for fatty acid oxidation and ketogenesis might be related to the carnitine status. Yeh et al (1985) noted a lack of ketogenic response to lipid infusion in 1-week-old, parenterally-alimented infants and speculated that this may be related to their decreased plasma carnitine concentrations. However, this relationship could not be proven because the control group (1–3-day-old term infants receiving regular oral feedings) was not comparable.

More recently, Christensen et al (1989) showed that premature infants who had received TPN for longer than 4 weeks had increased plasma FFA and decreased plasma ketone bodies compared with premature infants receiving TPN for a shorter period of time. This was seen before as well as after a lipid infusion. They concluded that the older infants had impaired fatty acid oxidation due to tissue depletion of carnitine. However, an effect of postnatal age on ketogenesis unrelated to carnitine status could not be ruled out. Moreover, no ketogenic response to the lipid infusion was observed. This may have been due

TABLE I.

Studies of the effect of L-carnitine supplementation in parenterally-alimented newborn infants

Gestational age (weeks)	Postnatal age* (days)	Fat challenge	Glucose (g kg^{-1} per day)	L-carnitine (mg kg^{-1} per day)	Effects	Reference
30 ± 1	15–19	No	15	2 p.o. (12 days)	None	Curran et al (1983)
29–33	6 ± 1	Yes	None†	10 i.v. (5–7 days)	↓ FFA/KB	Schmidt-Sommerfeld et al (1983)
34–37	6 ± 1	Yes	None†	Same	None	Schmidt-Sommerfeld et al (1983)
32–40	7	Yes	Yes	100 bolus + 100/6 h i.v.	None	Orzali et al (1984)
27–40	46–299	Yes	8–10	10 p.o. (7 days)	↑ KB	Helms et al (1986)
37 ± 3	8 +	Yes	10% 5%	12 p.o. (7 days)	None	Coran and Drongowski (1986)
29–34	16–21	Yes	Breast milk	6 p.o. (7 days)	↑ KB	Melegh et al (1986)
32 ± 4	14–45(?)	Yes	10–12	8–16 i.v. (14 days)	↓ FFA/KB ↓ TG, ↑ N$_{ret}$, wt	Helms et al (1990)
27–32	5 +	No	10 Breast milk	10 i.v. (5 days)	(↑ KB)	Larsson et al (1990)

*At time of lipid parameter measurement; †During fat challenge. KB, ketone bodies; FFA, free fatty acids; TG, triglycerides; N$_{ret}$, nitrogen retention; wt, body-weight.

to a suppression of ketogenesis by the concurrent infusion of glucose.

The most valuable information regarding the metabolic consequences of deficient carnitine intake in infants stems from studies of L-carnitine supplementation during TPN. Table 1 summarizes eight such studies with regard to patient demographics, nutritional circumstances, dosage and mode of carnitine administration and metabolic or clinical effects observed. In all studies, higher plasma carnitine concentrations were achieved through either intravenous or oral carnitine administration. Most studies measured parameters of lipid metabolism (triglycerides, FFA, ketone bodies) in conjunction with an intravenous fat challenge. In all studies except one (Orzali et al, 1984), physiological dosages (comparable to intake from regular milk formulas) of L-carnitine were given chronically (for at least 5 days). Ketone body utilization which may also be affected by carnitine was not measured in any of the studies.

Curran et al (1983) did not find any effect of L-carnitine supplementation on plasma levels of BOB, FFA and triglycerides, on nitrogen balance or skinfold thickness in very low birth-weight infants receiving TPN. No lipid challenge was given and the rate of glucose infusion was high. Under these circumstances, suppression of fatty acid oxidation must be presumed.

In our own study (Schmidt-Sommerfeld et al, 1983), premature infants < 34 weeks of gestation who received i.v. L-carnitine supplementation exhibited a distinctly lower FFA/BOB ratio in plasma after a lipid challenge compared with infants of similar gestation who received no carnitine with their TPN (Figure 6.) No such effect was seen in infants of higher gestational age. Since the plasma FFA/BOB ratio has been proposed to be a useful indicator of the β-oxidation capacity, this study indicated impairment of fatty acid oxidation due to nutritional carnitine deficiency in the lower gestational age group. It must be pointed out, however, that this effect of L-carnitine supplementation was demonstrated during presumably high rates of fatty acid oxidation provoked by a fat challenge (1 g kg^{-1} Intralipid over 4 h) without concomitant glucose infusion.

In the study of Orzali et al (1984), a mixed population of term and pre-term infants received two 4-h i.v. infusions of fat. The first was given without L-carnitine. During the second fat infusion, i.v. L-carnitine was given as an initial bolus followed by a continuous infusion (100 mg kg^{-1}) over 6 h. Despite a dramatic increase in plasma free and short-chain acylcarnitine during L-carnitine administration, no significant differences in plasma FFA and BOB were noted between the two fat challenges, although plasma concentrations of BOB at the

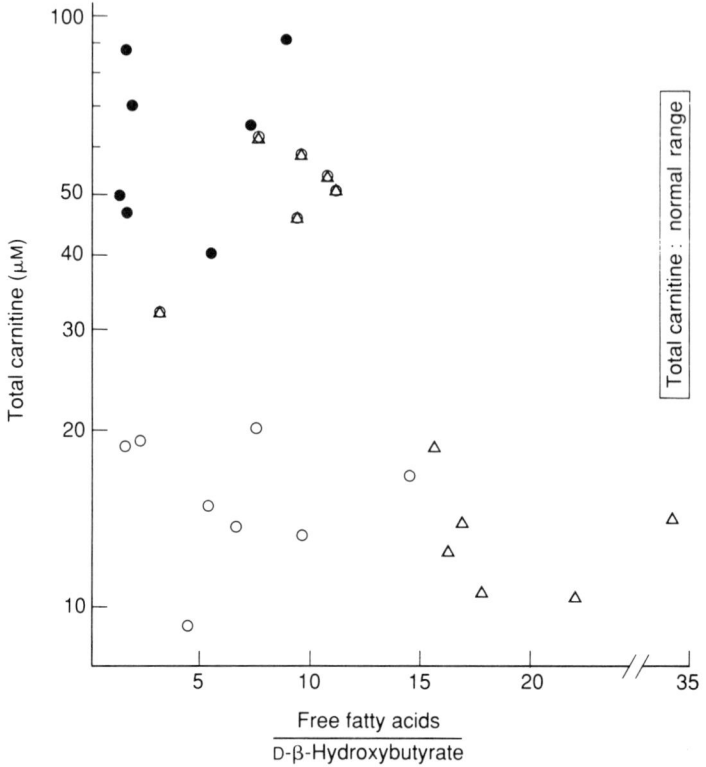

Figure 6. Relationship between total carnitine plasma concentrations before, and FFA/BOB ratios after, fat infusion in four groups of premature infants receiving TPN for 5–7 days: (●) carnitine-supplemented 34–37 weeks; (○) non-supplemented 34–37 weeks; (⬭) carnitine-supplemented 29–33 weeks; (△) non-supplemented 29–33 weeks of gestation. The lower gestational age group showed an improvement in fatty acid oxidation due to L-carnitine. From Schmidt-Sommerfeld et al (1983).

end of the lipid infusions tended to be higher with L-carnitine treatment. The lack of effect of L-carnitine on the measured lipid parameters could have been due to: (i) relatively preserved carnitine tissue stores as evidenced by only mildly depressed initial carnitine plasma concentrations, (ii) concomitant infusion of glucose, (iii) a treatment period too short to replete carnitine tissue stores and/or (iv) high (unphysiological) dose of L-carnitine which may have a different effect on fat metabolism than a physiological dose.

Helms et al (1986) studied oral L-carnitine supplementation in full-term and premature infants with various gastrointestinal diseases requiring long-term carnitine free TPN (mean duration 100 days).

These infants developed very low (mean 9.4 μmol l^{-1}) total carnitine plasma concentrations. The infants were randomized into carnitine supplemented and non-supplemented groups. No difference in ketone body levels after lipid infusion was found between the two groups before the supplementation protocol was started (pre-treatment, Figure 7). After 7 days of supplementation, a significantly higher ketogenic response to lipid challenge was found in the carnitine-supplemented group compared with the non-supplemented control group (post-treatment). Plasma FFA were not different. The conclusion from this study was that tissue carnitine depletion occurred after long-term TPN resulting in an inappropriate ketogenic response to a lipid challenge.

The concept that the duration of carnitine-free nutrition is an important factor in the development of nutritional carnitine deficiency in infants is supported by the study of Coran and Drongowski (1986) who did not find an effect of enteral carnitine supplementation on fatty acid oxidation parameters in a similar infant population receiving TPN over a much shorter period of time.

Melegh et al (1986) supplemented low birth-weight infants requiring combined parenteral and enteral (pooled breast milk) nutrition with oral L-carnitine for 7 days. The supplemented infants had higher basal plasma ketone body levels and their ketogenic responses following an intravenous lipid challenge were more pronounced than those of the non-supplemented control group. In contrast to all other studies, total carnitine plasma concentrations were normal in the control group and elevated in the supplemented group.

In a multicentre study by Helms et al (1990), infants receiving i.v. carnitine supplementation for 2 weeks had lower plasma FFA/ketone body ratios and lower plasma triglycerides after lipid infusion and also moderately higher nitrogen retention and better weight gain compared with the control group. This is the first report of a favourable effect of L-carnitine supplementation of TPN on nitrogen balance and weight gain in infants. Because of their potential clinical significance, these findings need to be confirmed. The authors also showed that 54% of the administered carnitine was retained. This is in agreement with our recent findings that children on TPN with low carnitine plasma concentrations have significant retention of intravenously-administered L-carnitine, whereas those with normal plasma carnitine levels retain carnitine poorly (Lyons and Schmidt-Sommerfeld, unpublished data). It supports the concept that low plasma carnitine levels during TPN reflect low carnitine tissue stores.

Most recently, Larsson et al (1990) studied premature infants receiving combined parenteral and enteral (breast milk) nutrition with and

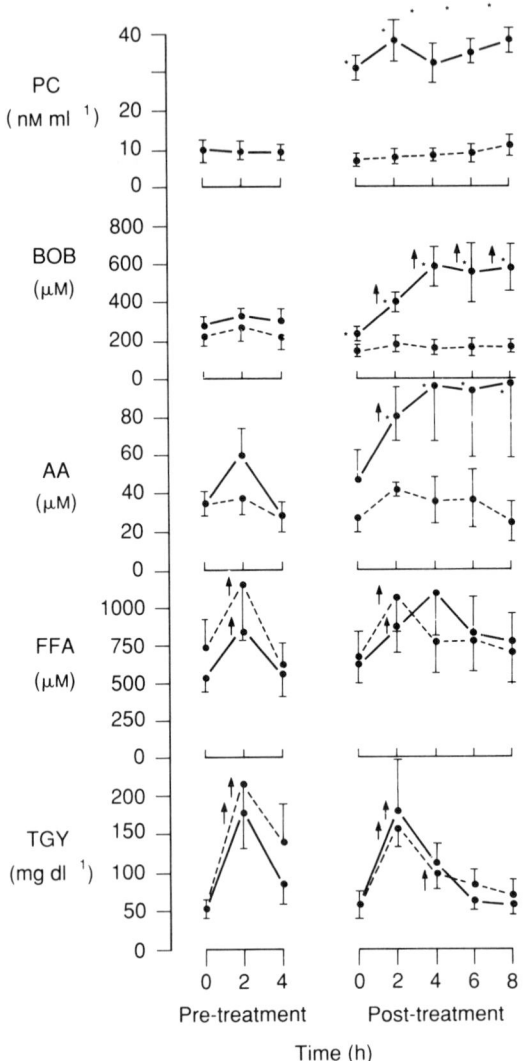

Figure 7. Response to 2-h lipid infusions in infants on long-term TPN before (pre-treatment) and after (post-treatment) receiving L-carnitine (●——●) or placebo (●- - -●). PC, total plasma carnitine; BOB, β-hydroxybutyrate; AA, acetoacetate; FFA, free fatty acids; TGY, triglycerides in plasma. *, significant differences in BOB and AA levels between the two groups were seen post-treatment but not pre-treatment. †, significant rises. From Helms et al (1986).

without L-carnitine supplementation. No fat challenge was performed. There was a higher plasma concentration of BOB in the supplemented group on day 2 but not on day 5 of L-carnitine supplementation. More than 50% of the carnitine taken in by the supplemented group was retained, whereas the non-supplemented group was in negative carnitine balance. The conclusion from this study was that despite significant carnitine uptake into tissues, only a temporary improvement of fatty acid oxidation was demonstrable with L-carnitine supplementation in a regular clinical setting.

Clinical symptoms due to deficient carnitine intake have not been established. It is not certain whether symptoms observed in patients with primary systemic carnitine deficiency, an entity which has recently been shown to be a congenital defect in carnitine transport (Treem et al, 1988), occur in infants receiving carnitine-free TPN. There are only anecdotal reports of muscle hypotonia, cardiomegaly or liver dysfunction which seemed to improve with L-carnitine supplementation of TPN in neonates (Tibboel et al, 1990). In general, the severe underlying clinical and metabolic condition of the infant dependent on TPN will make it difficult to attribute such symptoms solely to nutritional carnitine deficiency.

In adults, single cases of abnormal liver function, muscle weakness and hypoglycaemia occurring during long-term TPN have been attributed to carnitine deficiency (Worthley et al, 1983; Palumbo et al, 1987). However, most systematic studies did not reveal metabolic or clinical abnormalities due to deficient carnitine intake in adult patients.

Bowyer et al (1988) studied the effect of L-carnitine supplementation (1 g per day) in four adult patients receiving home parenteral nutrition for several years, who had developed low carnitine plasma and liver concentrations, abnormal liver tests and steatosis. After one month of supplementation, there was normalization of both plasma and liver carnitine levels, but no changes in liver tests, plasma FFA and triglycerides, hepatic FFA and triglyceride content or degree of microscopic steatosis were found.

The same group studied palmitate turnover and oxidation, ketone body and glucose production as well as leucine kinetics in four very similar patients after a short-term fast using radioactive and stable isotopes as tracers (Bowyer et al, 1989). An acute intravenous infusion of L-carnitine had no effect on the measurements. No consistent changes in fat, carbohydrate and protein metabolism were detected after a 1-month period of chronic i.v. L-carnitine supplementation. It was concluded that routine addition of L-carnitine to the TPN regimen is unnecessary. However, while this is an elegant study, the number of subjects is too small to allow a final conclusion. It must also be pointed out that the baseline plasma carnitine concentrations of these patients were only borderline-low indicating that they may not have been carnitine-deficient.

Pichard et al (1988, 1989) studied resting energy expenditure, respiratory quotient (RQ), nitrogen balance and parameters of fat metabolism in normocarnitinaemic adult patients on short-term (11 days) TPN post-operatively. No consistent differences in these measurements were found between the carnitine-supplemented and non-supplemented groups. The carnitine balance remained negative during carnitine supplementation indicating that little uptake of exogenous carnitine in tissues occurred.

In conclusion, impaired fatty acid oxidation due to deficient carnitine intake during TPN has been demonstrated in infants under the following circumstances: (i) after infusion of lipids with no or limited amounts of glucose; (ii) during short-term TPN in very premature infants; (iii) during long-term TPN irrespective of gestational age.

Improvement in nitrogen balance and weight gain was found in one recent study. With customary TPN regimens where rates of fatty acid oxidation are low, no metabolic disturbances due to deficient carnitine intake could be demonstrated in infants. No metabolic abnormalities due to deficient carnitine intake have been found in adult patients receiving TPN. Reports of clinical symptoms related to deficient carnitine intake during TPN remain anecdotal at the present time.

ANIMAL EXPERIMENTS

The role of carnitine in TPN has been studied in rats and pigs. Tao et al (1981) treated adult rats with TPN containing no or various pharmacological doses of DL-carnitine for 14 days. Carnitine plasma concentrations were only mildly depressed in the group receiving no carnitine and elevated only in the group receiving the highest dose (100 mg 100 g^{-1} body-weight per day). Urinary carnitine excretion in the group receiving no carnitine was not different from that in the orally-fed control group. The supplemented animals excreted 90–100% of the administered carnitine. Carnitine concentrations in muscle and liver were not different among the experimental groups and controls. Only heart carnitine concentrations were decreased in the group receiving carnitine-free TPN compared with controls. The authors concluded that carnitine tissue stores, except for the heart, are maintained by endogenous carnitine biosynthesis in the parenterally alimented adult rat. These results should be interpreted with caution, however, since the racemic mixture of DL-carnitine was given. It has been shown that D-carnitine interferes with L-carnitine transport (Rebouche, 1977). Nitrogen balance was improved in the groups receiving 10 and 100 mg, but not in the one receiving 50 mg 100 g^{-1} body-weight DL-carnitine. The authors provided no explanation for these discrepancies. They also noted that the fat content in the liver was inversely related to the administered carnitine dose. However, steatosis was not eliminated by carnitine supplementation suggesting that other factors are involved in the pathogenesis of the steatosis observed in rats receiving TPN. Other investigators have found no effect of supplementary DL-carnitine on fatty acid oxidation or nitrogen retention in parenterally-alimented rats (Hall et al, 1983).

Böhles et al (1983) studied the effect of low dose (1.5 mg kg^{-1} per day) L-carnitine supplementation in parenterally-alimented mini-pigs. The animals were studied during three sequential 48-h periods of TPN containing (i) amino acids and glucose, (ii) amino acids, glucose and lipids, (iii) amino acids, glucose, lipids and carnitine. During the period of carnitine supplementation, an increase in lipolysis and fatty acid oxidation was detected by RQ changes and by changes in plasma concentrations of triglycerides, FFA and BOB compared with the preceeding infusion periods. Nitrogen retention was also improved. The authors speculated that the latter was caused by enhanced lipid utilization during carnitine supplementation. It has been suggested by others that the observed effects may have been due to continuing adaptation to the lipid infusion during the last infusion period rather than to the carnitine supplement (Hall, 1984). However, Böhles (1983) later reported that the nitrogen retention in a control group without carnitine supplementation was lower than that in the supplemented animals during the same infusion period. The same authors also found decreased concentrations of taurine and GABA in brain cortex of pigs receiving carnitine-free TPN compared with carnitine-supplemented animals (Böhles et al, 1984). The significance of these findings remains speculative.

More recently, Böhles and Akretin (1987) reported a decrease of RQ, plasma FFA and liver triglyceride content and an increase in plasma BOB and nitrogen balance in rats receiving 1 mg 100 g^{-1} per day L-carnitine during a 3-day period of TPN. This effect was not seen with a higher dose (10 mg 100 g^{-1} per day). The authors concluded that the lower (more physiological) dose of L-carnitine may have a ketogenic, while the higher dose may have an antiketogenic effect.

Vasquez et al (1988) studied the effect of carnitine on protein metabolism in rats receiving TPN for 7 days. Supplementation of TPN with 5.5 mg 100 g^{-1} body-weight per day L-carnitine caused a two- to three-fold increase of carnitine levels in plasma, but no significant change in liver and muscle concentrations. Ninety percent of the administered dose was lost in the urine. There was no effect of carnitine supplementation on plasma concentrations of branched-chain amino acids and branched-chain ketoacids, whole body leucine oxidation, leucine turnover and incorporation into muscle and liver proteins, protein content of liver, muscle and kidney or nitrogen balance. The authors concluded that carnitine supplementation of short-term TPN may not be necessary.

It must be pointed out that in all the above cited animal studies, no decrease in carnitine tissue stores was demonstrated during carnitine free TPN. Therefore, the results cannot be extrapolated to a situation where impairment of endogenous carnitine biosynthesis, as e.g. during early development, may result in functionally significant tissue depletion of carnitine.

To our knowledge, no information is yet available on the effect of carnitine supplementation of TPN in neonatal animals. We have preliminary data to suggest that the newborn piglet may be a useful animal model to study nutritional carnitine deficiency during TPN (Penn and Schmidt-Sommerfeld, unpublished data). Newborn piglets receiving only 1 week of TPN had carnitine plasma and muscle concentrations that were about 50% of those in carnitine-supplemented or sow-fed animals of the same age. Urinary carnitine excretion decreased dramatically in the carnitine-deprived group. The plasma FFA/BOB ratio following a lipid bolus was higher and the rate of FFA clearance from plasma was slower in the carnitine-deprived compared with the carnitine-supplemented animals. Moreover, animals receiving no carnitine had significant hepatic steatosis 4 h after bolus lipid infusion. Fatty changes in the liver of carnitine-supplemented animals were minimal under the same conditions. These preliminary findings suggest that carnitine-free TPN may adversely affect the metabolism of exogenous lipid in newborn pigs.

In conclusion, although metabolic effects of L-carnitine were noted, there is no evidence that short-term TPN in the adult animal results in nutritional carnitine deficiency associated with abnormalities in fat or protein metabolism. Further investigation is needed to establish whether such a deficiency can be produced in newborn animals receiving TPN.

SHOULD PAEDIATRIC TPN SOLUTIONS BE SUPPLEMENTED WITH L-CARNITINE?

Early in life, the capacity for endogenous carnitine biosynthesis may be limited. Young children may become carnitine-depleted during prolonged TPN especially if they are prematurely born with low carnitine reserves. Their capacity for β-oxidation may be impaired partly due to nutritional carnitine deficiency. The accumulated evidence suggests that carnitine may be an essential nutrient for this patient population. However, evidence that nutritional carnitine deficiency causes clinical symptoms, impairs growth or has adverse metabolic consequences during customary TPN is not conclusive. Thus, while L-carnitine supplementation of TPN appears to be physiologically meaningful in young pediatric patients, its clinical relevance is uncertain at the present time.

REFERENCES

Bargen-Lockner C, Hahn P & Wittmann B (1981) *Am. J. Obstet. Gynecol.* 140: 412–414.

Berner YN, Larchian WA, Lowry SF et al (1990) *J. Parenter. Enter. Nutr.* 14(3): 255–258.

Böhles H (1983) *Infusionstherapie* 10: 142–143.

Böhles H & Akcetin Z (1987) *Am. J. Clin. Nutr.* 46: 47–51.

Böhles H, Segerer H & Feki W (1983) *J. Parenter. Enter. Nutr.* 8: 9–13.

Böhles H, Michalk D, Brandl U et al (1984) *J. Nutr.* 114: 671–676.

Bowyer BA, Fleming CR, Ilstrap D et al (1986) *Am. J. Clin. Nutr.* 43: 85–91.

Bowyer BA, Miles JM, Haymond MW & Fleming CR (1988) *Gastroenterology* 94: 434–438.

Bowyer BA, Fleming CR & Haymond MW (1989) *Am. J. Clin. Nutr.* 49: 618–623.

Cederblad G, Schildt B, Larsson J & Liljedahl S (1983) *Metabolism* 32(4): 383–389.

Cederblad G, Nikalasson A, Rydgren B et al (1985) *Acta Paediatr. Scand.* 74: 500–504.

Christensen ML, Helms RA, Mauer EC & Storm MC (1989) *J. Pediatr.* 115: 794–798.

Coran AG & Drongowski RA (1986) *Nutr. Int.* 2: 172–176.

Curran JS, Williams PR, Kanarek KS et al (1983) *Acta Chir. Scand.* 517 (supplement): 157–164.

Davis AT (1989) *J. Nutr.* 119: 262–267.

Davis AT (1990) *J. Nutr.* 120: 846–856.

Hahn P, Skala JP, Secombe DW et al (1977) *Pediatr. Res.* 11: 878–880.

Hahn P, Allardyee DB & Frolich J (1982) *Am. J. Clin. Nutr.* 36: 569–572.

Hall RI (1984) *J. Parenter. Enter. Nutr.* 8(5): 589.

Hall RI, Ross LH, Grant JP et al (1983) *Surg. Forum* 34: 71–74.

Helms RA, Whitington PF, Mauer EC et al (1986) *J. Pediatr.* 109: 984–988.

Helms RA, Mauer EC, Hay WW et al (1990) *J. Parenter. Enter. Nutr.* 14(5): 448–453.

Iapichino G, Radrizzani D, Colombo A & Ronzoni G (1988) *J. Parenter. Enter. Nutr.* 12(1): 35–36.

Larsson LE, Olegard R, Ljung BML et al (1990) *Acta Anaesthesiol. Scand.* 34: 501–505.

Melegh B, Kerner J, Sandor A et al (1986) *Acta Paediatr. Hung.* 27: 253–258.

Nakano C, Tasashima S & Takeshita K (1989) *Early Hum. Dev.* 19: 21–27.

Nanni G, Pittirut M, Giovannini I & Boldrini G (1985) *J. Parenter. Enter. Nutr.* 9(4): 483–490.

Novak M, Wieser PB, Buch M & Hahn P (1979) *Pediatr. Res.* 13: 10–15.

Novak M, Monkus EF, Chung D & Buch M (1981) *Pediatrics* 67: 95–100.

Olson AL & Rebouche CJ (1987) *J. Nutr.* 117: 1024–1031.

Orzali A, Maetzke G, Donzelli F & Rubaltelli FF (1984) *J. Pediatr.* 104: 436–440.

Palumbo JD, Schnure F, Bistrian BR et al (1987) *J. Parenter. Enter. Nutr.* 11: 88–92.

Penn D, Schmidt-Sommerfeld E & Wolf H (1980) *Early Hum. Dev.* 4: 23–34.

Penn D, Ludwigs B, Schmidt-Sommerfeld E & Pascu F (1985) *Biol. Neonate* 19: 21–27.

Pichard C, Roulet M, Rossle C et al (1988) *J. Parenter. Enter. Nutr.* 12(6): 555–562.

Pichard C, Roulet M, Schutz Y et al (1989) *Am. J. Clin. Nutr.* 49: 283–289.

Rebouche CJ (1977) *Biochim. Biophys. Acta* 471: 145–155.

Rebouche CJ & Paulson DJ (1986) *Annu. Rev. Nutr.* 6: 41–66.

Rebouche CJ, Bosch EP, Chenard CA et al (1989) *J. Nutr.* 119: 1907–1913.

Schäfer J & Reichmann H (1990) *J. Neurol.* 237: 213–215.

Schiff D, Chan G, Secombe D & Hahn P (1979) *J. Pediatr.* 95: 1043–1046.

Schmidt-Sommerfeld E, Penn D & Wolf H (1981) *Early Hum. Dev.* 5: 233–242.

Schmidt-Sommerfeld E, Penn D & Wolf H (1982) *J. Pediatr.* 100: 260–264.

Schmidt-Sommerfeld E, Penn D & Wolf H (1983) *J. Pediatr.* 102: 931–935.

Schmidt-Sommerfeld E, Penn D, Sodha RJ et al (1985) *Pediatr. Res.* 19: 700–706.

Schmidt-Sommerfeld E, Penn D, Bieber LL et al (1990) *Pediatr. Res.* 28(2): 158–165.

Scholte HR & Stinis JT (1978) *N. Engl. J. Med.* 299: 1079–1080.

Shenai JP & Borum PR (1984) *Pediatr. Res.* 18: 679–681.

Smith RB, Sachan DS, Plattsmier J et al (1988) *J. Parenter. Enter. Nutr.* 12(1): 37–42.

Tao RC, Peck GK & Yoshimura NN (1981) *J. Nutr.* 111: 171–177.

Tibboel D, Delemarre FMC, Przyrembel H et al (1990) *J. Pediatr. Surg.* 25(4): 418–421.

Treem WR, Stanley CA, Finegold DN et al (1988) *N. Engl. J. Med.* 319(20): 1331–1336.

Vazquez JA, Harbhajan PS & Siamak AA (1988) *Am. J. Clin. Nutr.* 48: 570–574.

Worthley LG, Fishlock RC & Snoswel AW (1983) *J. Parenter. Enter. Nutr.* 7: 176–180.

Worthley LIG, Fishlock RC & Snoswell AM (1984) *J. Parenter. Enter. Nutr.* 8: 717–719.

Yeh YY, Cooke RJ & Zee P (1985) *J. Pediatr. Gastroenterol. Nutr.* 4: 795–798.

Part IIb

Primary deficiencies

8

TREATMENT WITH L-CARNITINE OF THE INFANTILE AND ADULT FORM OF PRIMARY CARNITINE DEFICIENCY

C. Angelini, A. Martinuzzi and L. Vergani

Since the initial report by Engel and Angelini (1973), carnitine deficiency has been linked to an increasing number of clinical syndromes, either systemic (Karpati et al, 1975) or limited to the skeletal muscle. In recent years several cases, initially diagnosed as having carnitine deficiency, have been carefully investigated through assays following the various enzymatic steps of β-oxidation. It was possible in this way to identify patients in whom low carnitine levels are secondary to defects of acyl CoA dehydrogenases (Stanley, 1987; Zierz et al, 1988).

Many cases of systemic carnitine deficiency, however, show normal activities of β-oxidation enzymes and should, therefore, still be considered primary carnitine deficiencies (Engel, 1986). The mechanism of the carnitine deficiency in these cases is most likely due to a

139

L-Carnitine and Its Role in Medicine:
From Function to Therapy. ISBN 0–12–253940–0

defective carnitine uptake and/or inappropriate renal handling.

Recently some cases of systemic carnitine deficiency, who presented a remarkably similar clinical phenotype characterized by infantile Reye's episodes with cardiomyopathy, have been associated with a defect of high affinity carnitine uptake (Eriksson et al, 1988; Treem et al, 1988; Tein et al, 1990).

The form of carnitine deficiency limited to skeletal muscle was the first to be described, but appears to be rare. Criteria to fit a patient in this category (Table 1) are: low muscle carnitine with normal or only slightly decreased plasma carnitine, and in vitro correction by carnitine of impaired muscle β-oxidation (Engel and Angelini, 1973; Engel, 1986). This in vitro experiment was carried out in a few cases, and stimulation of carnitine on β-oxidation was observed. The aetiology of muscle carnitine deficiency remains elusive, but the hypothesis of a muscle-specific carnitine carrier defect is the most convincing (Rebouche and Engel, 1984).

The treatment of primary carnitine deficiency is based on carnitine supplementation; the success of the therapy however is not always predictable, and the use of corticosteroids or low fat diet may be necessary in order to achieve the maximal benefit.

We will address the rationale for the various therapeutic approaches in human primary carnitine deficiency, limiting our review to the cases in which the clinical and biochemical criteria delineated in Table 1 have been met.

TABLE I.

Clinical and biochemical criteria for primary carnitine deficiency syndromes

---

Muscle carnitine deficiency
Episodes of fluctuating muscle weakness
Low carnitine concentration in muscle
Carnitine and its esters have normal concentration in plasma and liver
Stimulation by L-carnitine of in vitro palmitate oxidation

Systemic carnitine deficiency
Autosomal recessive
Episodes of hypoketotic coma
Cardiomyopathy, hepatomegaly
Low carnitine concentration in plasma, liver and muscle
Renal leak of carnitine
Defect in high affinity carnitine uptake in fibroblasts

CARNITINE THERAPY IN SYSTEMIC CARNITINE DEFICIENCY AND CARDIOMYOPATHY

The most dramatic successes with carnitine therapy have been reported in the cases of systemic carnitine deficiency (SCD) associated with cardiomyopathy (Figure 1) (Chapoy et al, 1980; Tripp et al, 1981; Waber et al, 1982; Eriksson et al, 1988; Rodrigues Pereira et al, 1988; Treem et al, 1988; Tein et al, 1990), where an almost complete and stable clinical remission has been achieved.

The disorder appears to be autosomal recessive, since many instances of affected siblings have been reported, and intermediate values of carnitine uptake are described in fibroblasts of patients' parents. The typical presentation includes recurrent episodes of hypoketotic hypoglycaemic coma (Reye's syndrome like), cardiomyopathy, fatty liver (Figure 1c), muscle hypotonia and weakness (Figure 1a), and delayed psychomotor development. There is a low concentration of carnitine in serum (4–10% of control), and tissue (liver, muscle), abnormal renal carnitine handling, and dicarboxylic aciduria is usually absent.

The SCD syndrome should be differentiated from a similar clinical presentation of X-linked cardiomyopathy, muscle weakness, neutropenia and low carnitine concentration (Barth et al, 1983; Ino et al, 1988) which is associated with dicarboxylic aciduria and is probably due to abnormal mitochondrial function.

In all cases described the administration of oral L-carnitine progressively resolved the cardiac symptomatology and induced the normalization of ECG, echocardiogram, and emodinamic parameters. L-Carnitine treatment prevents the episodes of hypoketotic hypoglycaemic coma, and improves muscle strength (Figure 1b). The other neurological disturbances (mental retardation, seizures, ataxia) are also improved, albeit slightly, probably due to irreversible nervous system damage during the episodes of coma or cardiac arrest (Chapoy et al, 1980; Treem et al, 1988).

The therapy is free of collateral effects at the doses used in these cases (100–150 mg kg^{-1} per day). No side-effects were reported in one case with doses as high as 1 g kg^{-1} per day (Rodrigues Pereira et al, 1988), but in other cases at doses higher than 170 mg kg^{-1} per day diarrhoea and trimethylamine-like body odour occurred (Waber et al, 1982).

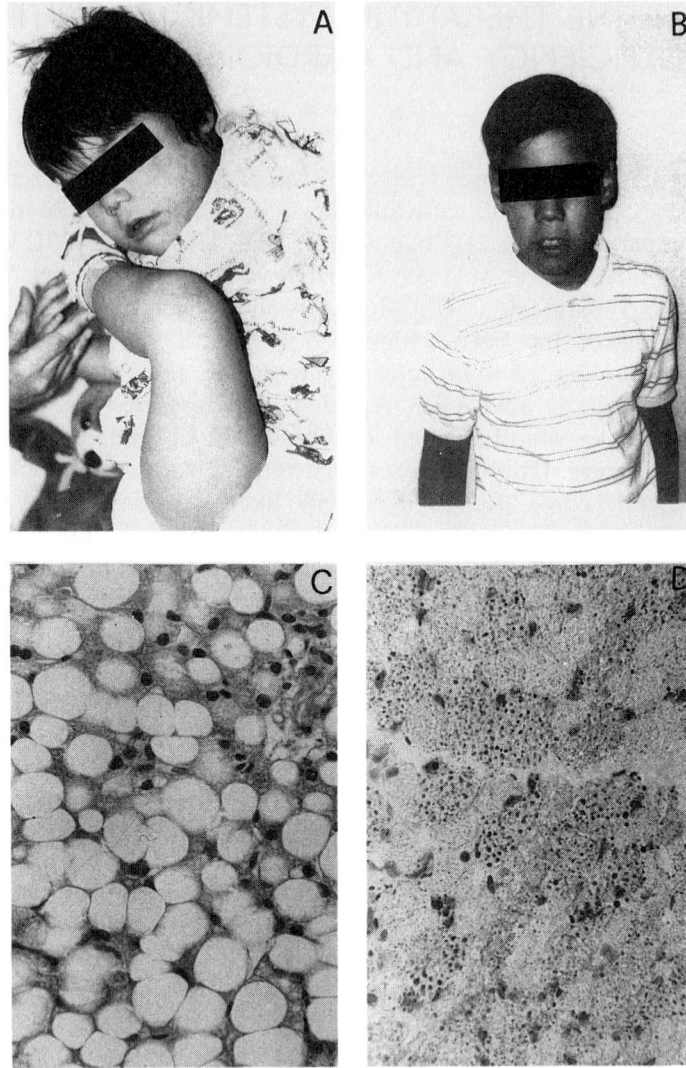

FIGURE 1. Case of systemic carnitine deficiency with cardiomyopathy and hepatomegaly. (a) Patient aged 4, presenting with hypotonia; (b) patient aged 12 after long-term L-carnitine therapy, with recovery of muscle strength and cardiac function; (c) liver biopsy at age 4 showing fatty infiltration; (d) oil red O stain of muscle biopsy at age 4 showing lipid storage.

CARNITINE THERAPY IN MUSCLE CARNITINE DEFICIENCY

In the cases of muscle carnitine deficiency, the beneficial effect of carnitine therapy has been less constant, and often associated treatment with corticosteroids was necessary. This was not only the case in the first patient described (Engel et al, 1974) (who was first treated with steroids because polymyositis was suspected, and then with diet and carnitine supplementation) but also true for a patient followed for several years in our centre.

Case report

A female child had negative family history for consanguineity. Both parents and her brother had normal strength. She had normal psychomotor development until age 7, when she started having difficulty climbing stairs and a waddling gait. Serum enzyme concentrations were elevated. The patient was diagnosed as having muscular dystrophy and was treated with vitamin tablets. She also had physiotherapy and improved during the following year. The mother states that she could walk but still had marked weakness. At age 8, after an episode of tachycardia, she was admitted to our hospital with anorexia, loss of weight and increased weakness (Angelini et al, 1986).

The patient had a considerable lumbar lordosis, and the Gowers sign was positive. She was unable to raise her arms straight (Figure 2a). The neck flexor and extensor muscles were thin and weak, and there was considerable weakness of triceps, scapular rotator, ileopsoas and thigh abductor muscles.

In the muscle biopsy, there was lipid excess and a vacuolar myopathy affecting type I fibres (Figures 2c and 2d). Muscle carnitine was 0.81 mmol per mg non-collagen protein (NCP) in the patient, and 7.75 mM mg NCP^{-1} in her mother (normal values 11–22 mmol mg NCP^{-1}). Serum carnitine level was 32 nmol ml^{-1} before treatment (normal values 36.2–72.9).

The patient was treated with 3 g per day oral L-carnitine, and was put on a low-fat diet with medium-chain triglycerides (MCT) oil. She rapidly recovered her strength. A muscle biopsy 8 months later showed a reduction of the lipid storage.

The child grew in size and muscle bulk in the following years (Figure 2b). At age 16, after discontinuing physiotherapy, the patient

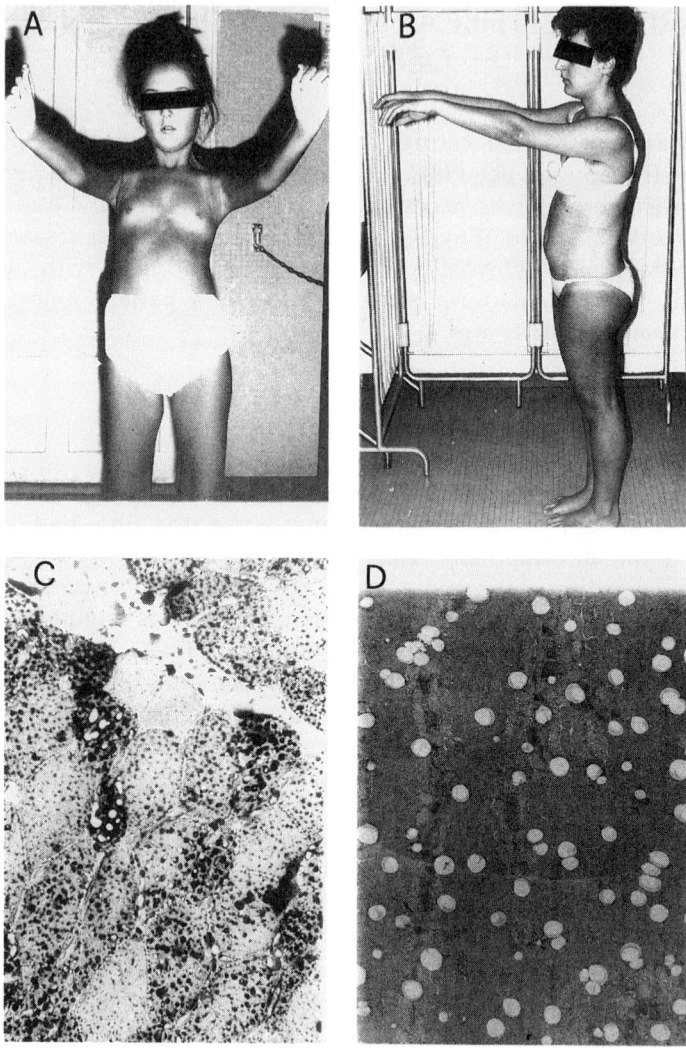

FIGURE 2. Case of muscle carnitine deficiency. (a) Patient aged 8 presenting with hypotrophy and muscle weakness of upper and lower girdle; (b) patient after L-carnitine therapy showing marked improvement of strength and muscle trophism; (c) Sudan black B stain of muscle biopsy taken at age 8 showing lipid storage within type I fibres; (d) electron micrograph of the same muscle biopsy displaying numerous lipid droplets.

had a relapse of weakness, and oral L-carnitine was increased to 5 g per day. Muscle strength did not increase, however, and she was again admitted to our hospital. The patient was very weak (she was not able to keep her arms above her head), serum enzymes were elevated (CPK was 465 mU ml^{-1}, normal values <60 mU ml^{-1}), and respiratory function was decreased.

To evaluate carnitine penetration in tissues, after informed consent, 50 μC of ^{3}H-L-carnitine was infused. A liver and muscle biopsy was obtained after 24 h. ^{3}H-Free carnitine was 3.82 nmol mg NCP^{-1} in the liver, and 3.21 μM mg NCP^{-1} in the muscle. The tritiated carnitine disappeared quickly from the blood (Figure 3). Given the limited penetration of L-carnitine into muscle, we changed our therapy to L-acetylcarnitine 2.5 g per day. The patient recovered and did well in the following years. Maximal tubular reabsorption was within control range (Figure 4).

At the age of 24 the patient married and wanted genetic counselling. A third muscle biopsy was done, and 1-^{14}C-palmitate oxidation was studied in the muscle homogenate with and without the addition of

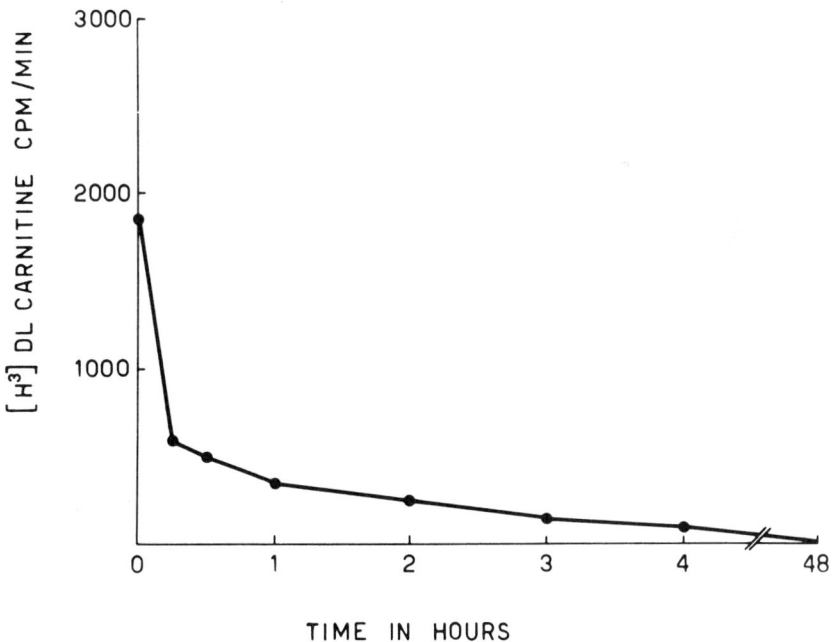

FIGURE 3. Infused tritiated carnitine disappears quickly from the plasma of a patient with muscle carnitine deficiency (see text for details of infusion).

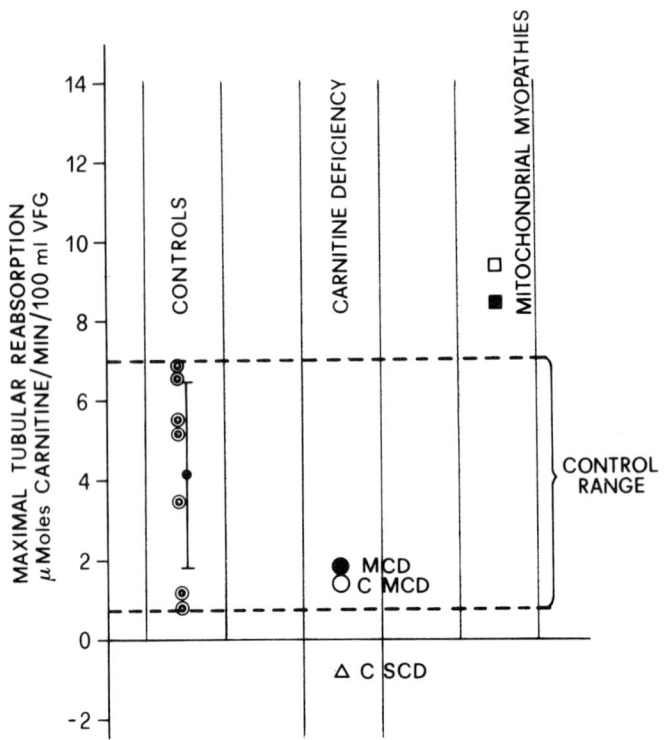

FIGURE 4. Maximal carnitine tubular reabsorption in muscle carnitine deficiency (MCD) and a parent of MCD (C-MCD), a sibling of a systemic carnitine deficiency patient (C-SCD), controls, and mitochondrial myopathies.

0.75 mM L-carnitine, recovering both CO_2 and perchloric acid-soluble products. Palmitate oxidation was low compared with the control (44%), and doubled after carnitine addition (Table 2). In a similar experiment with muscle from a patient with secondary carnitine deficiency, palmitate oxidation was not affected by carnitine addition. Carnitine however did not completely normalize the rate of $1\text{-}^{14}C\text{-}CO_2$ production.

At the age of 26 the patient started a weight-reducing diet, and became irregular in her feeding habits. She again developed increasing weakness and elevated serum enzymes. Total plasma carnitine was 58.5 nmol ml^{-1} (normal values 36.2–72.9), with no increase in short- and long-chain acylcarnitines. Acetylcarnitine was discontinued, and

TABLE 2.

Effect of L-carnitine addition on in vitro I-^{14}C palmitate oxidation in muscle homogenates from muscle carnitine deficiency patient (MCD) and secondary carnitine deficiency patient (SCD)

Muscle homogenate	−L-Carnitine	+ 0.75 mM L-Carnitine
MCD	23.05 ± 2.89	53.66 ± 10.69
SCD	8.63 ± 2.94	9.70 ± 2.10
Controls	52.62 ± 4.49	101.38 ± 10.58

Methods are as described elsewhere (Engel and Angelini, 1973). Values are expressed as pmol min^{-1} mg protein^{-1} of palmitate oxidized ± SD.

she was put on 30 mg alternate-day steroid (deflazacort) and supplemented with 3 g per day L-carnitine. She quickly recovered and since then has done well.

This case demonstrates that muscle carnitine deficiency can easily be improved with carnitine or acetylcarnitine supplementation. Low-fat diet and MCT oil are useful aids in therapeutic strategies. However, relapses frequently occur, and can be managed with modulation of supplementation therapy, or with steroid treatment.

CARNITINE SUPPLEMENTATION

Physiopathological considerations

The limiting factors in carnitine therapy include the bioavailability of the compound, the saturability of intestinal absorption (when the oral route is chosen), and the different capacity for tubular reabsorption in different patients. Only the L-carnitine isomer should be used in carnitine therapy, since D-carnitine competes with its L-isomer for intracellular uptake, and only the L-isomer is biologically active (Rebouche, 1977; Bremer, 1983). Intravenous or oral L-carnitine administration is followed by raised plasma carnitine concentration, and increased renal carnitine excretion. The pharmacokinetics of a bolus of L-carnitine in healthy subjects (Harper et al, 1988) show that intestinal absorption and tubular reabsorption is saturated by 2 g L-carnitine, and that the peak plasma carnitine concentration (50–60% above normal) is reached after about 4–5 hours (Bach et al, 1983).

Approximately 70% of an initial L-carnitine dose given orally to rats undergoes bacterial degradation in the gastrointestinal tract (Rebouche and Engel, 1984; Seim et al, 1985), and is recovered as trimethylamine-N-oxide and butyrobetaine. The same loss probably occurs in humans, greatly limiting carnitine bioavailability.

Once L-carnitine reaches the blood stream and the extracellular fluid, its transport within the cells in various tissues is limited by their different uptake capacities. L-Carnitine is imported into cells through an active, specific and saturable transport system (Bremer, 1983) with different kinetic parameters in various tissues. Apparent K_m values of carnitine uptake in fibroblasts (2–5 μM) are quite different from the apparent K_m of muscle (60 μM), kidney (90 μM), and brain or liver (2 and 5 mM, respectively). The stereospecificity of the process is also different in various tissues, with a high isomer specificity in the brain, and a very low specificity in the kidney. All these data suggest the presence of tissue-specific carnitine carriers.

Experiments in kidney cortex slices have shown that two active carnitine transport systems coexist in this tissue (Huth and Shug, 1980). Similarly, two transport systems have been described in human cultured fibroblasts and skeletal muscle (Rebouche and Engel, 1982; Vergani et al, 1990). The two transport systems described in cultured cells have very different K_ms (5–7 μM versus 150–200 μM) and are therefore designated as high-affinity and low-affinity active transport systems (Vergani et al, 1990) (Figure 5). Besides active transport, carnitine might reach the cells through non-saturable passive diffusion (V_{max} of 0.18 pmol min^{-1} mg protein^{-1} in cultured muscle or fibroblasts).

Clinical aspects

When considering carnitine therapy in a case of primary carnitine deficiency the following parameters should be kept in mind:

1. degree of carnitine deficiency in the various tissues;
2. amount of renal and intestinal carnitine loss;
3. amount of bioavailable carnitine delivered;
4. efficiency of the carnitine carrier in the target tissues;
5. possible modulation of the defective carrier with other drugs.

Plasma carnitine concentration is an indirect index of the carnitine concentration in other tissues such as liver and skeletal muscle, and this correlation might be completely lost in patients with primary

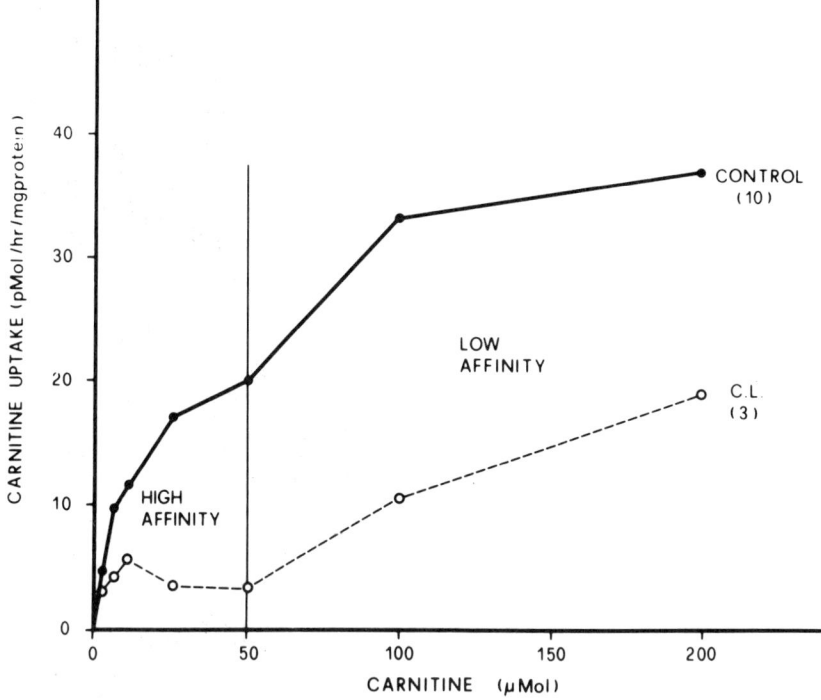

FIGURE 5. High and low affinity carnitine uptake in human muscle cultured for 20 days. Controls (●), and cultures from a patient with systemic carnitine deficiency (SCD) and high affinity uptake defect (○).

carnitine deficiency undergoing carnitine therapy. In patients affected by systemic or muscle carnitine deficiency undergoing carnitine therapy, plasma and liver carnitine levels returned to normal, but muscle carnitine concentration, though higher than in the pre-treatment muscle biopsy, remained much lower than in controls (Scarlato et al, 1977; Carrol et al, 1980; Tripp et al, 1981; Chapoy et al, 1980; Treem et al, 1988; Tein et al, 1990).

Although the muscle carnitine concentration is not substantially changed, there is usually a remarkable clinical improvement, and morphological evidence of decreased muscle lipid storage after long-term carnitine therapy has been found. In some of these cases a defect in carnitine uptake was demonstrated (Tein et al, 1990), and in others it was postulated. We hypothesize that the higher plasma carnitine concentration is enough to induce an increased intracellular carnitine pool. The small increase in carnitine flux inside the cells might then

be sufficient to cause a change in several metabolic parameters (i.e.
β-oxidation, CoA/acyl CoA ratio, pyruvate dehydrogenase (PDH)
complex) and be able to correct the morphological and the clinical
abnormalities.

The pathogenetic sequence of events in the patients with carnitine
leak would be as follows:

1. A defect of high affinity carnitine transport in most cells,
   including renal tubular cells, which are involved in a process
   of transluminal uptake; a small amount of carnitine reaches
   muscle, heart and kidney cells through the low affinity uptake.
2. The uptake defect impairs the cells' ability to concentrate
   carnitine against a steep concentration gradient, carnitine renal
   clearance increases, and plasma carnitine concentration drops.
3. With a severely reduced plasma carnitine concentration, low-
   affinity uptake becomes impossible, and thus the cells are
   forced to rely solely on the high-affinity uptake, which is
   faulty.
4. The intracellular carnitine pool drops below the threshold at
   which biochemical damage becomes apparent. A vicious circle
   is set up with increasing acyl CoA concentrations.
5. The accumulation of long-chain acyl CoAs inhibits several
   mitochondrial enzymes (Stumpf et al, 1985), causing further
   reduction of the cell's oxidative potential and loss of acylcarnitines.

The high doses of carnitine (2–4 g per day) that we use in the initial
therapy of carnitine deficiency syndromes may benefit cell metabolism
at three levels:

1. Replenishing the carnitine pool and compensating the amount
   lost in stools and urine.
2. Increasing plasma carnitine concentration, making possible
   low affinity uptake and passive diffusion, and thus allowing
   some carnitine to enter the cell.
3. Inducing the synthesis of a greater number of carnitine carriers
   (Molstad et al, 1978) (in the patients in which the protein
   carrier is not absent).

The inappropriate renal carnitine reabsorption seems the most
important factor in causing the rapid fall in plasma carnitine concentration observed upon temporary suspension of therapy (Waber et al,
1982). The critical role of renal carnitine reabsorption in the pathogenesis of carnitine deficiency is also confirmed by the reports of dramatic

clinical deterioration of patients with carnitine deficiency during pregnancy (Boudin et al, 1976; Cornelio et al, 1977). In pregnancy, a higher carnitine clearance has been demonstrated in normal women (Cederblad et al, 1986). Besides, the exposure to high oestrogen and progesterone concentrations (Vergani et al, 1989) causes a decrease in V_{max} of carnitine uptake in cultured cells.

CORTICOSTEROIDS

Corticosteroids have been used in carnitine deficiency syndrome both alone and in association with carnitine supplementation. They are known to decrease lipogenesis and to promote fatty acid mobilization (Littwack and Singer, 1972), but we speculate that the beneficial effect in patients may be due to a more specific action on carnitine transport. Induction of carnitine transport by corticosteroids was shown in the CCL27 cell line (Molstad and Bohmer, 1979). This increase in uptake appears to be due to a higher number of carriers, since the apparent K_m does not change. This effect was observed uniformly with various types of corticosteroids (prednisolone, triamcinolone, dexamethasone) and was dose-related. In the carnitine-deficient patients treated with corticosteroids, however, there was no correlation between the dosage of medication and the clinical improvement, nor were tissue carnitine concentrations raised.

Good results have also been obtained with corticosteroids associated with oral L-carnitine (2–4 g per day). Prednisone is the most widely used steroid, its posology in most cases was 1–1.5 mg kg^{-1} day^{-1}, reducing to as low as 10 mg day^{-1} in some. We also observed, in the MCD case described above, benefits with deflazacort (a new synthetic steroid) 30 mg on alternate day, associated with L-carnitine 3 g day^{-1} and a low-fat diet.

LOW-FAT DIET, MEDIUM-CHAIN TRIGLYCERIDES (MCT)

Fatty acids within the cell form esters with carnitine and reach the mitochondrial matrix as acylcarnitines. This transfer is essential to make long-chain acyl CoAs available for β-oxidation. Medium-chain and short-chain fatty acids are able to cross the mitochondrial membrane without the help of carnitine. Therefore, a low-fat diet poor in long-chain triglycerides and rich in medium and short-chain triglycerides can decrease intracellular lipid storage and assure at the same time adequate fuel for β-oxidation.

A low-fat diet supplemented with medium-chain triglycerides oil (MCT) has been tried on patients with lipid storage and low carnitine levels since 1976 (Smyth et al, 1975), and is still used by the authors in association with L-carnitine alone or L-carnitine plus steroids in patients with muscle carnitine deficiency. Engel and Askanas (1986) reported a patient in whom a high dose of oral L-carnitine (up to 12 g day^{-1}) and 100 mg day^{-1} of prednisone failed to produce a beneficial effect. The entire diet of the patient was then substituted by 'Portagen' (a synthetic formula containing MCT), protein powder, folate, vitamin E and B12, and raw vegetables. The patient had a complete and sustained remission of his muscle symptoms.

Low compliance, nausea and diarrhoea are the most frequent problems with the dietetic approach. An important note of caution in patients with systemic carnitine deficiency is to avoid prolonged fasting tests, since impaired ketogenesis in these patients might lead to a life-threatening crisis of hypoglycaemic coma (DiDonato et al, 1980).

CONCLUSIONS

A correct therapeutic approach in primary carnitine deficiency requires two steps: (i) to identify the exact biochemical diagnosis, and (ii) to adopt therapeutic measures to prevent a metabolic crisis. It is important that, in patients with low plasma or muscle carnitine levels, accurate and extensive biochemical investigations differentiate primary from secondary carnitine deficiency. Such distinction is not always easy, and may require sophisticated assays. L-Carnitine therapy may also be beneficial in dubious cases where the precise biochemical defect is uncertain, and it has been proved a safe and effective measure in patients having 'carnitine insufficiency' secondary to other biochemical defects (Stumpf et al, 1985; Engel, 1986; Stanley, 1987). However, in patients with low carnitine levels secondary to short-chain acyl CoA dehydrogenase deficiency, carnitine supplementation is sometimes ineffective, while dramatic improvement may be achieved with riboflavin therapy (30–100 mg day^{-1}) (DiDonato et al, 1989).

REFERENCES

Angelini C, Lucke S & Cantarutti F (1976) *Neurology* 26: 633–637.
Bach AC, Schirardin H, Sihr MO & Storck D (1983) *Diabetes Metabol.* 9: 121–124.
Barth PG, Sholte HR, Berden JA et al (1983) *J. Neurol. Sci.* 62: 327–355.
Boudin G, Mikol J, Guillard A & Engel AG (1976) *J. Neurol. Sci.* 30: 313–325.
Bremer J (1983) *Physiol. Rev.* 63: 1421–1480.
Carrol JE, Brooke MH, DeVivo DC et al (1980) *Neurology* 30: 618–626.
Cederblad G, Fahraeus L & Lindgren K (1986) *Clin. Nutr.* 44: 379–383.
Chapoy PR, Angelini C, Brown WJ et al (1980) *N. Engl. J. Med.* 303: 1389–1394.
Cornelio F, DiDonato S, Peluchetti D et al (1977) *J. Neurol. Neurosurg. Psychiatry* 40: 170–178.
DiDonato S, Peluchetti D, Rimoldi et al (1980) *Clin. Chim. Acta* 100: 209–214.
DiDonato S, Gellera C, Peluchetti et al (1989) *Ann. Neurol.* 25: 479–484.
Engel AG (1986) In Engel AG & Banker B (eds) *Myology*, pp 1663–1696 New York: McGraw-Hill.
Engel AG & Angelini C (1973) *Science* 179: 899–902.
Engel WK & Askanas V (1986) *Neurology* 36: 94.
Engel AG, Angelini C & Nelson R (1974) In Milharad AT (ed.) *Exploratory Concepts in Muscular Dystrophy* pp 601–618. New York: Elsevier.
Eriksson BO, Lindsted S & Nordin I (1988) *Eur. J. Pediatr.* 147: 662–663.
Harper P, Elwin CE & Cederblad G (1988) *Eur. J. Pharmacol.* 35: 555–562.
Huth PJ & Shug AL (1980) *Biochim. Biophys. Acta* 602: 621–634.
Ino T, Sherwood GF, Cutz E et al (1988) *Clin. Lab. Observ.* 113: 511–514.
Karpati G, Carpenter S, Engel AG et al (1975) *Neurology* 25: 16–24.
Littwack G & Singer S (1972) In Littwack G (ed.) *Biochemical Action of Hormones* vol. 2, p 114. New York: Academic Press.
Molstad P & Bohmer T (1979) *Biochim. Biophys. Acta* 585: 94–99.
Molstad P, Bohmer T & Hovig T (1978) *Biochim. Biophys. Acta* 512: 557–565.
Rebouche CJ (1977) *Biochim. Biophys. Acta* 471: 145–155.
Rebouche CJ & Engel AG (1982) *In Vitro* 18: 495–500.
Rebouche CJ & Engel AG (1984) *J. Clin. Invest.* 73: 857–867.
Rodriguez-Pereira R, Sholte HR, Luyt-Houwen IEM & Vaandrager-Verduin MHM (1988) *Eur. J. Pediatr.* 148: 193–197.
Scarlato G, Albizzati MG, Bassi S et al (1977) *Eur. Neurol.* 16: 222–229.
Seim H, Schultze J & Strack E (1985) *Biol. Chem.* 366: 1017–1021.
Smyth DPL, Lake BD, MacDermot J & Wilson J (1975) *Lancet* i: 1198–1199.
Stanley CA (1987) *Adv. Pediatr.* 34: 59–88.
Stumpf DA, Parker WD & Angelini C (1985) *Neurology* 35: 1041–1045.
Tein I, DeVivo DC, Bierman F et al (1990) *Pediatr. Res.* 28: 247–255.
Treem WR, Stanley CA, Finegold DN et al (1988) *N. Engl. J. Med.* 319: 1331–1336.
Tripp ME, Katcher ML, Peters HA et al (1981) *N. Engl. J. Med.* 305: 385–390.
Vergani L, Martinuzzi A, Rosa et al (1989) *Ital. J. Neurol. Sci.* 10: 237.
Vergani L, Martinuzzi A, Rosa et al (1990) *J. Neurol. Sci.* 98: 191.
Waber LJ, Valle D, Neill C et al (1982) *J. Pediatr.* 101: 700–705.
Zierz S, Engel AG & Romshe CA (1988) *Advances in Neurology* 48: 231–237.

9

PRIMARY SYSTEMIC CARNITINE DEFICIENCY MANIFESTED BY CARNITINE-RESPONSIVE CARDIOMYOPATHY

I. Tein and S. DiMauro

Over the past 10 years, there has been much difficulty in assessing the role of carnitine deficiency in both genetic and acquired defects of fatty acid oxidation, and in the past 3 years, it has become apparent that only a few disorders can be unequivocally attributed to primary carnitine deficiency.

Carnitine deficiency was first described in 1973 (Engel and Angelini, 1973) and patients have been divided into two groups. Those with 'systemic carnitine deficiency' had recurrent episodes of hypoglycae-mic, hypoketotic encephalopathy ('Reye-like' syndrome) beginning in

L-Carnitine and Its Role in Medicine:
From Function to Therapy. ISBN 0–12–253940–0

infancy or early childhood and had low concentrations of carnitine in serum, muscle and liver. Those with 'myopathic carnitine deficiency' had progressive lipid storage myopathy beginning in childhood or later in life and the carnitine deficiency was confined to skeletal muscle (DiMauro, 1979; Rebouche and Engel, 1983; Angelini et al, 1987).

In the mid-1970s, there were improvements in methods to identify abnormal fatty acid metabolites in urine (using gas chromatography and mass spectroscopy) and the introduction of more sensitive methods to measure acyl CoA dehydrogenase (through an electron-transfer flavoprotein (ETF)-linked assay) and respiratory chain activities. These allowed many previously diagnosed cases to be attributed to different defects of β-oxidation or the respiratory chain with secondary carnitine deficiency (Stanley, 1987). For example, medium-chain acyl CoA dehydrogenase (MCAD) deficiency was the underlying biochemical defect in many cases initially diagnosed as carnitine deficiency (Coates et al, 1984; Hale et al, 1985). Other inborn errors of fatty acid or amino acid oxidation resulting in a secondary carnitine deficiency include long-chain acyl CoA dehydrogenase (LCAD), short-chain acyl CoA dehydrogenase (SCAD), and multiple acyl CoA dehydrogenase (MAD) deficiencies, isovaleric acidaemia, methyl malonic aciduria, propionic acidaemia, β-hydroxy-β-methyl glutaryl CoA lyase and glutaryl CoA dehydrogenase deficiency (Stanley, 1987). In these disorders there is a block in the oxidation of one or more of the acyl CoA compounds that are normally esterified to carnitine. Most of these conditions seem to share some abnormalities seen in MCAD deficiency, including low plasma concentrations of total carnitine, increased ratio of esterified carnitine to total carnitine, and low tissue concentrations of total carnitine.

In the 'myopathic' form of carnitine deficiency it is presumed that the defect involves the carnitine transporter in skeletal muscle. However, some patients were shown to have other defects, such as SCAD deficiency (Turnbull et al, 1984; Coates et al, 1988). An important and still controversial issue in patients with secondary carnitine deficiency is whether carnitine therapy is beneficial in either the acute or chronic situations (Stanley, 1987).

Primary carnitine deficiency should be defined by the following criteria: (i) the metabolic disorder is caused directly by inadequate carnitine; (ii) it is accompanied by impaired fatty acid oxidation; (iii) it is corrected when carnitine concentration is restored to normal; and (iv) it is not secondary to a defect of mitochondrial β-oxidation (Table 1, after Treem et al, 1988).

A number of possible aetiologies for primary carnitine deficiency

TABLE 1.
Criteria defining primary carnitine deficiency. Adapted from De Vivo and Tein 1990 with permission of editor

1.	The condition is caused by inadequate tissue concentrations of carnitine
2.	The carnitine deficiency results in an impairment of fatty acid oxidation
3.	The condition is corrected when carnitine concentrations are restored to normal
4.	There is no evidence of a primary defect in intramitochondrial β-oxidation

have been proposed: (i) defective biosynthesis and dietary intake; (ii) defective intestinal absorption; (iii) defective transport affecting uptake and/or release of carnitine from tissues; (iv) renal loss due to decreased tubular reabsorption or increased excretion; (v) increased degradation. In several patients with 'systemic' carnitine deficiency there was no evidence of defective carnitine biosynthesis (Rebouche and Engel, 1980), defective absorption or excessive degradation (Rebouche and Engel, 1984) but these patients were later found to have MCAD deficiency.

The first evidence for a defect in the cellular uptake of carnitine was offered in 1988 (Eriksson et al, 1988, 1989; Treem et al, 1988), and four more patients have been reported (Tein et al, 1990) with a defect of the carnitine transporter resulting in primary systemic carnitine deficiency.

These cases were characterized clinically by carnitine-responsive cardiomyopathy with or without weakness, hypoglycaemic hypoketotic encephalopathy, and failure to thrive. Laboratory tests showed anaemia, low plasma and tissue concentrations of carnitine, lipid storage in muscle and liver, and severe renal leak of carnitine. Five other cases in the literature can be included in this group on the basis of indirect but compelling evidence including:

1. very low serum and tissue concentrations of carnitine;
2. cardiomyopathy;
3. rapid and dramatic response to carnitine therapy or, if no carnitine was given, family history of a similarly affected sibling with carnitine-responsive cardiomyopathy; and
4. lack of abnormal dicarboxylic aciduria (the laboratory hallmark of secondary carnitine deficiencies due to defects in β-oxidation), or lack of carnitine repletion in tissues despite oral carnitine supplementation (Tein et al, 1990).

These patients were also different from the cases of X-linked cardiomyopathy with neutropenia, short stature, abnormal carnitine metabolism and dicarboxylic aciduria (Neustein et al, 1979; Barth et al, 1983; Ino et al, 1988).

In this chapter we will outline the key clinical and biochemical features of 11 cases of true primary systemic carnitine deficiency manifested by carnitine-responsive cardiomyopathy and we will discuss the potential underlying pathophysiological processes. The importance of an accurate diagnosis of this potentially fatal disorder lies in its eminent treatability through lifelong oral carnitine supplementation.

DEMOGRAPHIC FEATURES

Sex distribution was equal with five males and six females affected. Siblings were affected in 8 of 11 families and parents were asymptomatic, suggesting an autosomal recessive pattern of inheritance, though consanguinity was documented in only one family. The patients had diverse ethnic backgrounds including Irish–American, East Indian, Italian, Yugoslavian, Mexican, Norwegian and German, suggesting that the defect is genetically widely distributed. Age of onset was under 4 years, with six patients presenting in the first year of life. The presenting feature was cardiomyopathy in eight cases, hypoglycaemic encephalopathy in two cases, and weakness or hypotonia in two cases (Table 2). Even when this was not present at onset, all patients developed a cardiomyopathy. Over time, weakness became manifest in six cases, episodes of hypoglycaemic encephalopathy in four cases (with seizures in two), developmental delay in three cases, and failure to thrive in four cases (where information was available). Two of the 11 children have died.

CARDIAC FEATURES

Cardiomyopathy was present in all cases. Depending upon the age at diagnosis and the stage of the disease, the echocardiogram may show increased left ventricular posterior wall thickness, left ventricular hypertrophy or biventricular hypertrophy, dilatation of left and right ventricles and left atrium with increased diastolic and systolic

TABLE 2.
Major clinical features in cases of primary systemic carnitine deficiency—literature review

Reference	Sex	Affected siblings	Consanguinity	Age of onset (months)	Presenting feature	Clinical spectrum	Failure to thrive
Chapoy et al (1980)	M	+(1)	–	3	E/C	W/S/D	+
Tripp et al (1981)	#1 F	+(3)	–	11	C		
	#2 M*	+(3)	–	26	C		
Waber et al (1982)	M	+(1)	+	40	C	W	–
Eriksson et al (1988)	#1 F	+(1)		<48	C		
	#2 M*	+(1)		<18	C		
Treem et al (1988)	F			3.5	E	C/S/D	–
Tein et al (1990)	#1 F	+(1)	–	1	C	W	+
	#2 M	–	–	17	W	C/D	+
	#3 F	–	–	1	H	C/W/E	–
	#4 F	+(1)	–	2	C	W/E?	+

C, cardiomyopathy; W, weakness or motor delay; E, hypoglycaemic encephalopathy; S, seizure; H, hypotonia; D, developmental delay; *deceased.

dimensions, decreased velocity of circumferential fibre shortening with decreased left ventricular ejection fraction, and variable degrees of mitral regurgitation (Table 3). The hallmark of the electrocardiography is the bizarre enlargement or peaking of the T-waves, but findings may include left or biventricular hypertrophy and various disturbances of rhythm, such as mild first degree heart block, sinus tachycardia, nodal escape rhythms and sinus arrest.

Many of these children developed end-stage congestive heart failure despite the institution of classic anti-failure medication regimens (Tripp et al, 1981; Waber et al, 1982; Tein et al, 1990). In contrast, the response to carnitine supplementation has been dramatic, specific, and evident within the first month of therapy (Tein et al, 1990), eliminating the need for other medications, such as digoxin and diuretics in two cases (Waber et al, 1982; Tein et al, 1990).

This prompt response to carnitine therapy occurred in eight cases. Of the remaining three children, two died during an acute episode (Tripp et al, 1981), presumably before a diagnosis was made and carnitine therapy instituted (Eriksson et al, 1988). In the last child, the diagnosis was made at 3.5 months and carnitine therapy was started when cardiac features were limited to increased thickness of the left ventricle and septum with normal-sized ventricle during systole and diastole, and normal shortening fraction (Treem et al, 1988).

The efficacy of carnitine therapy has been particularly well documented in four cases. The patient of Chapoy et al (1980) was a 6-month-old boy with biventricular hypertrophy and a minimal atrial septal defect (ASD) on cardiac catheterization. After 3 months on oral carnitine (approximately 100–120 mg kg^{-1} day^{-1}), there was marked improvement in the cardiothoracic ratio (before therapy 0.67, after therapy 0.57; normal <0.55), diastolic (before 37 mm, after 32 mm; normal <32 mm) and systolic chamber dimensions (before 37 mm, after 22 mm; normal <24 mm), left ventricular wall thickness (before 12 mm, after 9 mm; normal 5–7 mm), velocity of circumferential fibre shortening (before 0.8 s, after 1.3 s; normal 0.9–1.5 s) and percentage of shortening (before 18%, after 31%; normal 21–48%). The EKG showed ventricular hypertrophy before therapy and shortened PR interval after therapy.

One of the cases described by Tripp et al (1981), an 11-month-old girl, had poor myocardial contractility and concentric biventricular hypertrophy on cardiac catheterization. At 6 years, EKG showed bizarre T-wave enlargement, and at 9 years mitral regurgitation was diagnosed and she was treated with digitalis. Oral carnitine administration caused dramatic improvement in cardiac size and function. Left atrial and left

TABLE 3.

Cardiac features in primary systemic carnitine deficiency

Reference	Sex	Age at diagnosis (months)	Findings on cardiac echogram						EKG	
			Predominant feature	↑ LV wall thickness	↑ Diastolic and systolic dimensions	Decreased velocity circumferential fibre-shortening	↓ LV ejection fraction	Other	Peaked T-waves	Other
Chapoy et al (1980)	M	6	BVH	+	+	+		ASD min.		VH
Tripp et al (1981)	#1 F	11	BVH	+	+	+		MR	+	Sinus arrest nodal escape
	#2 M	26	BVH							
Waber et al (1982)	M	40	LVH	+	+		+		+	LVH
Treem et al (1988)	F	3.5		+	-	-				Sinus tachycardia
Tein et al (1990)	#1 F	48	LV + LA dilatation		+	+	+	MR	+	
	#2 M	90	Dilatation						+	
	#4 F	76	LV + RV dilatation	+	+	+		MR mild	+	BVH mild first degree heart block

BVH, biventricular hypertrophy; LVH, left ventricular hypertrophy; LV, left ventricle; LA, left atrium; RV, right ventricle; ASD, atrial septal defect; MR, mitral regurgitation.

ventricular systolic and diastolic dimensions were respectively 80% (percentile), >90%, and 90% before therapy and decreased to 40%, 85% and 70% after 2.5 months of therapy, and to 25%, 60% and 50% after 6 months of therapy. The percentage of myocardial fractional shortening, which was 19% before therapy, increased to 27% and 34% 2.5 and 6 months after therapy.

In the report of Waber et al (1982), a 4.5-year-old boy suffered from left ventricular hypertrophy and dilatation with severely decreased left ventricular ejection fraction (39%; normal 60–80%). After only 1 month of carnitine therapy, the ejection fraction had increased to 75% and, by 5 months, the cardiac echogram demonstrated only mild left ventricular wall thickening with good contractility and an ejection fraction of 69%. Digoxin and diuretic therapy could be discontinued after only 2 months of carnitine therapy. In case no. 1 of Tein et al (1990), a cardiac murmur was first noted at 1 month of age. This child suffered recurrent respiratory infections between 1 and 3 years of age: she had marked congestive heart failure with moderate-to-severe mitral regurgitation and marked left ventricular dilatation on cardiac echogram. The EKG demonstrated peaked T-waves in the anterolateral precordial leads (Figure 1). She was started on digoxin and diuretics and was in end-stage congestive heart failure by 4 years of age, when she was found to have very low concentrations of carnitine in serum and muscle. Oral carnitine therapy was started at 1 g 3 times daily and dramatic improvement in cardiac function became evident by 1 week (Table 4; Figure 2). After 4 weeks, she had gained weight and showed increased tolerance to exercise; the EKG showed inversion of the formerly peaked T-waves (Figure 1). After 4 months, she had good exercise tolerance and cardiac end-diastolic and end-systolic dimensions had markedly improved (Figure 2). Digoxin and diuretics were discontinued at 6.5 years and, by 9 years of age, she was a competitive swimmer at school.

Heart has a very high concentration of carnitine and is highly dependent upon fatty acid oxidation as a source of energy. In addition to its key function as a transporter of long-chain fatty acids across the inner mitochondrial membrane, carnitine plays an important role in trapping toxic long-chain acyl CoA metabolites which may accumulate in ischaemia and lead to sarcolemmal membrane damage and arrhythmias. Using a model of ischaemia in rat heart, Subramanian et al (1987) showed that ischaemic myocardial damage was potentiated during reperfusion with excess free fatty acids (e.g. palmitate) and that those hearts that were treated with L-propionyl carnitine or propionyl carnitine taurine amide showed significant improvement in

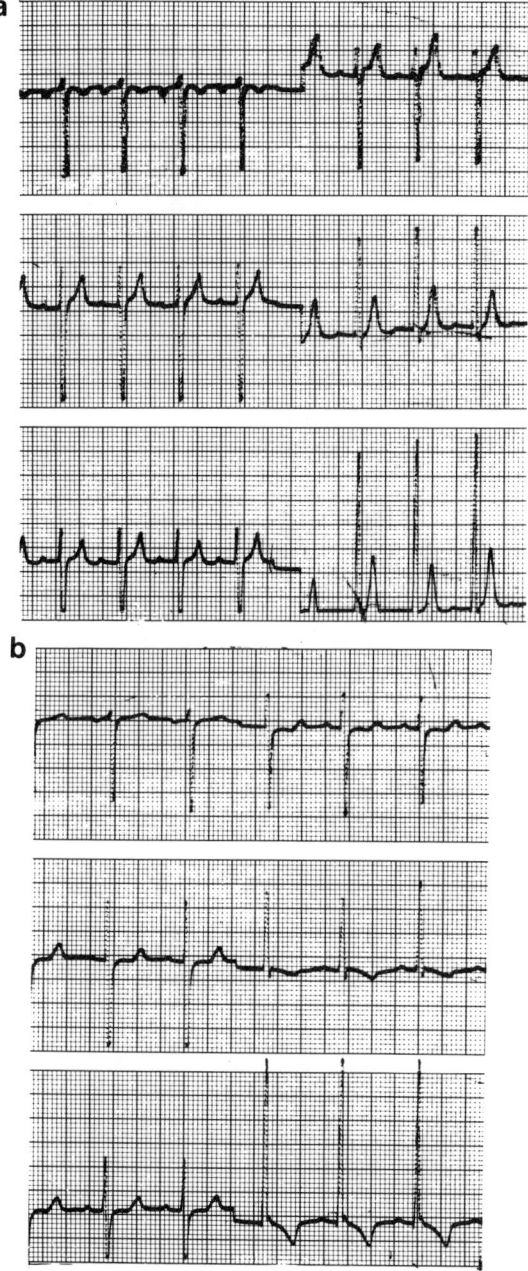

FIGURE 1. (a) Striking elevation of T-waves in midprecordium in case no. 1 of Tein et al (1990) immediately before oral carnitine supplementation (electrocardiogram from lead at half standard). (b) Inversion of T-waves 4 weeks after oral carnitine supplementation.

TABLE 4.
Cardiac parameters before and after carnitine therapy (Patient #1, Tein et al, 1990).

	Comment	LVEDD % Predicted	LVESD % Predicted	EKG	CXR
1 Day prior to treatment Age 4.25 years	(Stage 4 ventricle)	205	237	Peaked T-waves lateral precordial leads	Marked cardiomegaly + LAE
Post-treatment					
1 week		180	218		
2 weeks		166	203		
4 weeks	Moderate ↓ LV dimension ↑ LV function	163	174	Dramatic change in ST/T-wave segments, inversion of formerly peaked T-waves in V5/6 and II, III and AVF	
8 weeks	Improved LV dilatation				
16 weeks	↓ LV Systolic/diastolic dimension			Same	Notable ↓ in cardiomegaly
7 months	Moderate LV dilatation borderline low normal function	129	150	Same	
14 months	Same	127	135		
19 months				Non-specific ST/T-wave changes	
2 years	Mild LV dilatation	131	147	Same	Levocardia
3 years	Mild compensated MR	124	138		
3 years 8 months		126	143	Same	
4 years 2 months		126	128		

LV, left ventricle; LA, left atrium; LVEDD, left ventricular end diastolic dimension; LVESD, left ventricular end systolic dimension; MR, mitral regurgitation; LAE, left atrial enlargement; ↑, increase; ↓, decrease.

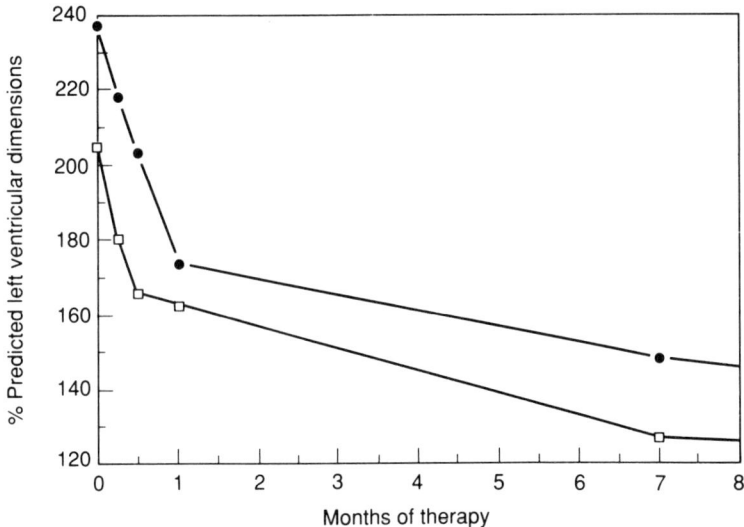

FIGURE 2. Left ventricular dimensions in case no. I of Tein et al (1990). Longitudinal follow-up of ratio between actual and percentage predicted left ventricular end diastolic (☐) and end systolic (●) dimensions after initiation of carnitine therapy. Accelerated response evident during 1st month of therapy persists toward a plateau by 8 months of treatment. From Tein et al (1990), with permission of editor.

recovery. They postulated that the protective action of these two compounds included increased myocardial extraction of free fatty acids, improved translocation of long-chain acyl CoA esters across membranes, and repletion of cellular carnitine stores. They also considered the possibility that treatment with propionyl carnitine might decrease free radical formation which may be involved in the peroxidation of membrane lipids. Conversely, Mak et al (1986) showed that pretreatment of isolated canine cardiac sarcolemmal membranes with palmitoyl CoA and palmitoylcarnitine potentiated free radical-induced lipid peroxidation injury. According to Siliprandi et al (1987), long-chain acyl CoAs may deform cellular membranes and potentiate the toxic effects of hydroperoxides, high Ca^{2+} concentrations or elevated temperatures on mitochondrial membranes. These toxic effects could be delayed by carnitine (Siliprandi et al, 1987). Therefore, carnitine appears to be a central compound in myocardial metabolism, as shown by the marked pathology noted in patients with primary carnitine deficiency and by the dramatic response to carnitine supplementation.

MYOPATHY

Weakness was documented in six cases, all of whom showed definite clinical improvement on carnitine therapy. Lipid storage was seen in muscle biopsies from eight patients and pre-treatment muscle carnitine concentrations ranged from 0.5 to 5.0% of normal mean values (Table 5). Though carnitine supplementation resulted in a three- to tenfold increase in muscle carnitine, the concentration remained well below normal, ranging from 2.6 to 13% of control mean values. Only one case (Chapoy et al, 1980) showed a relatively large increase of carnitine to 40% of normal (Table 6). In contrast to the incomplete correction of carnitine levels, clinical recovery was nearly complete and repeat muscle biopsies showed disappearance of the lipid storage (Chapoy et al, 1980; Tein et al, 1990).

In the case of Chapoy et al (1980), the proximal weakness of shoulder girdle and trunk musculature improved from 2/5 to 4/5 power and 3 weeks after therapy, the Gowers manoeuvre had disappeared, although the electromyography still showed some abnormal fibrillations. In case no. 4 of Tein et al (1990), there was a marked increase in strength, though this 7-year-old girl continued to have a degree of residual weakness (4/5) in the shoulder girdle after 5 months of carnitine therapy. In a 9-year-old girl (case no. 1 of Tein et al, 1990), persistence of a slightly myopathic facies and mild hypotonia were noted even after 5 years of carnitine therapy.

NEUROPATHY

Much attention has been focused on the myopathy of carnitine deficiency, and nerve conduction studies (NCS) were performed only in a few cases. Therefore, little information is available regarding the role of carnitine in peripheral nerve dysfunction. The young boy described by Chapoy et al (1980) had almost unmeasurable sensory nerve conduction velocities in the left peroneal nerve and showed neutral lipid storage on nerve biopsy. Both abnormalities were reversed with carnitine therapy. In case no. 1 of Tein et al (1990), a 9-year-old girl, motor NCS showed slightly prolonged distal latencies for both peroneal nerves, borderline-low motor unit action potentials for the right peroneal nerve and repetitive discharges on supramaximal stimulation of the right peroneal F-response. These changes were

TABLE 5.
Major laboratory features of cases of primary systemic carnitine deficiency—literature review

Reference	Sex	Decreased fasting ketogen	Anaemia	Decreased renal DCA reabsorption	Lipid storage in tissue	Plasma carnitine (total/free) (μmol l^{-1})	Carnitine levels % normal mean		
							Muscle	Liver	Heart
Chapoy et al (1980)	M	+		−	Muscle/liver/ nerve	4.8*	1.5	6	
Tripp et al (1981) #1 F			+	+		Muscle	4.8/3.6†	0.5		
#2 M			+	+		Liver/cardiac	4.5/3.5†	1	30	5
Waber et al (1982)	M	−	+	+	Muscle	4.2‡	2		
Eriksson et al (1988) F					+	Muscle	<3%	<1		<1
#2 M										
Treem et al (1988)	F	+	+	+	Muscle/liver	0–2.2§	<1	5	
Tein et al (1990) #1 F				+	+	Muscle	19.3/15.0‖	4		
#2 M				+	+	Muscle	1.2/1.2¶	5		
#3 F		+	−	+		0			
#4 F		+?	+		Muscle	9/5**	5		

N, normal values
*N = 35.5 ± 5.6 μmol l^{-1}
†N = 35–75 μmol l^{-1}
‡N = 20–80 μmol l^{-1}
§N = 37–58/28–47 μmol l^{-1}
‖N = 51.5 ± 11.6/40.0 ± 9.5 μmol l^{-1}
¶N = 45 ± 6.5/34 ± 8.8 μmol l^{-1}
**N = 35–56/29–45 μmol l^{-1}.

TABLE 6.

Beneficial response to carnitine therapy in cases of primary systemic carnitine deficiency—literature review

Reference	Sex	Plasma carnitine (total/free) (μM)	Muscle carnitine (% norm)	Motor function	Cardiac function	Growth	Anaemia	Cognitive function
Chapoy et al (1980)	M	/18.5*	40	+	+			−
Tripp et al (1981)	F	13.3–43.7/11.7–35.9†	5		+	+	+	
	M							
Waber et al (1982)	M	22–55‡		+	+			
Eriksson et al (1988)	F		low		+			
	M							
Treem et al (1988)	F	44/24§	2.6					
Tein et al (1990)	#1 F	25.6–60/17.2–33.5¶		+	+	+	+	+
	#2 M	9–28/9–17‖	13	+	+	+	+	−
	#3 F			++	++	++		
	#4 F			++	++	++		+

N, normal values
*N = 35.5 ± 5.6 μmol l⁻¹
†N = 35–75 μmol l⁻¹
‡N = 20–80 μmol l⁻¹
§N = 37–56/28–47 μmol l⁻¹
¶N = 51.5 ± 11.6/40.0 ± 9.5 μmol l⁻¹
‖N I 45 ± 6.5/34 ± 8.8 μmol l⁻¹.

present after 5 years of carnitine therapy. The borderline abnormalities in the peroneal nerve could have been a reflection of anomalous foot architecture (both extensores digitorum breves were absent), but they could also have represented early axonal changes related to partially treated carnitine deficiency. These cases underline the need for further NCS in future cases to define better the potential role of carnitine in peripheral nerve pathology.

CENTRAL NERVOUS SYSTEM

Coma occurred in four cases. This was most likely due to hypoglycaemia secondary to the inability of decreasing glucose consumption in the later stages of fasting, when ketone bodies generated from hepatic fatty acid oxidation became limited as a source of energy. Cognitive delay and pyramidal signs were noted in the cases of Chapoy et al (1980) and Treem et al (1988), which were probably attributable to hypoglycaemic encephalopathy, as well as to their respective cardiac and respiratory arrests. However, in the case of Chapoy, both pyramidal signs and ataxia disappeared 2 weeks after the institution of carnitine therapy. The speech disability and developmental delay, in contrast, did not improve at the same pace and improvement was considered only slight after 1 year of therapy, consistent with a static encephalopathy. Furthermore, CT scan of the head demonstrated marked enlargement of both lateral ventricles and of the sulci between the cerebral gyri.

Other unexplained central nervous system signs occurred in case no. 1 of Tripp et al (1981), a 9-year-old who had had no prior documented episodes of hypoglycaemic coma, but who had undergone an emergency tracheostomy at age 5 for croup, raising the possibility of an anoxic insult. She began having syncopal episodes at age 8, and at 9 years, had bilateral extensor plantar responses and minimal athetoid movements. Similarly, case no. 2 of Tein et al (1990), a 10-year-old boy, had moderate mental retardation in the absence of obvious predisposing factors by history. Unfortunately, cognitive function was not studied in all cases of primary carnitine deficiency. Therefore, the importance of carnitine *per se* in central nervous system function or development cannot be accurately assessed. Indirectly, however, carnitine plays a key protective role against the cardiomyopathy which may result in hypoxic ischaemic encephalopathy and against the impairment of hepatic fasting ketogenesis which may result in hypoglycaemic hypoketotic encephalopathy. In cases no. 1 and no. 4

of Tein et al (1990) and in the case of Waber et al (1982), affect and cognitive performance improved following carnitine therapy, but this may have been due to a general improvement in health and energy levels.

Carnitine concentration in the brain is relatively low (approximately 10% of the heart, muscle and liver concentrations) and the K_m for brain is very high (>1000 μM) (Bieber, 1988), though brain is one of the few tissues capable of endogenous carnitine biosynthesis. Both acetylcarnitine and γ-butyrobetaine (immediate precursor of carnitine) are normal constituents of mammalian brain tissue (Elliot and Jasper, 1959; Bergmeyer, 1974). The highest concentrations of carnitine in frozen canine brain are found in the cerebellum and the lowest levels in the hippocampus and pons (Shug et al, 1982).

The uptake of L-carnitine into brain has been demonstrated to occur by two mechanisms—non-saturable diffusion and active saturable energy and sodium-dependent, carrier-mediated transport. In synaptosomes isolated from guinea-pig cerebral cortex, this active process depends on $Na^+-K^+ATPase$ activity, is inhibited by oxidation phosphorylation uncouplers, and is saturated at 1–2 mM L-carnitine (Zoccarato et al, 1983). In rat brain slices, Huth et al (1981) demonstrated a saturable uptake for both L- and D-carnitine with K_ms respectively, of 2.85 mM and 10.0 mM and the same V_{max} of 1 μmol min^{-1} ml^{-1} of intracellular fluid. They also showed that L-carnitine uptake is competitively inhibited by γ-butyrobetaine (K_i = 3.22 mM), acetylcarnitine (K_i = 6.36 mM) and γ-aminobutyrate (GABA) (K_i = 0.63 mM), and suggested that carnitine and GABA may interact at a common carrier site. They therefore suggested that carnitine may modulate the transport of GABA, the major inhibitory CNS neurotransmitter. This is further supported by the observation that the levels of carnitine in cerebral cortex and CSF are much higher than those of GABA (Moroni et al, 1979; Shug et al, 1980). In mouse brain synaptosomes, Hannuniemi and Kontro (1988) have demonstrated that the GABA uptake system contains two saturable transport components, a high-affinity component which is competitively inhibited by carnitine, and a low-affinity component which shows a mixed pattern of inhibition by carnitine. Although they concluded that GABA and carnitine share the same carrier at synaptosomal membranes, they also pointed out that GABA is the preferred substrate and that the concentrations of carnitine which inhibited GABA uptake exceeded the physiological levels of carnitine in vivo.

Energetically, the brain is primarily dependent upon glucose and ketone bodies rather than on the mitochondrial oxidation of long-chain fatty acids. However, it has been suggested that carnitine may play a role in regulating the glycolytic flux through its effect on the mitochondrial matrix acetyl CoA/CoA ratio and the activity of carnitine acetyl transferase (CAT) (Bremer, 1977; Shug et al, 1980). Acetylcarnitine formed in the mitochondrial matrix by CAT and carnitine may provide a transport system for acetyl groups to the cytosolic cell compartment (Sugden et al, 1977) where they would be utilized for the synthesis of acetylcholine through the action of the enzyme choline–acetyl transferase, which is present only in the cytosol. Therefore, carnitine levels in the brain may stimulate glycolysis and acetylcholine formation (Shug et al, 1980) and, thus, affect pathways involved in excitatory function in the mammalian brain (Huth et al, 1981). However, carnitine probably does not act as a direct neurotransmitter; studies of Shug et al (1982) in rat brain slices failed to show changes in carnitine levels after in vivo stimulation of major afferent pathways in the caudate nucleus or K^+-stimulated release of carnitine.

Finally, L-acetylcarnitine has been shown to increase both spontaneous and evoked discharges in rat brainstem neurones and to potentiate cholinergic and serotonergic responses (Tempesta et al, 1985). It was suggested that acetylcarnitine had a stereospecific facilitatory action on the neuronal responses to acetylcholine and 5-hydroxytryptophan. This is another area that warrants further investigation.

ANAEMIA

An intriguing and unresolved question is the role of carnitine deficiency in the variegate anaemia noted in 6 cases (Table 7). In most, the anaemia was mild, but in case no. 2 of Tein et al (1990) the initial concentration (Hb) recorded for this 7.5-year-old boy was 5 g dl^{-1}. The earliest haemoglobin documentation of anaemia was at 15 days of age in a girl (Tein et al, 1990, case no. 4), but in most cases anaemia was discovered at the time that the cardiomyopathy was diagnosed. The red blood cell morphology on smear has varied from hypochromic (Tein et al, 1990, case no. 2) to macrocytic (Waber et al, 1982) to normocytic, normochromic (Tein et al, 1990, case no. 4). Family history has been positive for anaemia in four cases.

Depending upon the smear characteristics, these patients were subjected to different sets of investigations in search of the underlying aetiology, but with limited success. Both cases of Tripp et al (1981)

TABLE 7.

Features of anaemia in primary systemic carnitine deficiency

Reference	Sex		Hb (g dl⁻¹)	Age noted (months)	Characteristics	Positive family history	Hb concentration following carnitine therapy over time (months)	
Tripp et al (1981)	#1 F		Hct = 29	11		+	Hct = 35	2.5
	#2 M		mild ↓	12		+		
Waber et al (1982)	M		9.7	12	Macrocytic	+		
Tein et al (1990)	#1 F		10.2	48	Hypochromic		12.2	24
	#2 M		5.0	90	Normochromic		7.1–11.8	12
	#4 F		Hct = 28 (17 months)	15 days	normocytic	+		

Hb, haemoglobin; Hct, haematocrit; ↓, decrease.

(siblings of Norwegian and German descent) had mild anaemia, and one of these had a trial of iron therapy with no response. Waber et al (1982) documented an anaemia of 10.4 with mild macrocytosis in a 1-year-old boy in whom serum ferritin, folate, vitamin B_{12} and a bone marrow aspirate were normal. A male sibling of this child had died at 23 months of age with a cardiomyopathy and mild anaemia unresponsive to iron therapy. A 7.5-year-old Italian boy (case no. 2 of Tein et al, 1990) had marked hypochromic anaemia requiring blood transfusions (Hb 5 g dl^{-1}) as well as decreased serum iron of 25 µg dl^{-1} (normal 50–120 µg dl^{-1}). Thalassaemia was excluded. Finally, a girl of Mexican origin was found to have anaemia at 15 days of age and, at 7 months, the anaemia was characterized as normochromic and normocytic with a low reticulocyte count. Serum iron, total iron-binding capacity and ferritin were normal. Repeated work-ups for blood loss including an upper gastrointestinal (GI) series and stools for occult blood were negative. A bone marrow biopsy at 2 years 8 months was normal with the exception of slightly decreased iron stores for which she has been treated with iron supplementation. A haemoglobin electrophoresis was normal.

In the three patients in whom haemoglobin concentration was measured after carnitine therapy, there was a slight improvement, but it is uncertain whether this can be attributed to the supplemental carnitine. In two of these cases, iron therapy was also instituted though this was not felt to be helpful in one of the cases of Tripp et al (1981).

The concentration of carnitine in red blood cells (RBC) is 110 nmol g^{-1} of haemoglobin (Borum et al, 1985). Cooper et al (1988) also measured both carnitine and acetylcarnitine in RBC and found that carnitine concentration was comparable in RBC and plasma (30% of blood carnitine pool versus 60% in plasma). In contrast, acetylcarnitine was more concentrated in RBC (66% of blood acetylcarnitine pool versus 35% in plasma), and RBC carnitine and acetylcarnitine do not freely exchange with plasma pools (Cooper et al, 1988).

The role of carnitine in the RBC as well as the significance of carnitine palmitoyltransferase-1 (CPT-1) on the RBC membrane (Scholte et al, 1979) is not understood. It has been postulated that carnitine may protect the RBC from membrane damage by toxic fatty acyl CoA derivatives (Tripp et al, 1981; Gilbert, 1985). In support of this concept, Minshew et al (1981) using fluorescence spectroscopy, demonstrated a decrease in the rigidity of RBC membranes exposed to all concentrations of a sodium octanoate (medium-chain fatty acid) infusion ranging between 10^{-6} to 10^{-2} mol l^{-1}. However, none of the primary carnitine deficiency cases have shown overt haemolysis. Furthermore, RBC membranes have been shown to metabolize long-chain acylcarnitine esters in vitro (Wittels and Hochstein, 1967). Vacha et al (1983) have raised the question of whether L-carnitine improves lipid metabolism in the RBC membrane. This area warrants further investigation.

GASTROINTESTINAL PROBLEMS

The importance of carnitine for the bowel, another tissue highly dependent upon the oxidation of fatty acids, is raised by the 7.5-year-old Italian boy (Tein et al, 1990, case no. 2) who began having recurrent episodes of abdominal pain and diarrhoea for which cow's milk protein intolerance was excluded. It was, in fact, an episode of acute abdominal pain which precipitated his admission to the hospital at 7.5 years of age, when he was also found to have a dilatative cardiomyopathy. These episodes of abdominal pain resolved completely following the institution of carnitine therapy. None of the other reported cases of primary carnitine deficiency had this problem, but smooth muscle disorders (e.g. pyloric stenosis, recurrent stridor, and gastro-oeso-phageal reflux) were present in three of four children in the family described by Tripp et al (1981). Carnitine may play a role not only in ATP generation through the oxidation of long-chain fatty acids but also as a source and shuttle mechanism for acetyl units involved in cholinergic transmission in the gut.

LABORATORY FEATURES

Primary systemic carnitine deficiency is characterized by certain hallmark laboratory features (Table 5).

All of the children had very low plasma carnitine concentrations, usually <10% of normal plasma levels. Only case no. 1 of Tein et al (1990) had higher plasma concentrations which are difficult to explain. This differentiates the primary from the secondary carnitine deficiency cases in whom the plasma concentrations of carnitine generally range from 20 to 70% of normal (Stanley, 1987). In addition, in secondary disorders, the ratio of esterified carnitine to total carnitine is increased because the block in the oxidation of acyl CoA compounds increases their esterification to free carnitine to form acylcarnitines (Stanley, 1987). In primary carnitine deficiency, the ratio of esterified to total carnitine tends to remain normal. The absence of the abnormal dicarboxylic aciduria associated with most defects in intramitochondrial β-oxidation is another important distinguishing feature of primary carnitine deficiency. No abnormal dicarboxylic aciduria was documented in the six children tested. To explain this difference, it has been suggested that the dicarboxylic acids generated from microsomal ω-oxidation can be further oxidized by the mitochondria even in the absence of a carnitine-mediated transfer of fatty acids across the mitochondrial membrane when the β-oxidation pathway is intact (Treem et al, 1988).

Consistent with the low plasma concentrations of carnitine, carnitine concentrations in muscle and heart are also very low (<5% normal), while concentrations are variable in liver (5–30%), which, unlike muscle or heart, has the capability for endogenous carnitine biosynthesis. Tissue concentrations of carnitine tend to be lower than those reported in secondary carnitine deficiencies (Stanley, 1987).

A decrease in fasting ketogenesis has been documented in three children examined and has been elegantly demonstrated by Chapoy et al (1980) and Treem et al (1988) in detailed fasting studies. Treem et al (1988) also showed that 4 months of L-carnitine administration in their patient, who had presented at 3.5 months of age with hypoglycaemic encephalopathy, corrected the defect of hepatic fatty acid oxidation.

Finally, a renal leak of carnitine was demonstrated in the six children studied. This supports the concept of a carnitine transport defect resulting in an impairment of renal tubular reabsorption of carnitine leading to a decreased renal threshold.

PATHOPHYSIOLOGY AND TRANSPORT STUDIES

Studies of carnitine uptake in vitro support the concept that primary carnitine deficiency is due to a defect in the active transport of carnitine, as suggested by Treem et al (1988) and Eriksson et al (1988). Under normal conditions, the carnitine concentrations in tissues other than brain are twenty- to fiftyfold those in plasma (Stanley, 1987). Therefore, the uptake of carnitine occurs across a large concentration gradient and is maintained by a transport system driven by a large sodium potential across the plasma membrane (Bremer, 1983; Rebouche and Mack, 1984). Since carnitine is not degraded in the body, the kidney is primarily responsible for regulating body stores of carnitine and is capable of adjusting to wide variations in dietary carnitine because it has a threshold of 40 μmol l^{-1}, identical to the normal serum concentration (Engel et al, 1981). Decreased renal reabsorption of carnitine was demonstrated in all six patients in whom this was measured (Table 5). Furthermore, the concentration of carnitine in muscle did not return to normal in any of the five children in whom a repeat muscle biopsy was performed after plasma carnitine was raised through oral administration (Table 6). This suggests that transport into muscle is also impaired in these cases. In agreement with this concept, muscle carnitine concentrations were below 5% of normal in all nine children biopsied and below 2% in six of them, indicating severe tissue depletion.

Carnitine uptake studies in fibroblasts from normal controls have suggested the presence of a high-affinity, low-concentration, specific, carrier-mediated transport process, and a second, high-concentration, low-affinity transport or passive diffusion process (Figure 3) (Treem et al, 1988; Eriksson et al, 1989; Tein et al, 1990). The values for apparent K_m and maximal rate of uptake from different laboratories have been in close agreement. Treem et al (1988) found a K_m of 3.24 ± 0.58 μmol l^{-1} and a maximal rate of uptake of 1.67 ± 0.19 pmol min^{-1} mg protein^{-1} and Tein et al (1990) have determined a K_m of 5.5 ± 0.58 μmol l^{-1} and a V_{max} of 3.4 ± 0.36 pmol min^{-1} mg protein^{-1}. Similar values have been obtained in fibroblasts of children with secondary carnitine deficiency due to defects in MCAD or LCAD (Treem et al, 1988). In contrast, fibroblasts from the patient of Treem et al (1988) and from the four patients of Tein et al (1990) showed minimal or no uptake throughout the entire range of physiological concentrations of carnitine (Figure 3). In the four cases of Tein et al (1990), the negligible carnitine uptake precluded calculation of K_m and V_{max} values. For example, at a carnitine concentration of 5 μmol l^{-1}, the mean rate of uptake in the four children was 2% of controls. The parents of the four children showed intermediate maximal rates of carnitine uptake, 13–44% of control V_{max} values, whereas K_m values were normal (Table 8) (Tein et al, 1990). Normal K_m and reduced V_{max} values suggest the presence of a decreased number of normally functioning carnitine receptors, but this remains to be proven. At very high concentrations of carnitine (10 mM), patients, parents and controls had the same rate of carnitine uptake, reflecting common low-affinity, high-concentration, non-specific diffusion uptake.

In these children, other clinically affected tissues could have been depleted of carnitine because of the low serum concentration which, in turn, was due to impaired renal conservation. However, it has been

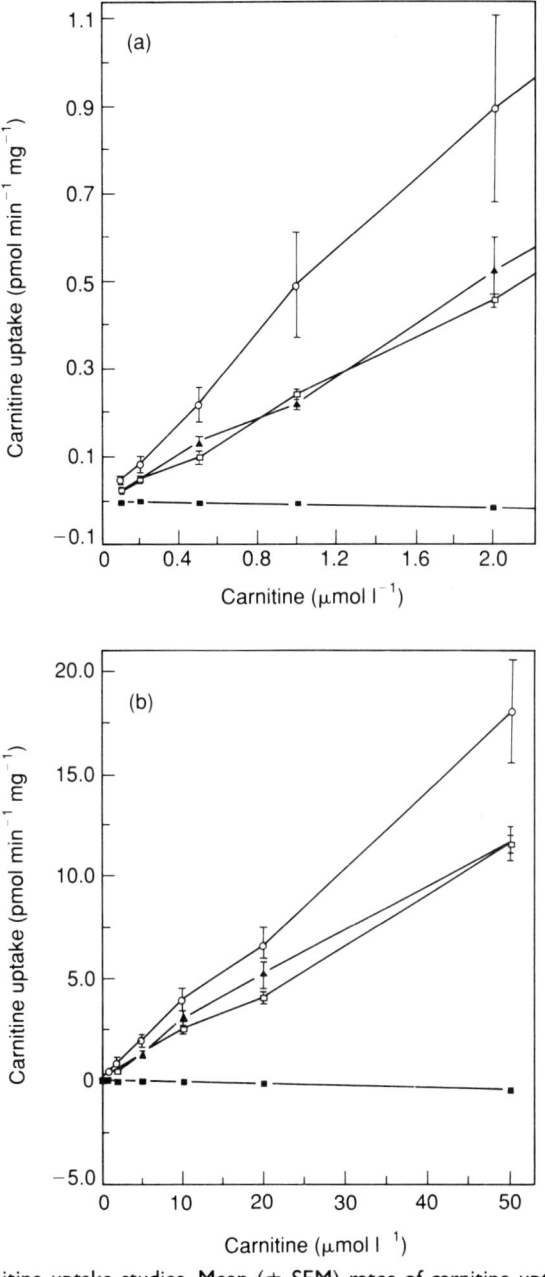

FIGURE 3. Carnitine uptake studies. Mean (± SEM) rates of carnitine uptake by cultured skin fibroblasts from case no. 1 (■) of Tein et al (1990), mother of case no. 1 (□), father of case no. 1 (▲) and six controls (○). The data represent two separate experiments (each performed in duplicate) in the patient and her parents and three to four separate experiments (each performed in duplicate) in each control. (a) Rates of uptake with extracellular carnitine concentrations ranging from 0.1 to 2.0 μmol l⁻¹. (b) Rates of uptake with extracellular carnitine concentrations ranging from 1.0 to 50 μmol l⁻¹. From Tein et al (1990), with permission of editor.

TABLE 8.

Carnitine uptake in cultured fibroblasts. From Tein et al (1990), with permission of editor

	K_m (10^{-6} mol l^{-1})		V_{max} Uptake (10^{-12} mol min^{-1} mg^{-1})		% Control V_{max}	
1. Normal controls (N = 6; 3F, 3M) (x ± SD)	5.5 ± 0.58		3.4 ± 0.36		100%	
2. Disease controls						
CPT deficiency	5.0		3.33		100%	
Methylmalonic acidaemia	5.0		1.67		50%	
Hyperinsulinism	6.6		3.00		88%	
Primary cardiomyopathy	6.6		2.00		59%	
3. Parents	Mother	Father	Mother	Father	Mother	Father
Case #1	5.0	5.0	1.33	1.33	40%	40%
Case #2	5.0	5.0	1.50	0.44	44%	13%
Case #3	5.8	5.8	1.33	0.75	40%	22%
Case #4	5.7	—	0.57	—	17%	—

CPT, carnitine palmitoyltransferase. x ± SD, mean ± standard deviation.

suggested that other tissues may share with fibroblasts the same defect in the specific plasma membrane carnitine transporter (Treem et al, 1988; Tein et al, 1990). This would better explain why carnitine concentrations failed to increase after carnitine replacement therapy. The therapeutic effect of carnitine administration may result from 'flooding' of the unaffected non-specific diffusion, low-affinity, high-concentration uptake mechanism, bypassing the specific carrier-mediated transporter.

In contrast to muscle, liver carnitine concentrations rose dramatically (from 5 to 400% and from 5 to 55% of normal, respectively) in two patients after oral supplementation (Chapoy et al, 1980; Treem et al, 1988). This suggested that the carnitine depletion in liver is due to low serum carnitine concentrations. Treem et al (1988) have proposed that their patient had a defect in a plasma membrane carnitine carrier shared by muscle, kidney, and fibroblasts but not by liver. Similar conclusions were suggested by case no. 2 of Tein et al (1990). It is unclear whether the severe cardiomyopathy is due to low serum carnitine or to a specific transporter defect, as no patient has had a repeat endocardial biopsy. Clarification of this issue could be provided by carnitine uptake studies in cultured skeletal muscle or heart cells from the patients. Circumstantial evidence that muscle, heart and fibroblasts may have a common or similar carnitine transporter arises from the observation that the K_m values for carnitine uptake in cultured human heart cells (4.8 ± 2.2 μM) (Bahl and Bressler, 1987) and muscle (1.90 ± 1.38 μM) (Rebouche and Engel, 1982) were similar to the K_m observed in cultured fibroblasts and very different from the K_m values found in human liver (500 μM) (Bieber, 1988) and brain (>1000 μM) (Bieber, 1988). This is an area that warrants further investigation.

GENETICS

Primary systemic carnitine deficiency has long been suspected to be inherited via an autosomal recessive gene. This has now been supported by the nearly equal sex distribution (six female, five male) in the 11 bona fide literature cases, by the history of affected siblings in eight cases, and by the fact that all parents were asymptomatic. Even more suggestive are the results of carnitine transport studies in skin fibroblasts from seven of the eight parents in the series of Tein et al (1990), showing V_{max} values in the heterozygote range (13–44% of control V_{max}) (Table 8). These data suggest that even a residual uptake of 13% is sufficient for normal function. Consanguinity has only been documented in one family and, as previously mentioned, the patients had diverse ethnic backgrounds. This would suggest that the defect is genetically widely distributed.

Compared with uptake studies, serum carnitine concentrations in the parents are not equally sensitive indicators of a decreased plasma membrane carnitine transporter. These have ranged from borderline-low to normal (Table 9) and do not correlate well with the results of uptake studies. For example, both parents of case no. 2 of Tein et al (1990) had low serum carnitine concentrations, but the father of case no. 1 had normal serum carnitine concentrations, despite a similarly decreased in vitro uptake. The variable serum concentrations probably reflect multiple factors, including dietary intake, biosynthetic capability and renal threshold. Thus, serum carnitine concentrations in the parents are a useful and simple screen, but in vitro cultured fibroblast uptake studies provide more definitive evidence of heterozygosity.

SUMMARY

Primary systemic carnitine deficiency is a specific entity characterized by carnitine-responsive cardiomyopathy with or without weakness,

TABLE 9.
Plasma carnitine concentrations in heterozygote parents

Reference	Plasma carnitine (total/free) (μmol l^{-1})		Controls (total/free) (μmol l^{-1})
	Mother	Father	
Chapoy et al (1980)	/ 24.6	/ 30.6	/34.95 ± 5.59
Tripp et al (1981)	38.7 / 28.0	39.9 / 29.3	35–75
Treem et al (1988)	20 / 15	38 / 35	37–58 / 28–47
Tein et al (1990)			
#1	35.7 / 27.8	60.9 / 54.7	51.5 ± 11.6 / 40 ± 9.5
#2	21 / 14	35 / 24	45 ± 6.5 / 34 ± 8.8

hypoglycaemic hypoketotic encephalopathy, failure to thrive, and anaemia with low plasma and tissue concentrations of carnitine, lipid storage in muscle, liver, nerve, and heart and severe renal leak of carnitine. Other associated features may include developmental delay, seizures, neuropathy, and smooth muscle disorders manifested by gastro-oesophageal reflux or recurrent abdominal pains. A rapid and dramatic improvement in cardiac function, strength, somatic growth, and a less marked improvement of the variegate anaemia follow the institution of oral carnitine supplementation despite incomplete restoration of tissue carnitine concentrations. Improvement of the dilatative and/or hypertrophic cardiomyopathy is particularly striking even within the first month of therapy. Exclusion of other defects in fatty acid oxidation is essential for the diagnosis of primary carnitine deficiency and is supported by the absence of an abnormal dicarboxylic aciduria characteristically seen in defects of fatty acid oxidation with secondary carnitine deficiency. The exquisite response to carnitine therapy and the severe decrease of carnitine in serum and various tissues also differentiate primary from secondary carnitine deficiency (Figure 4). The importance of accurate diagnosis of this potentially fatal entity lies in the eminently treatable nature of this disorder through lifelong oral carnitine supplementation.

The tissues most severely affected, namely muscle, heart, and liver, depend heavily on fatty acid oxidation. Carnitine depletion in liver may be due to the low serum carnitine secondary to impaired renal conservation, because liver carnitine returns to normal after replacement therapy. The lack of restoration of muscle carnitine with therapy suggests a specific transporter defect in muscle.

Studies of carnitine uptake in fibroblasts from affected children have demonstrated a defect in the specific, high-affinity, low-concentration, carrier-mediated uptake mechanism. Current evidence suggests that this defect is shared by muscle, kidney and fibroblasts, but not by liver. Whether the severe cardiomyopathy is due to low serum carnitine concentration or to a specific transporter defect awaits future investigation.

The equal sex distribution, history of affected siblings, and asymptomatic parents, and the finding of intermediate V_{max} values for carnitine transport in skin fibroblasts from parents, strongly suggest autosomal recessive inheritance.

Carnitine uptake studies in cultured skin fibroblasts are important for diagnosis and screening of siblings and heterozygote parents. Serum carnitine concentration in the parents are a useful and simple screen, but in vitro cultured fibroblast uptake studies provide more

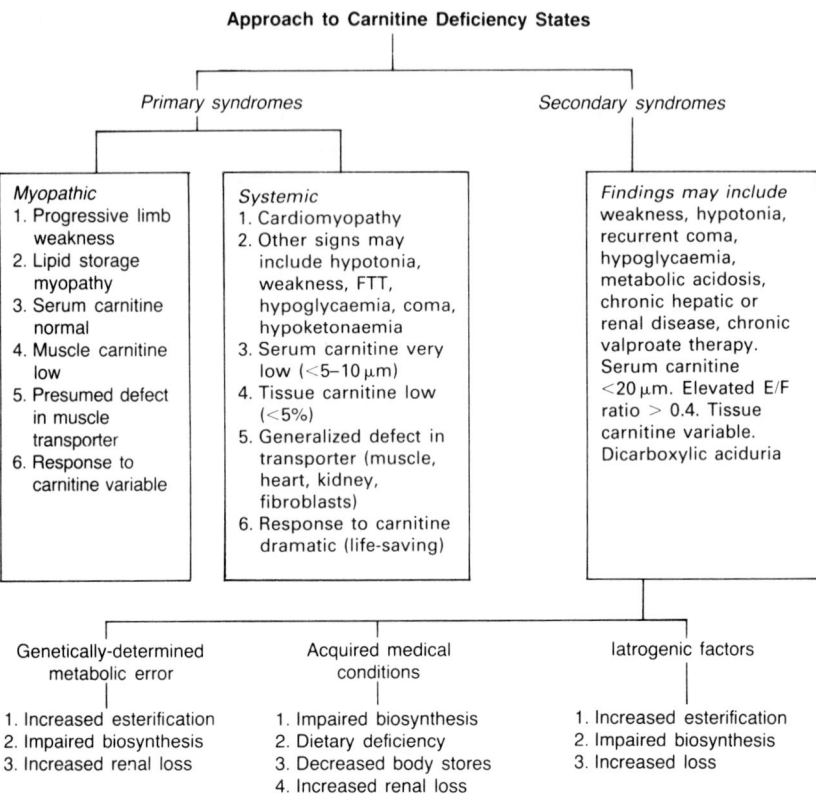

Approach to Carnitine Deficiency States

Primary syndromes   *Secondary syndromes*

Myopathic
1. Progressive limb weakness
2. Lipid storage myopathy
3. Serum carnitine normal
4. Muscle carnitine low
5. Presumed defect in muscle transporter
6. Response to carnitine variable

Systemic
1. Cardiomyopathy
2. Other signs may include hypotonia, weakness, FTT, hypoglycaemia, coma, hypoketonaemia
3. Serum carnitine very low (<5–10μm)
4. Tissue carnitine low ($<5\%$)
5. Generalized defect in transporter (muscle, heart, kidney, fibroblasts)
6. Response to carnitine dramatic (life-saving)

Findings may include weakness, hypotonia, recurrent coma, hypoglycaemia, metabolic acidosis, chronic hepatic or renal disease, chronic valproate therapy. Serum carnitine $<20 \mu$m. Elevated E/F ratio > 0.4. Tissue carnitine variable. Dicarboxylic aciduria

Genetically-determined metabolic error
1. Increased esterification
2. Impaired biosynthesis
3. Increased renal loss

Acquired medical conditions
1. Impaired biosynthesis
2. Dietary deficiency
3. Decreased body stores
4. Increased renal loss

Iatrogenic factors
1. Increased esterification
2. Impaired biosynthesis
3. Increased loss

FIGURE 4. An approach to the recognition of the primary and secondary disorders of carnitine metabolism. Certain clinical features are distinctive. The serum carnitine concentrations are normal in the myopathic form, markedly decreased in the systemic form and more variable in the secondary forms. Increased esterification and dicarboxylic aciduria are notable in the secondary forms. From De Vivo and Tein (1990), with permission of editor.

definitive evidence of heterozygosity. The finding of intermediate maximal rates of carnitine uptake but normal K_m values in the parents suggests that the heterozygotes have a reduced number of normal functioning carnitine transporters. Therefore these studies are also useful in understanding the pathogenesis and the molecular basis of this disease. Given the frequent history of previously unexplained sibling deaths in these families, the early identification of presymptomatic siblings with the institution of oral carnitine supplementation

(100–200 mg kg^{-1} day^{-1}) may decrease immediate and long-term morbidity and mortality.

Acknowledgements

Part of the work described here was supported by Center Grants from the National Institute of Neurological and Communicative Disorders and Stroke (NS 11766), the Muscular Dystrophy Association, the Colleen Giblin Foundation for Pediatric Neurological Research and by a generous donation from Libero and Graziella Danesi, Milano, Italy. Dr Tein was supported by a fellowship from the Muscular Dystrophy Association of America.

REFERENCES

Angelini C, Trevisan C, Isaya G et al (1987) *Clin. Biochem.* 20: 1–7.
Bahl JJ & Bressler R (1987) *Annu. Rev. Pharmacol. Toxicol.* 27: 257–277.
Barth PG, Scholte HR, Berden JA et al (1983) *J. Neurol. Sci.* 62: 327–355.
Bergmeyer HV (ed) (1974) *Methods of Enzymatic Analysis*, Volume 4, 2nd edition, pp 2290–2291. London: Academic Press.
Bieber LL (1988) *Annu. Rev. Biochem.* 57: 261–283.
Borum PR, York CM & Bennett SG (1985) *Am. J. Clin. Nutr.* 41: 653–656.
Bremer J (1977) *Trends in Biochemical Sciences* 2(3): 207–209.
Bremer J (1983) *Physiol. Rev.* 63: 1420–1480.
Chapoy PR, Angelini C, Brown WJ et al (1980) *N. Engl. J. Med.* 303(24): 1389–1394.
Coates PM, Hale DE & Stanley CA (1984) *J. Paediatr.* 105: 679.
Coates PM, Hale DM, Finocchiaro G et al (1988) *J. Clin. Invest.* 81: 171–175.
Cooper MB, Forte CA & Jones DA (1988) *Biochim. Biophys. Acta* 959: 100–105.
De Vivo & Tein (1990) *Int. Pediatr.* 5(2): 134–141.
DiMauro S (1979) In Vinken PJ & Bruyn GW (eds) *Handbook of Clinical Neurology, Vol. 41, Diseases of Muscle*, Part II, pp 175–234. New York: North Holland.
Elliot K & Jasper H (1959) Gamma-aminobutyric acid *Physiol. Rev.* 39: 383–406.
Engel AG & Angelini C (1973) *Science* 179: 899–902.
Engel AG, Rebouche CJ, Wilson DM et al (1981) *Neurology* 31: 819–825.
Eriksson BO, Lindstedt S & Nordin I (1988) *Eur. J. Pediatr.* 221: 662–663.
Eriksson BO, Gustafson B, Lindstedt S et al (1989) *J. Inher. Metab. Dis.* 12: 108–111.
Gilbert EF (1985) *Pathology* 17: 161–169.
Hale DE, Cruse RP & Engel A (1985) *Arch. Neurol.* 42: 1133.
Hannuniemi R & Kontro P (1988) *Neurochem. Res.* 13(4): 317–323.
Huth RJ, Schmidt MJ, Hall PV, Fariello RG & Shug AL (1981) *Journal of Neurochemistry* 36(2): 715–723.

Ino T, Sherwood WG, Cutz E et al (1988) *J. Pediatr.* 113(3): 511–514.
Mak IT, Kramer JH & Weglicki WB (1986) *J. Biol. Chem.* 261(3): 1153–1157.
Minshew NJ, Henderson AC & Pettegrew JW (1981) *Neurology* 31(2): 143.
Moroni T, Beralla T & Costa E (1979) In Krongfgaard P, Scheel-Kruger J, Larsen K & Kofod H (eds) *GABA Neurotransmitters,* pp 95–106. New York: Academic Press.
Neustein HB, Lurie PR, Dahms B et al (1979) *Pediatrics* 64(1): 24.
Rebouche CJ & Engel AG (1980) *Clin. Chim. Acta* 106: 295–300.
Rebouche CJ & Engel AG (1982) *In Vitro* 18(5): 495–500.
Rebouche CJ & Engel AG (1983) *Mayo Clin. Proc.* 58: 533–540.
Rebouche CJ & Engel AG (1984) *J. Clin. Invest.* 73: 857–867.
Rebouche CG & Mack DL (1984) *Arch. Biochem. Biophys.* 235: 393–402.
Scholte HR, Jennekens FGI & Bouvy JJBJ (1979) *J. Neurol. Sci.* 40: 39–51.
Shug AL, Hayes B, Thomsen JH et al (1980) In Frenkel R & McGarry JD (eds) *Carnitine Biosynthesis, Metabolism and Functions,* pp 321–340. New York: Academic Press.
Shug AL, Schmidt MJ, Golden GT et al (1982) *Life Sci.* 31: 2869–2874.
Siliprandi N, DiLisa F, Pivetta A et al (1987) *Z. Kardiol.* 5 (supplement): 34–40.
Stanley CA (1987) *Adv. Pediatr.* 34: 59–88.
Subramanian L, Plehn S, Noonan J et al (1987) *Z. Kardiol.* 76(5): 41–45.
Sugden PH & Newsholme EA (1977) *Comp. Biochem. Physiol.* 566: 89–94.
Tein I, De Vivo DC, Bierman F et al (1990) *Pediatr. Res.* 28(3): 247–255.
Tempesta E, Janiri L & Pirrongelli C (1985) *Neuropharmacology* 24(1): 43–50.
Treem WR, Stanley CA, Finegold DN et al (1988) *N. Engl. J. Med.* 319(20): 1331–1336.
Tripp ME, Katcher ML, Peters HA et al (1981) *N. Engl. J. Med.* 305(7): 385–390.
Turnbull DM, Bartlett K, Stevens DL et al (1984) *N. Engl. J. Med.* 311: 1232–1236.
Waber LJ, Valle K, Neill C et al (1982) *J. Pediatr.* 101(5): 700–705.
Wittels B & Hochstein P (1967) *J. Biol. Chem.* 242: 126–130.
Vacha G, Giorcelli G, Siliprandi N et al (1983) *Am. J. Clin. Nutr.* 38: 532–540.
Zoccarato F, Siliprandi N & Rugolo M (1983) *Biochim. Biophys. Acta* 734: 381–383.

Part IIc

Secondary deficiencies

10

DEFECTS OF
MITOCHONDRIAL
β-OXIDATION ENZYMES

M.J. Bennett and D.E. Hale

Inherited defects of intramitochondrial fatty acid β-oxidation enzymes are recent additions to the list of metabolic diseases. The first enzyme defect was that of medium-chain acyl CoA dehydrogenase (MCAD) deficiency. It was described by four groups in 1982–1983 (Kolvraa et al, 1982; Divry et al, 1983; Stanley et al, 1983; Rhead et al, 1983). This chapter reviews the central role of fats in fasting fuel homeostasis, describes the enzymes involved in this important metabolic pathway, compares and contrasts the clinical and laboratory features of the known β-oxidation enzyme defects, and discusses the secondary carnitine deficiency which is a common feature in all of the defects to date.

FUELS AND FASTING

To understand the consequences of a defect in an enzyme involved in β-oxidation, it is essential to recognize the central role that fatty

187

L-Carnitine and Its Role in Medicine:
From Function to Therapy. ISBN 0–12–253940–0

acids play in fasting adaptation. In the immediate post-prandial period, energy needs are primarily met by utilization of fuels absorbed from the gut (Figure 1a). Excess fuel is stored as glycogen or fat, and this process is primarily controlled by insulin. After about 2 hours, gut absorption is complete and endogenous fuel stores must be utilized for continued energy production. Initially, glycogen is the primary fuel. Endogenous muscle glycogen can be used by the muscle for

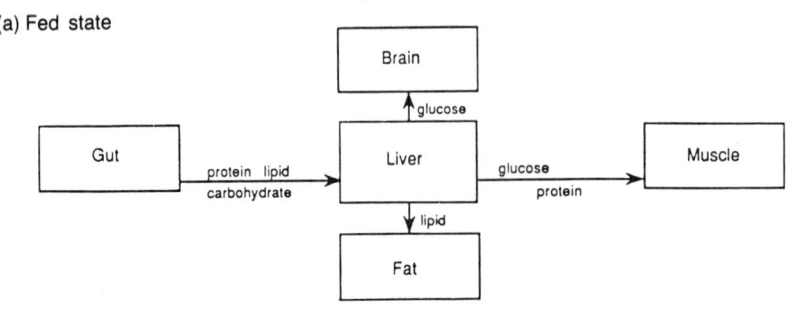

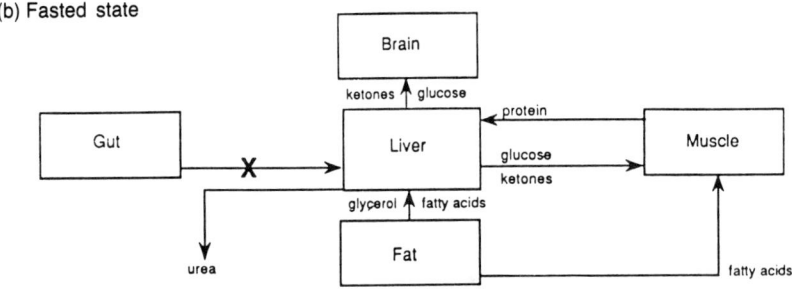

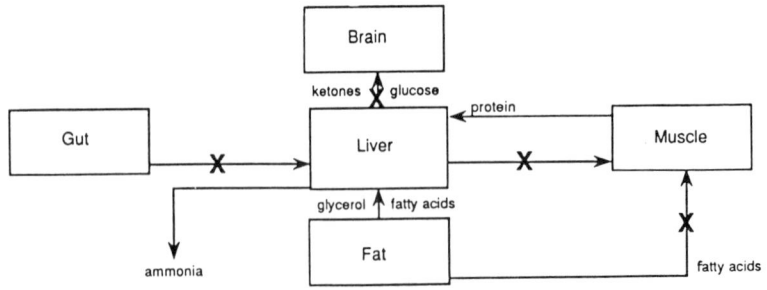

FIGURE 1. Energy substrate movements. X, metabolic block.

energy, but glucose cannot be exported because muscle lacks the requisite enzyme for glucose release, glucose-6-phosphatase. On the other hand, the liver can export glucose and serves as the primary supplier of fuels to glucose-dependent tissues, especially red blood cells and brain. Beyond 8–10 hours of fasting, glycogen reserves are depleted and alternative means of producing energy are activated including gluconeogenesis, fatty acid oxidation and ketogenesis.

The liver plays a central role in generating glucose from amino acids, lactate and glycerol. The breakdown of muscle protein results in the production of amino acids. These are transaminated within the muscle yielding alanine and glutamine which, in turn, are released and transported to the liver where they are the primary gluconeogenic precursors. Lactate resulting from the anaerobic metabolism of glucose is recycled via the gluconeogenic pathway. Glycerol, resulting from the release of fatty acid from triglyceride, is also utilized as a gluconeogenic precursor. Gluconeogenesis is an energy-requiring process and maximal rates of gluconeogenesis are only sustained if there is an abundant supply of intracellular ATP and NADH. In addition, the utilization of the carbon skeleton of the amino acid for gluconeogenesis results in increased production of ammonia and the consequent need for increased ureagenesis, another energy-requiring hepatic process.

As fasting is prolonged, fat is mobilized as an alternative fuel for those organs and tissues which can use fat, primarily muscle and heart. This significantly reduces the demand for glucose as well as preserving glucose for those tissues which have an absolute requirement for it (Figure 1b). Carnitine is a central requirement for the uptake of the predominantly long-chain fatty acids into mitochondria for β-oxidation and therefore any defect in carnitine availability has the potential for affecting the normal response to fasting. Fat is also utilized by the liver as the primary source of energy to drive both gluconeogenesis and ureagenesis. In addition, the end-product of fatty acid oxidation, acetyl CoA is the precursor for ketone body synthesis. Ketones are exported from the liver and are an important auxiliary fuel for many tissues, including the brain.

Thus, the overall scheme of fasting adaptation is the assurance of a constant supply of glucose for those organs which require it absolutely, the provision of an alternative fuel, fatty acids, for those tissues capable of utilizing it, and in certain tissues supplementation of both these fuels with ketones.

From this perspective, it is clear that individuals with disorders in the enzymes of fatty acid oxidation are likely to develop clinical symptomatology primarily when fasting. This symptomatology may reflect either inability to generate sufficient glucose (hypoglycaemia) or inability to utilize fat for energy by a specific tissue such as muscle or heart (Figure 1c). The onset of symptoms may occur with either decreased energy intake (fasting, intercurrent illness) or increased energy demand (vigorous exercise, concurrent viral illness). Infants and young children are at particular risk from these disorders for several reasons. First, basal energy needs in the infant are high due to the large surface area to mass ratio which necessitates significantly greater energy expenditure than older children or adults to maintain body temperature. Second, the infant brain is very large relative to infant mass and is highly dependent on glucose for its energy needs. Thus, there is a greater relative glucose requirement. Third, many of the enzymes involved in energy production from fat show developmental changes and, for instance, are at low levels in newborns relative to adult values (Hale, unpublished data); hence the infant's capacity to maintain fuel homeostasis is less efficient.

THE ENZYMES OF β-OXIDATION

The metabolic pathway and enzymes involved in the intramitochondrial β-oxidation of straight-chain fatty acids are shown in Figure 2. As described in detail in earlier chapters, long-chain fatty acids are transported through the inner mitochondrial membrane by the concerted actions of acyl CoA synthetase, carnitine palmitoyl transferase 1 and carnitine: acylcarnitine translocase. Carnitine palmitoyl transferase 2 which lies on the inner mitochondrial membrane serves to re-form acyl CoA, the activated substrate for β-oxidation. Medium-chain and short-chain fatty acids, which represent only a small proportion of the normally available fatty acids, pass through the inner mitochondrial membrane independently of this carnitine-requiring pathway (Beiber and Farrell, 1983; Bremer, 1983; Hoppel, 1990).

The first intramitochondrial step of the β-oxidation pathway involves the removal of two hydrogen atoms and the insertion of a double bond in the 2–3 position of the acyl CoA to form an enoyl CoA. The enzyme involved is acyl CoA dehydrogenase, an FAD-containing protein. In mammals, there are three acyl CoA dehydrogenases which have specificity for long-chain acyl CoAs (long-chain acyl-CoA dehydrogenase, LCAD), medium-chain acyl CoAs (medium-chain acyl CoA dehydrogenase, MCAD), and short-chain acyl CoAs (short-chain

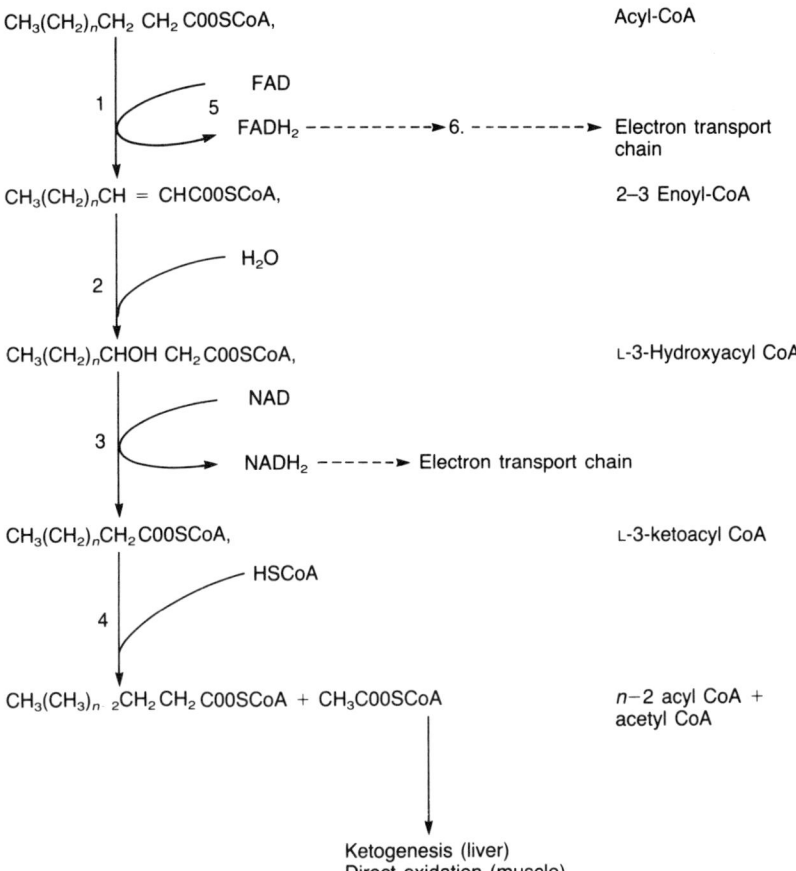

$$CH_3(CH_2)_nCH_2\,CH_2\,COOSCoA, \qquad\qquad\qquad Acyl\text{-}CoA$$

1, 5

FAD

$FADH_2$ ---------►6. --------► Electron transport chain

$$CH_3(CH_2)_nCH = CHCOOSCoA, \qquad\qquad\qquad 2\text{--}3\ Enoyl\text{-}CoA$$

2

H_2O

$$CH_3(CH_2)_nCHOH\,CH_2\,COOSCoA, \qquad\qquad\qquad L\text{-}3\text{-}Hydroxyacyl\ CoA$$

3

NAD

$NADH_2$ ------► Electron transport chain

$$CH_3(CH_2)_nCH_2\,COOSCoA, \qquad\qquad\qquad L\text{-}3\text{-}ketoacyl\ CoA$$

4

HSCoA

$$CH_3(CH_3)_{n\ 2}CH_2\,CH_2\,COOSCoA + CH_3COOSCoA \qquad\qquad n\text{--}2\ acyl\ CoA + acetyl\ CoA$$

Ketogenesis (liver)
Direct oxidation (muscle)

FIGURE 2. The enzymes of mitochondrial β-oxidation. 1, Acyl CoA dehydrogenase, 2, enoyl CoA hydratase, 3, L-3-hydroxyacyl CoA dehydrogenase; 4, L-3-ketoacyl CoA thiolase; 5, electron transfer flavoprotein; 6, electron transfer flavoprotein: coenzyme Q oxidoreductase.

acyl CoA dehydrogenase, SCAD) (Ikeda et al, 1985). The three enzymes are believed to operate sequentially as the initial long-chain acyl CoA is chain-shortened by the β-oxidation cycle. There is considerable overlapping chain-length specificity between MCAD and SCAD activity, at least when assayed in vitro (Hale et al, 1990a). Electrons are transferred from the acyl CoA to coenzyme Q in the respiratory chain through the action of FAD and two proteins, electron transfer flavoprotein (ETF), and electron transfer flavoprotein: coenzyme Q oxidoreductase (ETF:QO). ETF and ETF:QO are also electron acceptors for other mitochondrial acyl CoA dehydrogenases, including isovaleryl CoA dehydrogenase and glutaryl CoA dehydrogenase in the leucine and lysine degradation pathways, respectively (Frerman and Goodman, 1989).

The second reaction of the β-oxidation cycle involves the addition of water across the reduced 2–3 position of the enoyl CoA to produce an L-3-hydroxyacyl CoA. The enzyme involved is enoyl CoA hydratase. In mammals there are at least two hydratases, one specific for long-chain enoyl CoAs and the other for short-chain enoyl CoAs (Fong and Schulz, 1981). The short-chain-specific enzyme is also known as crotonase.

The third reaction reduces the L-3-hydroxyacyl CoA to form a 3-ketoacyl CoA compound. This is carried out by the NAD-requiring L-3-hydroxyacyl CoA dehydrogenase. There are at least two such enzymes in man, one mitochondrial matrix enzyme is specific for long-chain 3-hydroxyacyl-CoAs (LCHAD) and one soluble enzyme is specific for short-chain 3-hydroxyacyl CoAs (SCHAD) (El-Fakhri and Middleton, 1979). When assayed in vitro in cultured fibroblasts, there is considerable overlap in chain length specificities between LCHAD and SCHAD (Hale et al, 1990b).

The final step of the cycle involves the thiolytic cleavage of the 3-ketoacyl-CoA to form acetyl CoA and an acyl CoA species that has been chain-shortened by two carbons from the original acyl CoA. This re-enters the cycle until the fatty acid is converted entirely to acetyl CoA. The acetyl CoA is used to feed the tricarboxylic acid cycle in tissues such as skeletal muscle and is used for the generation of ketones by the liver through the 3-hydroxy-3-methyl-glutaryl-CoA pathway. There are at least two thiolase enzymes involved in mitochondrial β-oxidation of straight-chain fatty acids with long- and short-chain 3-ketoacyl CoA specificities (Middleton, 1975).

Two additional enzymes, an enoyl CoA isomerase and a dienoyl CoA reductase are required for the complete oxidation of unsaturated fatty acids, such as linoleic acid (Schulz and Kunau, 1987).

CLINICAL AND LABORATORY FEATURES OF DEFECTS OF β-OXIDATION ENZYMES

Since the initial enzyme description of MCAD deficiency in 1982 (Kolvraa et al, 1982) a total of five other intramitochondrial enzyme disorders have been well characterized. These include deficiencies of LCAD (Hale et al, 1985, 1990a), SCAD (Amendt et al, 1986; Coates et al, 1987), ETF and ETF:QO (Frerman and Goodman, 1985) and LCHAD (Wanders et al, 1989; Hale et al, 1990b; Duran et al, 1991). Of the remaining intramitochondrial enzymes there are individual case reports of SCHAD deficiency (Tein et al, 1991), and a patient who may have 2,4-dienoyl CoA reductase deficiency (Roe et al, 1990b). The other disorders including defects of the hydratase and thiolase steps of β-oxidation and the enoyl CoA isomerase of unsaturated fatty acid oxidation await characterization. Table 1 lists the known enzyme defects. MCAD deficiency appears to be the most prevalent of the fatty acid oxidation disorders, with greater than 100 cases in the literature. In caucasian populations of Northern European origin its frequency has been estimated to be of the order of 1 in 10 000 to 1 in 20 000 (Bennett et al, 1987; Blakemore et al, 1991). It is important to note that it is probably a rare disorder in other population groups. To date no patients with MCAD deficiency from Japanese or African American origin are known to the authors and only one Asian is known (in a family of closely-related parentage). The other enzyme disorders appear not to be related to specific ethnic groups.

All of the defects have in common certain specific clinical and laboratory findings including: acute metabolic decompensation associated with fasting, accumulation of fat in tissue, hypoketotic hypoglycaemia, deficiency of serum and tissue carnitine with altered degrees of

TABLE I.
Defects of intramitochondrial β-oxidation enzymes described to date

Enzyme	Cases in literature
Medium-chain acyl CoA dehydrogenase (MCAD)	100–200
Long-chain acyl CoA dehydrogenase (LCAD)	20
Short-chain acyl CoA dehydrogenase (SCAD)	3
Long-chain L-3 hydroxyacyl CoA dehydrogenase (LCHAD)	11
Electron transfer flavoprotein (ETF)	40
Electron transfer flavoprotein dehydrogenase (ETF:QO)	40
Short-chain L-3-hydroxy acyl CoA dehydrogenase (SCHAD)	2
2,4-Dienoyl CoA reductase	1

esterification of carnitine, and dicarboxylic aciduria associated with acute disease symptoms (Bennett, 1990). It is clear that a better understanding of the basic enzyme defects will allow us to understand the normal physiology and the pathophysiological mechanisms resulting in secondary carnitine deficiency. This chapter will now review the clinical features and biochemistry of the known enzyme defects in the β-oxidation pathway.

Shared clinical features of fatty acid oxidation disorders

Given the central role of fats in fuel homeostasis during fasting, it is not surprising that children with inborn errors of this pathway are most prone to clinically evident dysfunction during fasting; hence the children are more likely to be found comatose and unresponsive in the morning after an overnight fast. Factors which decrease oral intake such as intercurrent viral illness are likely to exacerbate this problem. A Reye-like syndrome has been reported in many affected children (Coates et al, 1985; Taubman et al, 1987). Similarly, increased energy expenditures such as fever or vigorous exercise may result in metabolic decompensation. Since there are clearly developmental aspects to fasting adaptation, younger children are more susceptible to clinical difficulties with fasting than are older children or adults. About 20% of children with known enzyme defects have originally been given the diagnosis of sudden infant death syndrome (SIDS) or 'near-miss' SIDS, and clearly any patient who dies suddenly and unexpectedly or who has an acute life-threatening event is at high risk of having one of those disorders (Howat et al, 1984, 1985; Duran et al, 1986; Harpey et al, 1986; Roe et al, 1986; Allison et al, 1988; Bennett et al, 1990a).

As fat is the primary source of fuel during prolonged fasting, a defect in this pathway has consequences for virtually all tissues. Tissues which normally use fat, including liver and muscle, cannot use this fuel effectively. Thus the tissue must obtain its energy from another source. Since ketones are not being produced, the only other source of fuel is glucose. Hence glucose cannot be reserved for those tissues which absolutely require it, such as brain. Since fat is mobilized during fasting and cannot be used by tissues for energy production, fats enter a variety of alternative pathways including storage as intracellular triglyceride, conjugation and excretion as carnitine esters (Roe et al, 1985, 1986, 1990; Schmidt-Sommerfeld et al, 1990) or glycine esters (Rinaldo et al, 1987, 1988, 1990; Bennett et al, 1990b) and excretion as dicarboxylic acids (Gregersen, 1985). Intracellular fatty acyl CoA compounds which accumulate secondary to fat dysmetabolism potentially interfere with many critical pathways, especially those which require CoA as a cofactor and may also interfere with transport systems including those which require carnitine as a cofactor. Any or all of these factors may result in multiple dysfunctions of fat-derived, energy-dependent tissues and result in both the accumulation of intracellular fat within these tissues and failure of energy-requiring pathways.

Table 2 lists the features that appear to be common to all of the intramitochondrial enzyme defects. Hypoketotic hypoglycaemia has been one of the more consistent features associated with the known fatty acid oxidation disorders, reflecting the central role of fats in fuel homeostasis and the accelerated rate of glucose utilization. Increased free fatty acids in the serum provide further evidence of impaired fat utilization and serve to rule out problems in fat mobilization such as hyperinsulinism. Acidosis has been found at the time of presentation in most affected children, though this has generally been less severe than the child's clinical condition would lead one to expect. In addition, lactic acidosis has been demonstrated in some individuals, perhaps reflecting poor perfusion of muscle or inhibition of critical enzymes by fatty acid intermediates.

Alterations in serum and tissue levels of carnitine have been associated with many defects in fatty acid and amino acid metabolism. All of the intramitochondrial fatty acid oxidation defects have demonstrated serum carnitine levels between 10 and 50% of normal. Tissue levels of carnitine have been more variable but are generally reduced. Tissue carnitine values have been far less frequently reported. In addition, regardless of the absolute amount of carnitine, all of the

TABLE 2.

Shared clinical pathological and biochemical features of β-oxidation enzyme defects

Clinical	Fasting intolerance
Pathological	Fat accumulation in tissues
Biochemical	Hypoglycaemia
	Hypoketonuria
	Serum fatty acid elevations
	Dicarboxylicaciduria
	(medium-chain with C_6, C_8, C_{10} dicarboxylic acids predominating)
	Secondary carnitine deficiency
	Increased esterified carnitine

NB When the patient is well the only features consistently present are the carnitine abnormalities.

children have had increased amounts of acylcarnitines and a consequent shift in the esterified/free carnitine ratio.

The presence of dicarboxylic acids, the microsomal ω-oxidation products of non-metabolized acyl CoAs, has been a consistent finding in the urine of affected children when they are unwell; however, these metabolic intermediates are not reliably present when the children are well or when the child has been receiving glucose intravenously. Figure 3 demonstrates a urine organic acid chromatogram from a patient with MCAD deficiency in a sample collected during the acute phase. Many abnormalities, including dicarboxylic aciduria can be easily seen. In contrast, Figure 4 shows a urine chromatogram collected from the same patient following restoration of euglycaemia and clinical recovery. This is clearly a normal profile. Since dicarboxylic acids are also seen when children are fed certain formulas (e.g. those containing MCT (medium-chain triglycerides oil), or have hormonal defects (e.g. diabetes mellitus), the amounts of these intermediates must be evaluated in relation to the quantity of ketones present. In the fatty acid oxidation disorders, the amount of dicarboxylic acids present in the acute sample usually significantly exceeds the amount of ketones. The presence of significant dicarboxylic acids tends to point toward an intramitochondrial enzyme defect and away from a fatty acid oxidation defect involving fatty acid or carnitine transport (e.g. CPT-1 deficiency, carnitine transport defects and carnitine: acylcarnitine translocase defects).

Unique features of specific enzymatic defects

In the course of delineating the defects in fatty acid oxidation, several clinical and laboratory features have been recognized which aid in distinguishing the various defects from each other. In some cases, these features may be unique and specific, though absolute certainty in this regard awaits the delineation of all potential defects in the fatty acid oxidation sequence. The differentiating clinical and biochemical features are described below and briefly summarized in Table 3.

As is clear from Table 3, careful analysis of organic acids in urine, acylglycine and acylcarnitines, provides the most helpful information in the localization of the site of defect. The elevated long-chain (C_{12}, C_{14}) dicarboxylic acids in LCAD deficiency remain to be fully evaluated, particularly in the well patient. MCAD deficiency is characterized by a number of markers some of which appear to be pathognomonic for instance, 3-phenylpropionylglycine, an unusual metabolite of the

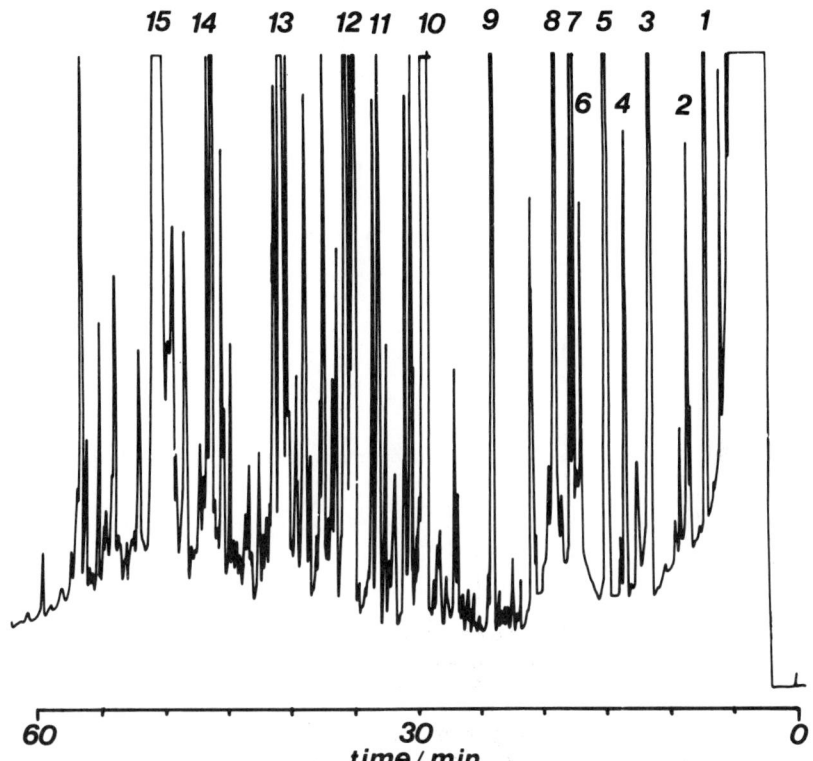

FIGURE 3. Organic acid chromatogram of urine from a 1-year-old patient with medium-chain acyl CoA dehydrogenase deficiency, collected on admission. Organic acids were extracted from salt-saturated, acidified urine into ethyl acetate and diethyl ether. After evaporating to dryness, trimethylsilyl derivatives were made and the mixture analysed by GC and GC/MS on a capillary column. The figure shows the flame ionization detector chromatogram after separation on a 50 m OV 101 column, temperature programmed from 70° C to 270° C at 4° C min^{-1}. The peak identities are: 1, lactate; 2, p-cresol; 3, 3-hydroxybutyrate; 4, acetoacetate (peak 1); 5, urea + acetoacetate (peak 2); 6, octanoate; 7, phosphate; 8, succinate; 9, 5-hydroxyhexanoate; 10, adipate; 11, hexanoylglycine; 12, unsaturated and saturated suberate; 13, unsaturated and saturated sebacate; 14, 3-hydroxy unsaturated and saturated sebacate; 15, suberylglycine and stearate (internal standard) in approximately equal amounts. Also identified but not shown were 3-phenylpropionylglycine and octanoylglucuronide. Reprinted with permission of the editors of *Annals of Clinical Biochemistry*.

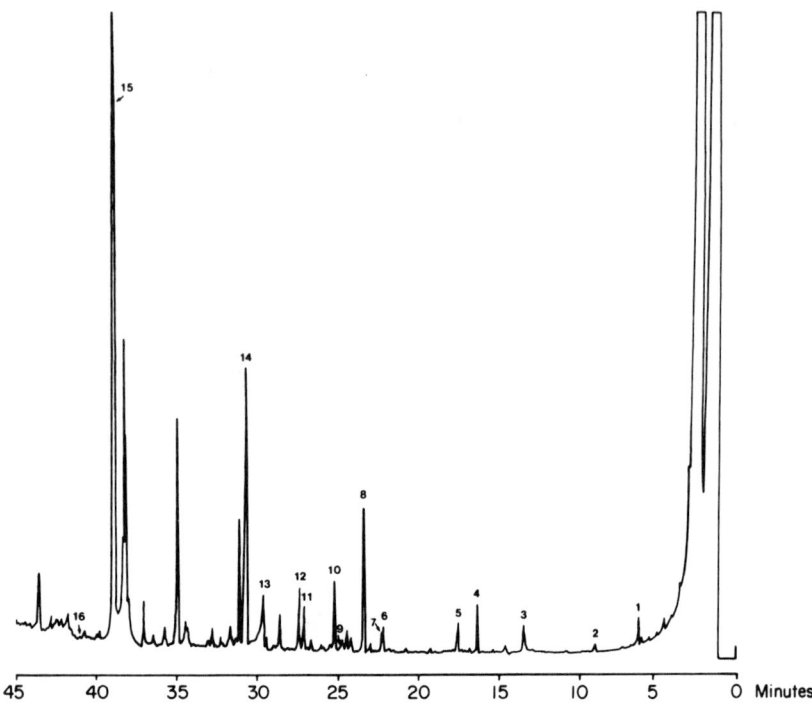

FIGURE 4. Organic acid chromatogram of urine from a 1-year-old patient with medium-chain acyl CoA dehydrogenase deficiency when well. The amount of urine extracted was identical to that in Figure 3. The urine was analysed on a 50 m BP 1 capillary column, using conditions similar to those described for Figure 3. Margaric acid (17:0) was added as internal standard in place of stearic acid (18:0) at the same concentration. The peak identities are: 1, lactate; 2, *p*-cresol; 3, 3-hydroxyisobutyrate (No 3-hydroxybutyrate); 4, urea: 5, phosphate; 6, malate; 7, adipate; 8, pyrogallol (solvent impurity); 9, hexanoylglycine + 3-hydroxy-3-methylglutarate; 10, *p*-hydroxyphenylacetate; 11, suberate; 12, aconitate; 13, hippurite; 14, citrate; 15, margarate (internal standard); 16, suberylglycine. Note the very small amounts of suberylglycine and hexanoylglycine whose presence can be confirmed only by mass spectrometry.
Reprinted with permission of the editors of *Annals of Clinical Biochemistry.*

bacterial product 3-phenylpropionic acid. This is normally metabolized to hippurate in man, following one cycle of β-oxidation and intramitochondrial glycine conjugation, and requires MCAD. 3-Phenylpropionylglycine excretion is a constant urinary finding in MCAD deficiency beyond infancy. Neonates apparently do not have the appropriate gut flora to produce 3-phenylpropionic acid (Bennett

TABLE 3.
Differentiation of known mitochondrial β-oxidation disorders

Enzyme defect	Unique clinical findings	Specific organic acid
LCAD	Cardiomyopathy, muscle weakness early age of onset for acute episodes	C12 and C14 dicarboxylic acids
MCAD	Onset variable; some patients asymptomatic; rare chronic problems	Phenylpropionyl glycine, hexanoylglycine, suberylglycine octanoylcarnitine
SCAD	Neuropathy, myopathy; few patients known	Ethylmalonic, methylsuccininic, butyrylglycine; butyrylcarnitine
LCHAD	Myopathy or cirrhosis as chronic problems; cirrhosis has bad prognosis	C8-C14-dicarboxylic acids
SCHAD	Only two patients reported; one with myopathy and the other in SIDS	Probably short-chain 3-OH intermediates
ETF	Neonatal hypoglycaemia and aciduria, odour of sweaty feet; chronic myopathy with episodic emapholopathy	Glutaric, 2-OH glutaric isovalerylglycine isobutyrylglycine, ethylmalonic acid, octanoyl; butyryl-isovaleryl- and glutarylcarnitine
ETF:QO	As above; renal cysts in some subjects in acute neonatal presentation	As above

and Hale, unpublished data). Octanoylcarnitine, particularly if a carnitine load is given, is another significant marker for MCAD deficiency. Butyrylglycine and butyrylcarnitine appear to be useful markers for SCAD deficiency, although presently too few patients have been evaluated. SCAD deficiency is the only β-oxidation enzyme defect in which an animal model, the Balb$c$/ byJ SCAD deficient mouse, is available for further study (Wood et al, 1990). LCHAD deficiency is characterized by the presence of medium (C_8)- to long (C_{14})-chain 3-hydroxydicarboxylic acids in urine and with 3-hydroxymonocarboxylic acids in blood. Caution must be taken, however, as many patients with 3-hydroxydicarboxylic aciduria do not have LCHAD deficiency. In a single case report and following a loading test of 3-phenylpropionic acid, 3-hydroxyphenylpropionic acid was reported in a patient with LCHAD deficiency (Wanders et al, 1989). This metabolite was presumably formed in a manner similar to the 3-phenylpropionylglycine formation in MCAD deficiency. The utility of 3-hydroxyphenylpropionic acid excretion clearly requires further evaluation.

Clinical differentiation of the various disorders is less satisfactory than biochemical differentiation based on metabolite analysis. However, certain clinical features are outstanding, including the chronic cardiomyopathy and myopathy in LCAD deficiency (Treem et al, 1991). Chronic myopathy also appears to be a feature of LCHAD deficiency (Hale et al, 1990b). LCHAD deficiency also has a clinical phenotype which includes a severe progressive liver damage which is frequently fatal. The mechanism for the liver damage is poorly understood as subjects with the same apparent enzyme defect do not all have this problem.

It should also be noted that MCAD deficiency may have a silent phenotype. A number of asymptomatic cases have been described in families where other individuals have had severe symptoms (Duran et al, 1986; Roe et al, 1986; Bennett et al, 1990c). These individuals were presumably spared the severe clinical consequences arising out of prolonged fasting in infancy.

Disorders affecting the electron transfer flavoprotein and its dehydrogenase, both referred to as glutaric aciduria type 2 may present as severe neonatal hypoglycaemia with the associated odour of 'sweaty feet'. Some of these cases may also present with dysmorphology, in particular with the presence of polycystic kidneys (Frerman and Goodman, 1989). Molecular analysis of ETF and ETF:QO is likely to provide an explanation of these findings. The defects in short-chain fatty acid oxidation have been poorly characterized, primarily because of the very few cases identified to date. There are only three documented cases of systemic SCAD deficiency for which there may be neuropathy and/or myopathy, and only two cases of SCHAD deficiency are known to the authors. One appears to be liver-specific (Hale and Bennett, unpublished data) in a patient with SIDS, the other appears to be muscle-specific (Tein et al, 1991) raising the possibility of tissue specificity of some of the enzymes of fatty acid oxidation. The appropriate studies to confirm tissue specificity are awaited.

DIAGNOSTIC APPROACHES AND SCREENING TOOLS

Approach to the investigation of the individual patient

The first line of investigation for the individual patient requires documentation of a failure to adapt satisfactorily to prolonged fasting. If this evidence is available and the child is well, analysis of urine for the characteristic metabolites to suggest ETF or ETF:QO deficiencies and for the specific carnitine and glycine conjugates associated with the MCAD and SCAD deficiencies is probably the easiest approach and the one likely to have the highest yield. Presently, and as discussed earlier there are no defined urinary abnormalities for well patients with LCAD deficiency and the L-3-hydroxydicarboxylic acids present in acute samples collected from patients with LCHAD deficiency have not been fully evaluated in well LCHAD-deficient patients.

Direct measurement of the serum total and free carnitine concentration is the next important step, since almost all of the patients identified to date have reductions in the amount of carnitine present and alterations in the degree of esterification even when they are well. The two potential exceptions to this rule are the very young child (less than 4 months of age) who is not yet carnitine-depleted and individuals with the CPT-1 deficiency where the total serum carnitine concentration may be in the high normal range.

Because dicarboxylic acids are byproducts of reduced fatty acid oxidation, they generally disappear from the circulation quickly once normoglycaemia is restored and fat mobilization ceases. For this reason, it is essential to collect urine for dicarboxylic acid analysis during an acute episode. If urine or plasma is recoverable from an acute episode, questions related to the integrity of biochemical pathways can be asked. If acute samples are not available then a specific fasting test should be undertaken in a very carefully controlled situation. The focus of the fasting test is to establish the probable site of defect based on the analysis of temporal changes in both substrates (glucose, free fatty acids, lactate) relevant hormones (growth hormone, cortisol, insulin) and metabolites (ketones, dicarboxylic acids). Children must be fasted to the point that they are significantly symptomatic or have a blood glucose level below 50 mg% (2–7 mmol l^{-1}). At this point, a significant dicarboxylic aciduria in the absence of a good ketotic response provides strongly presumptive studies which must be further guided by the organic acid, acylglycine and acylcarnitine analysis. The absence of dicarboxylic acids appear to point toward a defect involving the transport of fat into the mitochondria (carnitine uptake defect, translocase deficiency). The presence of predominantly long-chain intermediates suggests a defect of one of the enzymes involved with long-chain fatty acid oxidation, while the presence of short-chain intermediates points toward a defect in short-chain fatty acid oxidation. Unique localization of the site of defect, for example, the presence of 3-phenylpropionylglycine and octanoylcarnitine appears to be very specific for MCAD deficiency.

Since clinically useful molecular probes are only available for the MCAD deficiency (see below), specific enzymatic analysis for other enzymes must be undertaken. In most cases, these studies can be performed using cultured skin fibroblasts, although the question of whether or not some of the enzymes have tissue-specific isoforms remains to be answered.

Investigators should be aware that most 'standard metabolic screens' are not designed to identify inborn errors in fatty acid oxidation, particularly if samples are not obtained in the acute situation.

Population-based approaches

The association between inherited defects in fatty acid oxidation and sudden infant death syndrome has been well-established. Among more than 100 children now recognized to have enzyme-confirmed MCAD deficiency, almost 20% were originally given the diagnosis of SIDS or 'near miss' SIDS. In addition, more than 20 siblings of affected individuals have died unexpectedly, with the most common diagnosis being SIDS. Cases of children with each of the other recognized deficiencies initially diagnosed as SIDS have also been reported. Screening strategies for high-risk population rather than the entire newborn population is considerably easier to accomplish, primarily because of the smaller number of individuals involved. Whereas it is relatively easy to investigate individuals in a population such as SIDS there are many more practical problems, including the non-availability of urine. Direct enzymatic assay of all of the β-oxidation enzymes is not practical; several other approaches have therefore been advocated, including organic acid analysis of blood or vitreous humour, carnitine determination in tissue, or fat-specific staining of tissues. An increased incidence of fatty infiltration of liver has been documented in a prospectively gathered series of SIDS infants compared with controls. Carnitine measurements in post mortem tissues and organic acid analysis in other body fluids has not yet been reported.

Screening of a newborn population in a systematic fashion has not been undertaken, but may be justified for selected groups of individuals. As with the SIDS population, it is unclear as to the optimum method to use in the analysis. Several approaches to screening have been advocated including analysis of urine or newborn filter spot blood cards for specific metabolites, and most recently, molecular probes for one of the defects, the MCAD deficiency. To date approximately 90% of MCAD alleles investigated in MCAD deficient patients present with a single common mutation. An A to G nucleotide transition at position 985 in the cDNA results in a lysine to glutamate substitution at amino acid position 304 of the mature MCAD protein (Kelly et al, 1990; Matsubara et al, 1990; Yokota et al, 1990). This finding raises the possibility of a common ancestral heritage for this mutation and probably explains the high prevalence of MCAD deficiency in a single ethnic group. It also presents a strategy for population analysis. One study has been undertaken using the specific molecular probes for this common mutation leading to the MCAD deficiency. This study which looked at 456 consecutive neonatal blood spot cards in a northern English population, did not identify a homozygous affected patient but did demonstrate the carrier state for that single mutation to be about 1 in 68 (Blakemore et al, 1991). This data is in agreement with earlier metabolic data suggesting a common disorder in this population (Bennett et al, 1987). Population studies of other ethnic groups for this mutation are awaited.

TREATMENT

Once a diagnosis of a fatty acid oxidation is confirmed, the mainstay of treatment is the avoidance of prolonged fasting. The ability to fast is dependent on the age of the child, but generally should not exceed 12 h in affected children under 4 years of age. In the event of acute metabolic decompensation, intravenous glucose should be administered at rates sufficient to prevent fatty acid mobilization (8–10 mg kg^{-1} min^{-1}, usually 10% dextrose at 1 to $1\frac{1}{2}$ times maintenance rates) until the child is able to take oral feeds.

In patients with defects involving long-chain fatty acid oxidation, the use of MCT oil as a nutritional source of fat may be a useful adjunct as, theoretically, it bypasses the defect.

Uncooked corn starch, in doses similar to that used in the treatment of glycogen storage disease (2 g kg body weight^{-1} per dose), may be a useful way of prolonging the post-absorptive state and delaying the onset of fasting adaptation. This may be especially helpful in the older child who is exercising vigorously or in subjects with low fasting tolerance.

Riboflavin has been reported to be a useful adjunct to therapy in some patients with defects in the acyl CoA dehydrogenase step of the β-oxidation pathway. In at least one patient with a short-chain defect and ethylmalonic adipic aciduria, there was dramatic clinical improvement and resolution of the organic acid abnormalities while the patient was on riboflavin at a dose of 200–300 mg per day (Green et al, 1985). There are several less well-documented reports of clinical improvement in response to riboflavin. This response is thought to be related to a role for riboflavin in stabilizing a mutant acyl CoA dehydrogenase, or ETF.

Carnitine supplementation (50–100 mg kg^{-1}) has been tried in a number of the known fatty acid oxidation defects with variable results. Because of the increased capability of carnitine esters to cross cellular membranes, it is believed that carnitine serves to remove potentially toxic acyl intermediates from within the cell. In addition, the removal of the acyl groups releases CoA, a critical intracellular cofactor. In the case of children with the carnitine transport defect, normalization of carnitine levels has been accompanied by normalization of cardiac function and complete resolution of clinical disease (Stanley et al, 1990). In children with other fatty acid oxidation disorders, the provision of carnitine leads to increased excretion of esterified intermediates but clinical response has been difficult to judge, as the children appear normal between clinical attacks. Whether carnitine supplementation results in decreased clinical problems remains to be shown.

Because of the small numbers of patients with specific defects available at any one institution, it has not been possible to systematically evaluate any single treatment regimen or compare various treatments. The current approach to treatment continues to be avoidance of prolonged fasting and the benefits of carnitine, MCT or riboflavin supplementation must be judged on a case-by-case basis until objective parameters are established and careful clinical studies are undertaken.

REFERENCES

Allison F, Bennett MJ, Variend S & Engel PC (1988) *Br. Med. J.* 299: 1771–1773.
Amendt, BA, Greene C, Sweetman L et al (1986) *J. Clin. Invest.* 79: 1303–1309.
Beiber LL & Farrell S (1983). In Boyer PD (ed.) *The Enzymes*, 3rd edn, pp. 627–644. New York: Academic Press.
Bennett MJ (1990) *Ann. Clin. Biochem.* 27: 519–531.
Bennett MJ, Worthy E & Pollitt RJ (1987) *J. Inher. Metab. Dis.* 10: 241–242.
Bennett MJ, Allison F, Pollitt RJ & Variend S (1990a) In Tanaka K & Coates PM (eds) *Fatty Acid Oxidation. Clinical, Biochemical and Molecular Aspects* pp. 349–364. New York: Alan R. Liss.
Bennett MJ, Coates PM, Hale DE et al (1990b) *J. Inher. Metab. Dis.* 13: 5707–5715.
Bennett MJ, Pollitt RJ, Taitz LS & Variend S (1990c) *Clin. Chem.* 36: 1695–1697.
Bremer J (1983) *Physiol. Rev.* 63: 1420–1480.
Blakemore A, Singleton H, Pollitt RJ et al (1991) *Lancet* i: 298–299.
Coates PM, Hale DE, Stanley CA et al (1985) *Pediatr. Res.* 19: 671–676.
Coates PM, Hale DE, Finnocchiaro G et al (1987) *J. Clin. Invest.* 81: 171–175.
Divry P, David M, Gregersen N et al (1983) *Acta Paediatr. Scand.* 72: 943–949.
Duran M, Holkamp M, Rhead WJ et al (1986) *Pediatrics* 78: 1052–1057.
Duran M, Wanders RJA, de Jager et al (1991) *Eur. J. Pediatr.* 150: 190–195.
Editorial (1988) *Lancet* ii: 1073–1075.
El-Fakhri M & Middleton B (1979) *Biochem. Soc. Trans.* 7: 392–393.
Fong JC & Schulz H (1981) *Methods Enzymol.* 71: 390–398.
Frerman FE & Goodman SI (1985) *Proc. Natl Acad. Sci. USA* 82: 4517.
Frerman FE & Goodman SI (1989) In Scriver CR, Beaudet AL, Sly WS & Valle D (eds) *The Metabolic Basis of Inherited Disease*, 6th edn, pp 915–931. New York: McGraw-Hill.
Green A, Marshall TG, Bennett MJ et al (1985). *J. Inher. Metab. Dis.* 8: 67–71.
Gregersen N (1985) *Scand. J. Clin. Lab. Invest.* 45 (supplement 174): 1–60.
Hale DE, Batshaw ML, Coates PM et al (1985) *Pediatr. Res.* 19: 665–671.
Hale DE, Stanley CA & Coates PM (1990a) In Tanaka K & Coates PM (eds) *Fatty Acid Oxidation. Clinical, Biochemical and Molecular Aspects* pp 303–311. New York: Alan R. Liss.
Hale DE, Thorpe C, Braat K et al (1990b) In Tanaka K & Coates PM (eds) *Fatty Acid Oxidation. Clinical, Biochemical and Molecular Aspects* pp 503–510. New York, Alan R. Liss.
Harpey J-P, Charpentier C & Paterneau-Jouas M (1986) *Lancet* ii: 1332.
Harpey J-P, Charpentier C & Paterneau-Jouas M (1987) *J. Pediatr.* 110: 881–884.
Hoppel CL (1990) In Tanaka K & Coates PM (eds) *Fatty Acid Oxidation. Clinical, Biochemical and Molecular Aspects* pp 435–450. New York, Alan R. Liss.
Howat AJ, Bennett MJ, Shaw L & Variend S (1984) *Br. Med. J.* 288: 976.
Howat AJ, Bennett MJ, Variend S et al (1985) *Br. Med. J.* 290: 1771–1773.
Ikeda Y, Okamura-Ikeda K & Tanaka K (1985) *J. Biol. Chem.* 260: 1311–1325.
Kelly DP, Whelan AJ, Odgen ML et al (1990) *Proc. Natl Acad. Sci. USA* 87: 9236–9240.
Kolvraa S, Gregersen N, Christensen E & Holbolth N (1982) *Clin. Chim. Acta* 126: 53–67.
Matsubara Y, Narisawa K, Miyabayashi S et al (1990) *Lancet* i: 1598.
Middleton B (1975) *Methods Enzymol.* 35: 128–136.

Rhead WJ, Amendt BA, Fritchman KS & Felts SJ (1983) *Science* 221: 73–75.

Rinaldo P, O'Shea JJ & Tanaka K (1987) *Lancet* ii: 1158.

Rinaldo P, O'Shea JJ, Coates PM et al (1988) *N. Engl. J. Med.* 319: 1308–1313.

Rinaldo P, O'Shea JJ, Welch RD & Tanaka K (1990) In Tanaka K, Coates, PM (eds) *Fatty Acid Oxidation. Clinical, Biochemical and Molecular Aspects* pp 411–418. New York: Alan R. Liss.

Roe CR, Millington DS, Maltby DA et al (1985) *Pediatr. Res.* 19: 459–466.

Roe CR, Millington DS, Maltby DA & Kinnebrew P (1986) *J. Pediatr.* 108: 13–18.

Roe CR, Millington DS, Kahler SG et al (1990a) In Tanaka K & Coates PM (eds) *Fatty Acid Oxidation: Clinical Biochemical, and Molecular Aspects* pp 383–402. New York: Alan R. Liss.

Roe CR, Millington DS, Norwood DL et al (1990b) *J. Clin. Invest.* 85: 1703–1704.

Schmidt-Sommerfeld E, Penn D, Kerner J & Beiber LL (1990) In Tanaka K & Coates PM (eds) *Fatty Acid Oxidation; Clinical, Biochemical and Molecular Aspects* pp 403–409. New York: Alan R. Liss.

Schulz H & Kunau W-H (1987) *Trends Biochem Sci.* 12: 403–406.

Stanley CA, Hale DE, Coates, PM et al (1983) *Pediatr. Res.* 17: 877–894.

Stanley CA, Treem WR, Hale DE & Coates PM (1990) In Tanaka K & Coates PM (eds) *Fatty Acid Oxidation: Clinical Biochemical and Molecular Aspects* pp 457–464. New York: Alan R. Liss.

Tein I, DeVivo DC, Hale DE et al (1991) *Ann. Neurol.* (in press).

Taubman B, Hale DE & Kelley RI (1987) *Pediatrics* 79: 382–385.

Treem W, Stanley CA, Hale DE et al (1991) *Pediatr.* 87: 328–333.

Wanders RJA, Duran M, Ijlst L et al (1989) *Lancet* ii: 52–53.

Wood PA, Amendt BA, Rhead WJ et al (1990) In Tanaka K & Coates PM (eds) *Fatty Acid Oxidation: Clinical, Biochemical and Molecular Aspects* pp 427–454. New York: Alan R. Liss.

Yokoto I, Indo Y, Coates PM & Tanaka K (1990) *J. Clin. Invest.* 86: 1000–1003.

Part IId

Other considerations

11

CARNITINE DEFICIENCY IN PAEDIATRICS: EXPERIENCE AT VALLEY CHILDREN'S HOSPITAL, FRESNO, CALIFORNIA

Susan C. Winter, W. Hugh Vance,
Elinor M. Zorn, Carol K. Vance,
Kenneth Jue, Grzegorz Opala,
Lawrence Linn, Anne Szabo,
Howard Winter and Maria Bakas

INTRODUCTION TO INVESTIGATIONS

In September 1983 we began to use L-carnitine for treatment of carnitine deficiency at Valley Children's Hospital in Fresno, California. Since that time, we have treated over 700 patients for carnitine-related

L-Carnitine and Its Role in Medicine:
From Function to Therapy. ISBN 0–12–253940–0

problems and have expanded our knowledge and understanding of the uses for this natural substance in treating a variety of paediatric disorders.

Our first patient was a newborn male infant with methylmalonic aciduria due to deficient activity of the apoenzyme, methylmalonyl CoA mutase. In 1983, the reported prognosis for this disorder was death or severe neurological dysfunction (Matsui et al, 1983). Conventional dietary therapy was begun and for the first 5 months of life his general health was good with adequate weight gain; only a few episodes of acidosis required hospitalization and other milestones were normal. However, over the next 4 months, he rapidly deteriorated with severe bouts of acidosis, chronic neutropenia with resultant infections, failure to thrive, muscle-wasting, hypotonia, and developmental delay. The change in clinical status seemed inexplicable simply on the basis of his enzymatic deficiency since he had done so well in the first 5 months of life. Therefore, we reasoned that a secondary problem must be leading to his deterioration.

Our search for the reason for this deterioration led to carnitine after a colleague reported he had heard of a case of carnitine deficiency in a child with isovaleric aciduria. Virtually nothing was reported about L-carnitine for the treatment of organic acidurias. Plasma carnitine levels on our patient showed a severe deficiency of both total and free carnitine and elevated carnitine esters.

At 9 months of age, the patient began therapy with L-carnitine (Sigma Tau Pharmaceuticals) at the dose of 50 mg kg^{-1} day^{-1}. His clinical status improved slightly but his plasma carnitine concentrations remained deficient. When he reached a carnitine dose of 200 mg kg^{-1} day^{-1}, a sudden improvement in activity level, infection frequency, weight, hypotonia and developmental delays was noted. The rest of his therapy had remained unchanged and the only explanation appeared to be the addition of L-carnitine therapy.

This sudden improvement was difficult to ignore and raised many significant questions in our minds concerning the clinical implications of carnitine deficiency states. Reviewing 34 cases reported in the literature between 1975 and 1984, we found carnitine deficiency described as a primary disorder due to the genetic deficiency of carnitine biosynthetic enzymes. This implied our patient should have two genetic disorders, methylmalonyl CoA mutase deficiency and deficiency of a carnitine synthetic enzyme. This seemed possible but unlikely. To add to our confusion, we determined carnitine levels in other patients with metabolic disorders and found several more to be carnitine-deficient. Given the exceedingly low incidence of primary carnitine deficiency, it did not seem reasonable that our hospital would have such a large number of children with carnitine synthetic defects.

The signs and symptoms of carnitine deficiency reported in literature case reports were similar to those found in our initial patients: progressive muscle weakness with a lipid storage myopathy, acute encephalopathy, hepatic dysfunction, cardiomyopathy, and non-ketotic hypoglycaemia. Of 34 patients described, 30 were of children and there was a 30% mortality rate (Karpati et al, 1975; Cornelio et al, 1979; Scholte et al, 1979; Chapoy et al, 1980; Glasgow et al, 1980; Tripp et al, 1981; Waber et al, 1982; Rebouche and Engel, 1983; Slonim et al, 1983; Cannon 1984; DiDonnato et al, 1984; Roe et al, 1984.)

By September 1986, we had treated 51 patients with carnitine deficiency and submitted our first publication describing the clinical syndrome of plasma carnitine deficiency (Winter et al, 1987). We had decided that our patients did not have a genetic defect of carnitine synthesis (primary carnitine deficiency) but rather that another cause had led secondarily to the carnitine deficiency. We decided that the causes of secondary carnitine deficiency must be numerous and be due to several possible mechanisms: decreased intake of carnitine in the diet (especially in the young infant), decreased stores of maternal carnitine either due to maternal carnitine deficiency or prematurity, malabsorption of carnitine associated with severe diarrhoea or cystic fibrosis, decreased synthesis of carnitine secondary to an inborn error of metabolism limiting substrate for synthesis, decreased renal reabsorption of carnitine, and increased loss of carnitine in the ester form as seen in organic acidurias and during valproic acid therapy.

These patients shared signs and symptoms similar to those reported in the literature: muscle weakness (40/51), cardiomyopathy (10/51), encephalopathy (9/51), non-ketotic hypoglycaemia (8/51), frequent infections (33/51) and failure-to-thrive (33/51). We reported improvement of symptoms on carnitine therapy including all patients with cardiomyopathy resolving their cardiac dysfunction, and nearly one half of the patients with failure to thrive gaining weight. No patients had a recurrence of their hypoglycaemia or encephalopathy on therapy and infection frequency decreased.

As we identified and treated more and more patients with carnitine deficiency, our interest and that of others, focused on what specific disorders and symptoms appeared to respond to L-carnitine therapy. Certainly, we had a large number of patients with inborn errors of metabolism and the patients were easier to manage, and experienced less episodes of metabolic decompensation, on carnitine therapy. The most dramatic improvements were in muscle strength and tone, and in growth. These patients, like our first patient, required larger doses of L-carnitine to restore carnitine concentrations to normal. They also had persistently raised concentrations of plasma carnitine esters, reflecting the role of carnitine in removing the specific organic acids that accumulated due to the metabolic disorder (DiDonato, 1984a; Roe, et al, 1984).

Another group of patients were being treated with valproic acid for seizure disorders. Valproic acid therapy had been reported to cause hyperammonaemia which resolved on initiating carnitine therapy (Ohtani et al, 1982: Stumpf et al, 1983; Coulter, 1984; Laub et al, 1986; Matsuda et al, 1986). A specific acylcarnitine species, valproyl carnitine was identified in the urine of patients on valproic acid therapy (Millington et al, 1985).

The third group of patients were affected with cardiomyopathy. There are many reports of carnitine deficiency being associated with cardiomyopathy, with suggestions of a cause–effect relationship in some instances. A few reported cases of dramatic clinical improvement prompted us to investigate this treatment with our cardiomyopathy patients (Tripp and Shug, 1981; Waber, 1982; Kudo et al, 1983; Tripp et al, 1984; Ino et al, 1988).

In recent years, the role L-carnitine plays in the modulation of the mitochondrial acyl CoA to free CoA ratio has been delineated. It is the removal of acylcarnitine derivatives from the mitochondria and their excretion in the urine that leads to the improvement in patients with organic acidopathies, fatty acid oxidation defects and mitochondrial defects. In such disorders, the absolute value of free carnitine may not truly reflect sufficiency of carnitine to meet the metabolic demand. Therefore, the ratio of esterified to free carnitine (E/F) appears to be the best indicator of altered carnitine states (Coates and Roe, 1989).

Serious clinical consequences can result from metabolic conditions that produce an increase of acyl CoA derivatives in the mitochondria and an alteration of the acyl CoA to free CoA ratio where the production of free CoA is decreased. This increased ratio can result in decreased fatty acid metabolism, decreased gluconeogenesis, decreased pyruvate metabolism with lactate accumulation and decreased production of adenosine triphosphate due to the secondary effects on many mitochondrial pathways. Since fatty acid metabolism is the primary energy source for cardiac and skeletal muscle and is a necessary energy source during fasting and stress, a decrease in fat metabolism can result in a variety of clinical signs and symptoms. These are similar to those described in patients with carnitine deficiency including: muscle weakness and hypotonia, failure-to-thrive, cardiomyopathy, hepatic dysfunction and encephalopathy (Coates and Roe, 1989).

OVERALL CASE EXPERIENCE:

Of more than 700 patients treated with L-carnitine between September 1983 and October 1990, a cohort of 612 patients were identified. Criteria for inclusion in this cohort were a free carnitine concentration having been taken prior to therapy, and the inclusion of L-carnitine in therapy. A retrospective evaluation and abstraction of the medical records was conducted in order to assess the reason for carnitine therapy, the signs and symptoms of the carnitine-related disorder and response to therapy. Patients were assessed as being carnitine-deficient if their plasma carnitine concentration was ≤ 20 μmol l^{-1} and carnitine insufficient if their plasma E/F ratio was 0.4 or greater. Occasionally, tissue carnitine concentrations were available and deficiency was identified if the free carnitine level was lower than 2 standard deviations below the laboratory mean. All plasma and tissue samples were sent to Metabolic Analysis Laboratory in Madison Wisconsin for analysis of total, free and esterified carnitine concentrations.

We conducted a study of plasma carnitine concentrations in 145 normal paediatric patients in order to define normal values as controls for our own work, as well as for comparison with normal values from other centres. These values are summarized in Table 1. Carnitine concentrations during the first week of life are lower than in adults and then quickly rise into the range of normal adult values.

The following information was obtained during the chart review: age, carnitine start and stop dates, primary diagnosis, aetiology of

TABLE I.
Plasma carnitine concentrations by age group (μmol l^{-1})

Age group	n	Total	Free	Ester
<5 days	23	29.4 ± 6.7	20.2 ± 5.1	8.9 ± 4.1
I week–I year	17	51.1 ± 9.2	40.2 ± 6.1	10.9 ± 5.6
>I year	105	45.4 ± 9.9	35.7 ± 9.1	8.9 ± 5.4

carnitine deficiency, pre-treatment carnitine level, signs and symptoms of carnitine deficiency, adverse events, and response to therapy for failure-to-thrive, muscle weakness and cardiomyopathy.

There were 250 girls and 362 males in the study ranging in age at the start of carnitine therapy from birth to 20.7 years. Two hundred and eighty-two patients had carnitine deficiency, 307 had carnitine insufficiency and 185 had both insufficiency and deficiency. Patients in the group with insufficiency and deficiency combined are also counted in the separate categories of deficiency and insufficiency throughout this chapter. Of the 282 patients with carnitine deficiency, the aetiology of the carnitine deficiency state was due to a metabolic disorder in 56 cases, valproic acid therapy in 87 patients, prematurity and poor carnitine stores in 54 cases, dietary deficiency in 61 cases, and was unknown in 24 patients.

Signs and symptoms of carnitine deficiency and/or insufficiency included 147 with decreased muscle tone and strength, 38 with cardiomyopathy, 168 with failure-to-thrive, 45 with frequent infections, 70 with encephalopathy, 33 with increased seizure frequency, 25 with hepatic dysfunction, 24 with developmental delay, 17 with dicarboxylic aciduria, 1 with neutropenia, 15 with hypoglycaemia, 12 with decreased stamina, 12 with decreased appetite, and 36 with acidosis.

CARNITINE TREATMENT REGIMEN

We use 100 mg kg^{-1} day^{-1} of L-carnitine in oral solution or in tablets to treat simple deficiency with no evidence of an ongoing loss such as occurs in the renal Fanconi syndromes or inborn errors of metabolism. If there was no ongoing loss and deficiency seemed to be only dietary in origin, carnitine therapy was continued for up to 6 months and then discontinued, with a carnitine concentration being measured one month after stopping therapy.

In cases with an ongoing loss, as in the renal Fanconi syndromes or organic acidurias, we began with an oral dose of 200 mg kg^{-1} day^{-1} L-carnitine and increased it to as high as 800 mg kg^{-1} day^{-1}, using both clinical response and free carnitine concentrations to guide our dosage regimen. Recently, we have paid more attention to the E/F ratio and raise carnitine dosage in an attempt to normalize these ratios.

Please note that the exact dosage of L-carnitine needed to treat a deficient or insufficient patient has not been clearly demonstrated. The doses quoted here have resulted in free carnitine concentrations in the normal range for the majority of the cases.

Side-effects from carnitine therapy were mainly gastrointestinal with 19 patients experiencing diarrhoea and one with vomiting. Three patients had abdominal cramping. Increased body odour was seen in seven patients and hair loss, transient in nature, in seven patients. In all, 7.68% of patients experienced a side-effect from carnitine therapy.

CARNITINE RESPONSE

Two hundred and fifteen patients presented with hypotonia and were treated with carnitine. One hundred and forty-seven of them had either carnitine deficiency or insufficiency: 105 were carnitine-deficient, 114 were insufficient and 72 were both insufficient and deficient. A total of 93 of these 147 patients showed improvement of tone on therapy. Of these, 64 were carnitine-deficient, 74 insufficient and 45 were both deficient and insufficient.

Failure to thrive was seen in 230 patients and, of these, 168 had either carnitine deficiency or insufficiency. Of these 168 patients, 104 showed improvement of growth with weight going from below to above the 5th percentile for age. Of these 104 patients showing resolution of their failure-to-thrive, 59 were carnitine-deficient, 68 were insufficient and 45 were both deficient and insufficient.

INBORN ERRORS OF METABOLISM

Eighty-two patients had a metabolic aetiology for their carnitine deficiency or insufficiency (Table 2). Of these, 51.2% experienced an improvement in either muscle tone and strength or failure-to-thrive, compared with 29.5% of the patients who did not have an underlying metabolic aetiology leading to an altered carnitine state. This supports the hypothesis that one of the main functions of carnitine is to remove acyl CoA derivatives such as those building up during organic acidopathies.

Thirty-nine of these patients were examined in more detail with regard to response to therapy in light of the initial esterified to free carnitine ratio. If carnitine's role is modulation of the acyl CoA/free CoA ratio, one would expect an improved response to therapy in those

TABLE 2.
Metabolic diagnoses of patients with carnitine deficiency

Methylmalonic/propionic aciduria	11
Mitochondrial disorder	10
Fatty acid oxidation defect	14
Glutaric aciduria, Type II	12
Peroxisomal defect	6
Diabetes	5
Betaketothiolase deficiency	2
Isovaleric acidaemia	1
Cystinosis	1
5,10-Methylene tetrahydrofolate reductase deficiency	1
Ornithine transcarbamylase deficiency	1
Maple syrup urine disease	1
Glucose-6-phosphatase deficiency	1
Other	16
Total	82

patients with an increased acyl CoA load as reflected by an increase in the esterified to free (E/F) carnitine ratio.

There were 34 patients with decreased muscle tone and stength and 18 (52%) improved, 35 with delayed motor milestones with 16 (46%) improving, 19 with increased infection frequency with 7 (36%) improving, 7/15 (47%) with failure-to-thrive improved and 13/19 (45%) with altered mental status.

There were eight patients with an E/F ratio greater than 1.0 and 31 with a ratio less than 1.0. Three of the eight patients (37.5%) with the E/F ratio greater than 1.0 demonstrated a life-saving effect of L-carnitine therapy, whereas only two of 31 (6.5%) with an E/F less than 1.0 responded. Five out of eight patients (62.5%) with an E/F ratio greater than 1.0 had failure-to-thrive, and four of these five (80%) resolved the failure-to-thrive on carnitine therapy. While 10 of 31 (32%) of the patients with E/F ratios below 1.0 had failure-to-thrive, only four of the 10 (40%) of these patients showed resolution of their growth problem on carnitine therapy.

We believe the findings of improved clinical response in patients with increased esterified to free carnitine ratios strongly supports the role of carnitine as a detoxifier of mitochondrial acyl CoA derivatives.

CARDIOMYOPATHY

Of 51 patients with cardiomyopathy, 33 improved with carnitine therapy. Of those patients who improved, the pre-treatment carnitine concentration was deficient in 20 patients and insufficient in 18 patients and both deficient and insufficient in 14 patients. Of those patients who did not improve, eight of 18 were carnitine-deficient and 11 of 18 were insufficient and 6 of 18 were both deficient and insufficient.

A more detailed chart review was carried out on 33 of these 55 cardiomyopathy patients who had documented echocardiograms and carnitine concentrations recorded prior to carnitine therapy. Thirty-one of the patients had dilated cardiomyopathy and two had hypertrophic cardiomyopathy. Five of the patients had a normal plasma free carnitine concentration ($>20 \ \mu$mol l^{-1}) and seven had normal free carnitine concentrations but carnitine insufficiency with an E/F ratio of greater than 0.4. Twenty-one patients had carnitine deficiency and 14 of these had insufficiency as well.

In order to quantify the impact of carnitine therapy on cardiomyopathy, we grouped the patients with regard to possible causes of carnitine deficiency/insufficiency and scored them according to overall outcome. Scores of 1, 2 and 3 indicate no change, improved, and resolved, respectively. Of 11 newborns (eight premature) the average score was 2.81 with two deaths. Of seven patients with dietary deficiency, on parenteral nutrition or unsupplemented formulas, the average score was 2.43. Seven patients with identified or suspected metabolic disorders had an outcome score of 1.86 with four deaths; this included two glutaric aciduria type II, two lipid storage myopathy, one mitochondrial myopathy, one generalized myopathy and one familial cardiomyopathy with mental retardation and optic atrophy. In general, the metabolic cardiomyopathies fit into the general category of mitochondrial myopathies with suspected disorders of electron transport. Of the seven patients in whom no aetiology for a carnitine deficiency or insufficiency state could be found, the outcome score was 1.2.

VALPROIC ACID THERAPY

Of the 126 patients treated with L-carnitine because of therapy with valproic acid, 87 were carnitine-deficient, 67 insufficient, and 52 both deficient and insufficient. Signs and symptoms of carnitine deficiency included: 30 with encephalopathy, 28 with seizures, 13 with hepatic dysfunction, nine with decreased strength, seven with recurrent infections, six with failure-to-thrive, six with developmental delay, three with decreased appetite, two with decreased stamina, one with hypoglycaemia, and one with cardiomyopathy. Twelve of 30 (40%) patients with hypotonia and decreased muscle strength, and nine of 29 of the patients with failure-to-thrive improved (31%) while on carnitine therapy.

Several subsets of our valproic acid patients were studied in more detail. One hundred and thirty-five patients on valproic acid with or without other anticonvulsant drugs were compared with 89 patients from our control population. The mean total carnitine concentration was $33.1 \mu mol \, l^{-1}$ for the valproate group versus $45.5 \, \mu mol \, l^{-1}$ for the normal group. The free plasma carnitine concentration for the valproate group was $24.1 \, \mu mol \, l^{-1}$ versus $36.7 \, \mu mol \, l^{-1}$ for the normal patients and the E/F ratio for the valproic acid group was 0.44, compared with 0.25 for the controls. All values were significantly different at the level of $p < 0.0001$. A group of 43 patients on other anticonvulsant medications did not show any significantly different carnitine concentrations from the controls (Opala, 1991).

Additional analysis of these patients showed that free plasma carnitine concentrations in patients on valproic acid are lowest in the patients less than 2 years of age and that they increase with age. This is of particular interest because it is the child under the age of 2 who is at greatest risk of developing a hepatic dysfunction with valproic acid. Carnitine's role in the aetiology of this hepatoxicity remains to be elucidated.

Another cohort of 66 patients on valproic acid therapy and carnitine therapy were examined for the effect of carnitine therapy in improving valproic acid-induced side-effects. Twenty-two of the patients were neurologically symptomatic for valproic acid side-effects and had records that allowed us to score changes in mental status, school performance, seizure frequency and muscle strength. Of 15 patients with altered mental status, 11 improved and four resolved. Of 13 patients with deterioration in school performance, 11 improved and two returned to pre-therapy levels. Six experienced improvement in seizure frequency. Of seven with decreased muscle strength, all improved with two changing from non-ambulatory to a condition of mildly- or moderately-decreased strength.

DIABETES

The similarity of diabetes mellitus to inborn errors of metabolism with a build-up of acyl CoA derivatives due to the increased fatty acid breakdown with insulin deficiency, prompted us to study children attending a summer camp for diabetics for plasma carnitine deficiency and insufficiency. They were asymptomatic for carnitine deficiency.

A total of 54 children participated in the study with 31 boys and 23 girls aged from 7 to 10 years. Thirteen patients had a plasma free carnitine concentration below 20 μmol l^{-1} and when comparing our patient population with a group of 20 control patients, the diabetic patients had a significantly elevated (p <0.001) E/F ratio (Winter et al, 1989).

SUMMARY

We have studied the clinical symptoms and response to carnitine therapy in 612 patients. The aetiologies of the secondary carnitine deficiency were multiple and varied but fit into two main groups: decreased synthesis or intake of carnitine and increased loss in the urine. Urine loss occurs as esterified carnitine in the organic acidurias or valproic acid therapy or loss of free carnitine in the renal Fanconi syndromes.

Carnitine deficiency was defined as a free plasma carnitine concentration of equal to or below 20 μmol l^{-1} and carnitine insufficiency as a plasma esterified carnitine/free carnitine of greater than or equal to 0.4. These values are distinctly abnormal from a group of normal children living in our community and are applicable after the age of 1 week.

Carnitine deficiency and insufficiency are associated with many signs and symptoms with most related to alterations of mitochondrial metabolism that occur during states of carnitine deficiency or insufficiency. Children present with muscle weakness, hypotonia, failure to thrive or cardiomyopathy and failure to recognize the need for carnitine therapy could result in death. Hepatic dysfunction and encephalopathy, so-called Reye's syndrome, can also be associated with carnitine deficiency and insufficiency. Frequent infections with metabolic decompensations and hospitalizations are also a hallmark of the carnitine-deficient or insufficient patient, especially if the underlying aetiology is an inborn error of metabolism.

Treatment with L-carnitine results in improvement of some sign or symptom in at least 50% of the patients with insufficiency or deficiency. The most obvious areas of improvement are in muscle tone, strength and bulk with resultant improvement in failure-to-thrive.

The main role of carnitine appears to be the modulation of the acyl CoA to free CoA ratio within the mitochondria via the removal of the derivatives attached to the CoA moiety and excretion of these derivatives as an acyl carnitine in the urine. The specific species of acyl carnitines identified in the urine are those expected for each metabolic disorder and can be used as a diagnostic tool for these disorders (DiDonato, 1984a; Roe, 1984; Millington, 1985).

Alterations of carnitine concentrations reflect altered mitochondrial metabolism and may also result in alteration of the metabolism due to the inability to modulate the acyl CoA/free CoA ratio and inhibition of the tricarboxylic acid cycle, fatty acid oxidation, pyruvate metabolism and gluconeogenesis. Failure to recognize the need for carnitine therapy during such a metabolic crisis could result in a life-threatening episode and disability or death.

One should investigate for carnitine deficiency and insufficiency and consider therapy in patients presenting with one or more of the following signs or symptoms: hypotonia, muscle weakness, failure-to-thrive, cardiomyopathy, hepatic dysfunction, recurrent illness or infections, non-ketotic hypoglycaemia and encephalopathy. In addition in any child with a predisposing condition such as known poor dietary intake, prematurity, inborn error of metabolism or renal Fanconi syndrome, carnitine deficiency or insufficiency should be suspected. It must be remembered that carnitine deficiency and insufficiency are secondary problems and once diagnosed must be followed by a thorough investigation into the cause. The investigation should include metabolic testing and often a referral to a metabolic specialist.

In our experience, treatment with L-carnitine appears safe and has minimal side-effects. In cases of severe alterations of mitochondrial metabolism, as evidenced by the signs and symptoms outlined above, carnitine treatment can be started while awaiting the metabolic work-up and can be life-saving. Freezing 10–60 cm^3 of urine and 2–10 cm^3 of plasma for future metabolic studies would be advisable prior to treatment so that further metabolic studies can be performed if needed.

Based on our experience, an elevated esterified/free carnitine ratio appears to be the best indicator for success with carnitine treatment and reflects the detoxification role of carnitine conjugation.

REFERENCES

Cannon RA (1984) *Hosp. Pract.* 19: 139F.

Chapoy PR, Angelini C, Brown WJ et al (1980) *N. Engl. J. Med.* 303: 1389–1394.

Coates P & Roe CR (1989) In Scriver CK, Beauder D, Sly WS & Valle D (eds) *The Metabolic Basis of Inherited Diseases*, vol. 1, 6th edn. New York: McGraw-Hill.

Coulter DL (1984) *Lancet* ii, 689.

Cornelio F, DiDonato S, Peluchetti D et al (1979) *Perspectives in Inherited Metabolic Diseases* 3, 128–150.

DiDonato S, Rimoldi M, Garavaglia B et al (1984a) *Clin. Chim. Acta* 139: 13–19.

DiDonato S, Peluchetti D, Rimoldi M et al (1984b) *Neurology* **34**: 157–162.

Glasgow AM, Eng G & Engel AG (1980) *J. Pediatr.* 96: 889–891.

Ino T, Sherwood WG, Benson LN et al (1988) *J. Am. Coll. Cardiol.* 11: 1301–1308.

Karpati G, Carpenter S, Enge AG et al (1975) *Neurology* 25: 15–24.

Kudo Y, Shoji T et al (1983) *Jpn. Circ. J.* 47: 1391–1397.

Laub MC, Paetzke-Brunner I & Jaeger G (1986) *Epilepsia* 109: 131–134.

Matsuda I, Ontani Y & Ninomiya N (1986) *J. Pediatr.* 109: 131–134.

Matsui SM, Mahoney MJ & Rosenberg LE (1983) *N. Engl. J. Med.* 308: 857F.

Millington DS, Bohan TP et al (1985) *Clin. Chim. Acta.* 145: 69–76.

Ohtani Y, Endo F & Matsuda I (1982) *J. Pediatr.* 101: 782–785.

Opala G, Winter S, Vance C et al (1991) *Am. J. Dis. Child.* (in press).

Rebouche CJ & Engel AG (1983) *Mayo Clin. Proc.* 58: 533–540.

Roe CR, Millington DS, Malthy DA et al (1984) *J. Clin. Invest.* 73: 1785–1788.

Scholte HR, Meijer AEFH, Van Wijngaarden GK et al (1979) *J. Neurol. Sci.* 42: 87–101.

Slonim AE, Borum PR, Mrak RE et al (1983) *Neurology* 33: 29–33.

Stumpf DA, Parker WD & Haas R (1983) *J. Pediatr.* 103: 175–176.

Tripp ME & Shug AL (1984) *Biochem. Med.* 32: 199–206.

Tripp ME, Katcher ML, Peters HA et al (1981) *N. Engl. J. Med.* 305: 385–390.

Waber LJ, Valle D, Neill C et al (1982) *J. Pediatr.* 101: 700–705.

Winter SC, Szabo-Aczel S, Curry CJR et al (1987) *Am. J. Dis. Child.* 141: 660–665.

Winter SC, Simon M, Zorn EM et al (1989) *Am. J. Dis. Child.* 143: 1337–1339.

12

PLASMA CARNITINE
EVALUATION IN CHILDREN
WITH CARDIOMYOPATHY

C. Dionisi Vici, M. Bevilacqua, A.B. Burlina,
G.M. Gagliardi, G. Sabetta and E. Bertini

Cardiomyopathies (CMPs) are a heterogeneous group of rare disorders in children. In most cases it is difficult to establish a precise aetiological diagnosis and thus the pathogenetic mechanism is often considered to be 'idiopathic'. On the other hand, several inborn errors of metabolism may cause cardiomyopathy (Kohlschutter and Hausdorf, 1986). These inherited conditions can be roughly divided in two main groups: (i) 'large' molecule diseases (storage disorders, i.e. glycogen storage diseases, lysosomal storage diseases); (ii) 'small' molecule diseases (i.e. organic acidurias, β-oxidation defects, and disorders of the respiratory chain) (Applegarth et al, 1989).

In the first group of diseases, the clinical phenotype and the multi-organ involvement are helpful for the differential diagnosis, while in the second group, specific biochemical investigations are needed to define the underlying enzymatic defect.

In addition to the intramitochondrial transport of long-chain fatty acids, carnitine plays a crucial role in the regulation of intramitochondrial acyl CoA/CoA ratio (Siliprandi et al, 1989). Because of this 'buffer' function, secondary carnitine deficiency has been associated with

223

L-Carnitine and Its Role in Medicine:
From Function to Therapy. ISBN 0–12–253940–0

organic acidurias, β-oxidation defects and some cases of respiratory chain disorders (Dionisi Vici et al, 1988; Roe et al, 1990).

Primary carnitine deficiency, caused by a specific multi-organ membrane transport defect, is also responsible for a carnitine-responsive CMP in children (Eriksson et al, 1988; Treem et al, 1988; Tein et al, 1990).

In order to define a useful approach for the differential diagnosis of CMP, we have screened plasma carnitine levels and evaluated its importance in 53 children.

MATERIALS AND METHODS

Fifty-three children (age range: 3 days to 16 years) affected by CMP were observed in the last 4 years at the Department of Cardiology of the Bambino Gesu' Hospital. All underwent clinical examination, electrocardiography, two-dimensional heart ultrasonography, heart gallium and/or tallium scintigraphy, and most of them had cardiac catheterization with endomyocardial biopsy. By the use of this protocol, 33 patients were classified as dilated CMP, eight as hypertrophic CMP, two as restrictive CMP and 11 as CMP secondary to histologically demonstrated myocarditis. Eleven patients underwent heart transplantation and were excluded from the follow-up. Thirteen children died during the follow-up period. Laboratory investigations included routine haematological examination (glucose, ammonia, transaminases, creatine kinase), viral antibody concentrations, HLA phenotypes, T-lymphocyte subpopulations. Biochemical studies included determination of plasma carnitine, and blood concentrations of lactate and pyruvate. Urine organic acid GC/MS screening was performed in 33 patients and muscle biopsy in 24. Muscle carnitine levels were measured in five patients and heart carnitine in one. Total and free carnitine was determined radioenzymatically (McGarry and Foster, 1976). Organic acids in urine were detected by GC/MS (Burlina, 1986). Muscle biopsies were performed following standard techniques (Dubowitz, 1985). Age-matched controls for plasma carnitine levels consisted of 19 healthy children.

RESULTS

Of the 43 patients with CMP, 35 were classified as 'idiopathic', four as secondary to small molecule disease (two with long-chain

3-hydroxyacyl CoA dehydrogenase (LCHAD) deficiency, one with a combined deficiency of complex I and complex IV of the mitochondrial respiratory chain, and one with undefined primary lactic acidosis), three as secondary to large molecule disease (two acid maltase deficiency, one undefined multisystemic glycogen storage disease), and one with primary carnitine deficiency.

In the idiopathic group, mean plasma total and free carnitine concentrations were significantly elevated compared with controls (Table 1), and to myocarditis ($p < 0.05$ for total and free respectively). The acyl/free carnitine ratio did not show significant differences between patients and controls. Total carnitine concentration was above normal in 25 children (71%), normal and low–normal in 7 (20%) and reduced in 3 (9%). Free carnitine was above normal in 15 children (43%), normal in 17 (48%) and reduced in 3 (9%). All three children with reduced carnitine levels showed marked growth retardation with signs of malnutrition.

Muscle carnitine levels were normal in five idiopathic CMP patients and showed no correlation with the corresponding plasma carnitine levels. In the only case (patient 22) in whom myocardial carnitine concentration was measured, we found markedly reduced levels (total: 3.9 μmol per g non-collagen protein; controls 9.9 ± 0.8 [Regitz et al, 1990]) despite high normal concentrations of plasma carnitine.

As expected, all children with CMP secondary to small molecule disease showed markedly reduced levels of free carnitine, low–normal levels of total carnitine, and significant increase of acyl/free carnitine ratio (Table 2). Plasma carnitine values in children with CMP secondary to large molecule diseases were comparable to controls (Table 2). The mean plasma values of total carnitine ($50 ± 15$ μmol^{-1}) as well as of free carnitine ($34 ± 11$ μmol^{-1}) and the acyl/free carnitine ratio ($0.5 ± 0.2$) in children with CMP secondary to myocarditis were comparable to controls.

RELEVANT CASES

Primary carnitine deficiency

This child is patient #2 in Tein et al (1990) (see also Tein and Di Mauro, Chapter 9 in this book). The patient was born at term by a normal delivery to healthy and unrelated parents. Birth-weight was

TABLE I.

Individual plasma carnitine levels (μmol l^{-1}), and acyl/free carnitine ratio in patients with idiopathic cardiomyopathy and in 19 age-matched controls

Cardiomyopathy		Sex	Total	Free	Acyl/free
1.	Dilated		m	105	70	0.5
2.	Dilated	(t)	m	95	72	0.3
3.	Dilated	(+t)	f	95	65	0.5
4.	Dilated	(+)	m	93	66	0.4
5.	Dilated	(+t)	m	89	68	0.3
6.	Dilated	(t)	f	87	46	0.9
7.	Dilated		f	82	71	0.1
8.	Dilated	(+)	m	82	41	1.0
9.	Dilated	(+)	m	82	40	1.0
10.	Dilated		m	75	61	0.2
11.	Dilated	(t)	m	70	45	0.5
12.	Dilated		m	66	53	0.2
13.	Restrictive	(+)	m	65	51	0.3
14.	Dilated	(+)	f	65	26	1.5
15.	Dilated		f	62	41	0.5
16.	Dilated		f	61	31	1.0
17.	Dilated	(+t)	f	60	49	0.2
18.	Dilated	(+t)	f	60	43	0.4
19.	Dilated		f	60	40	0.5
20.	Dilated		m	59	39	0.5
21.	Dilated		m	57	40	0.4
22.	Dilated	(t)	f	56	51	0.1
23.	Hypertrophic		m	55	50	0.1
24.	Dilated		m	55	33	0.7
25.	Dilated		f	53	35	0.5
26.	Dilated		f	48	36	0.3
27.	Hypertrophic	(+)	m	48	30	0.6
28.	Dilated		f	44	31	0.4
29.	Dilated	(+)	f	41	35	0.2
30.	Dilated	(+t)	f	39	36	0.1
31.	Dilated	(t)	f	38	33	0.1
32.	Dilated		f	37	34	0.1
33.	Restrictive	(+t)	f	30	20	0.5
34.	Hypertrophic		m	29	20	0.4
35.	Dilated		m	25	19	0.3
Total patients		(#35)		62 ± 21*	43 ± 15†	0.4 ± 0.3‡
Controls				46 ± 6.5	34 ± 8.8	0.4 ± 0.19

(+), deceased; t, transplanted; *$p < 0.001$; †$p < 0.01$; ‡not significant.

TABLE 2.

Individual plasma carnitine levels (μmol I^{-1}) and acyl/free carnitine ratio in children with cardiomyopathy secondary to small and large molecule diseases and in 19 age-matched controls

		Total	Free	Acyl/free
Small molecule disease				
1.	Senger's syndrome	59	15	2.9
2.	Lactic acidosis	37	18	1.1
3.	LCHAD deficiency	33	8	3.1
4.	LCHAD deficiency	23	9	1.5
Total		38 ± 15†	12 ± 4.8*	2.1 ± 1.0*
Large molecule disease				
1.	Glycogenosis type II	68	37	0.8
2.	Glycogenosis (?)	43	31	0.4
3.	Glycogenosis type II	35	28	0.2
Total		49 ± 17†	32 ± 4.5†	0.4 ± 0.3†
Controls		46 ± 6.5	34 ± 8.8	0.4 ± 0.2

*$p < 0.0001$; † not significant.

3.5 kg. From the first months of life he showed delayed motor and intellectual development and from the age of 18 months he suffered recurrent episodes of abdominal pain. He was referred to our hospital aged 7.5 years because of cardiomegaly and severe hypochromic anaemia (haemoglobin 5 g dl^{-1}), requiring blood transfusion. Dilatative CMP was demonstrated by chest X-ray and two-dimensional heart ultrasonography. ECG showed a peculiar pattern with peaked T-waves. He had weakness and a positive Gower's manoeuvre. The IQ score was 67 (Wechler-R scale). Routine laboratory tests including glucose, lactate, ammonia, transaminases, creatine kinase, triglycerides, were normal. Thalassaemia was ruled out. Plasma total carnitine was extremely low (1.2 μmol l^{-1}) and the fractional tubular reabsorption was reduced to 52% (normal >95%). Urine organic acid profile was normal. Muscle biopsy showed lipid storage myopathy with apparently normal mitochondria. Muscle carnitine was also low (total 1.1 μmol per g non-collagen protein, controls 19.1 ± 7.7) and carnitine uptake in cultured skin fibroblasts was severely impaired. A dramatic improvement was observed a few days after the onset of carnitine supplementation (150 mg kg^{-1} day^{-1}). Cardiomegaly and the abnormal

ECG pattern normalized after 6 months and intellectual performances improved.

Senger's syndrome with multiple respiratory chain defects

This female infant was admitted to our hospital at the age of 3 months for CMP. Clinical examination showed generalized hypotonia, nystagmus and bilateral cataract. Echocardiography disclosed hypertrophic CMP. Brainstem evoked responses were abnormal and compatible with severe neurosensory deafness. Blood lactate was elevated to 54 mg dl^{-1} (normal ≤ 25) and plasma free carnitine was reduced with an increased acyl/free carnitine ratio (Table 2, patient 1). Urine organic acid profile showed increased excretion of lactate, α-oxoglutarate and succinate. Muscle biopsy showed subsarcolemmal accumulations of glycogen and mitochondria without typical red ragged fibres. Histoenzymatic reaction for cytochrome oxidase was absent in numerous fibres. Biochemically NADH cytochrome-C-reductase activity was reduced to 43% and cytochrome oxidase to 36% of the normal mean with a proportional decrease of immunoreactive cytochrome oxidase protein by ELISA (Servidei et al, 1990). The absence of mitochondrial DNA deletions suggested an abnormality of nuclear DNA-encoded subunits of both complex I and IV.

Long-chain 3-OH acyl CoA dehydrogenase deficiency

Patient 1 (Dionisi Vici et al, 1990): This girl was first admitted to another hospital at the age of 9 months for failure to thrive. Intellectual development was apparently normal while motor milestones were slightly delayed. The ophthalmological examination showed a pigmentary retinal degeneration. During hospitalization she had several episodes of fasting hypoketotic hypoglycaemia. Cow's milk protein intolerance was suspected. At 10 months of age the child was admitted to our hospital because, during an upper respiratory tract infection, she developed feeding refusal, vomiting, lethargy and generalized hypotonia. The diagnosis at admission was Reye-like syndrome with grade 1 coma. Liver edge was palpable 6 cm below the right costal margin, reflexes could not be elicited, heart rate was 140 per min, and she had a gallop rhythm with signs of cardiac failure. Laboratory investigations showed low blood glucose (38 mg dl^{-1}), increased lactate (63 mg dl^{-1}), creatine kinase (600 U l^{-1}), GOT (150 U l^{-1}), GPT (130 U l^{-1}), and mild hyperammonaemia. Plasma carnitine was reduced and the acyl/free carnitine ratio was increased (Table 2, patient 4). Ketones were absent in the urine. CSF lactate was 32 mg dl^{-1} (normal <12) and the intracranial pressure was slightly increased to 30 cm H$_2$O (normal <12). Screening of urine organic acids by GC/MS showed significant 3-OH-dicarboxylic aciduria. Chest X-ray showed cardiomegaly; two-dimensional heart ultrasonography disclosed hypertrophic hypokinetic CMP. The patient was treated with glucose infusion, insulin, mannitol, carnitine, and slowly recovered in two days. Severe sensory-motor polyneuropathy was detected by nerve conduction velocity studies. After 1 week, the clinical course rapidly worsened, with heart and liver failure and respiratory distress requiring mechanical ventilation, and the child died of cardiorespiratory arrest. Autopsy showed fatty infiltration of liver, muscle, heart, and kidney, brain oedema, slight atrophy of the thymus and hypoplasia of the bone marrow. Biochemical studies of cultured fibroblasts confirmed a defect of the mitochondrial LCHAD.

Patient 2 (Dionisi Vici et al, 1991): This boy was healthy until 13 months when he presented with lethargy and hypotonia following an upper respiratory infection. Creatine kinase was elevated (2850 U l^{-1}) as well as SGOT (193 U l^{-1}) and SGPT (385 U l^{-1}). Glucose was not measured. This episode resolved spontaneously. A few weeks later he was readmitted to hospital for evaluation of myopathy. Two-dimensional heart ultrasonography disclosed a hypertrophic CMP. The plasma free carnitine concentration was reduced (see Table 2, patient 3). During a controlled fast of 14 hours, the glucose fell to 54 mg dl^{-1}, the free fatty acids increased to 1.78 mmol l^{-1}, while ketone bodies remained low (3-hydroxybutyrate 0.19 mmol^{-1}; acetoacetate 0.13 mmol l^{-1}). Urinary organic acid analysis showed a significant 3-OH-dicarboxylic aciduria consistent with a defect in fatty acid oxidation. The response to an oral medium-chain triglyceride load was normal (plasma 3-hydroxybutyrate increased from 0.091 mmol l^{-1} to 0.754 mmol l^{-1}), suggesting that the proximal portion of the fatty acid oxidation pathway was intact. Muscle biopsy revealed fatty infiltration. Muscle total carnitine concentration was reduced (1.72 μmol per g non-collagen protein, controls 19.2 ± 7.7). Muscle CPT-1 and CPT-2 activities were normal (kindly performed by Dr H. Scholte, Rotterdam, The Netherlands). CMP resolved with the start of a low-fat diet and carnitine supplementation. Over the next few years, the boy presented with intermittent episodes of acute muscle weakness and pain induced by febrile illnesses associated with fasting for more than 12 h, prolonged motor activity, cold temperature, or psychological stress. These episodes were accompanied by high creatine kinase and transaminase levels and, since the fourth year of life, by frank myoglobinuria. The CMP has not recurred and his intellectual development remains normal. The acute episodes always responded to intravenous therapy with glucose and carnitine. Neurological examination at age 5 showed distal muscle weakness and stepping gait. Nerve conduction velocity studies were decreased. Enzymatic studies in fibroblasts showed a defect of the LCHAD.

DISCUSSION

Cardiomyopathies in children are a heterogeneous group of disorders requiring multidisciplinary diagnostic tools. Clinical features, including positive family history, early onset, and multisystemic involvement suggest the possibility of inborn errors of metabolism (Kohlschutter and Hausdorf, 1986).

In our series, measurement of plasma carnitine levels helped us identify one patient with primary carnitine deficiency. The pathogenesis of primary carnitine deficiency has been elucidated only recently and it has been attributed to a genetic defect of carnitine transport (Treem et al, 1988; Tein et al, 1990). Extremely low total carnitine levels in plasma (below 5 μmol l^{-1}) should suggest this disorder, which is responsive to carnitine supplementation.

Several disorders related to the metabolism of small molecules (organic acidurias, β-oxidation defects, respiratory-chain defects) are associated with CPM. This group of inherited metabolic disorders are generally familial, show intermittent episodes of metabolic decompensation with multi-organ involvement and may cause secondary carnitine deficiency (Chalmers et al 1980, 1984; Kohlschutter, 1983; Nhyan, 1988).

The mechanism of secondary carnitine deficiency is related to the intramitochondrial buffer function of carnitine which increases the shuttling of accumulated acyl CoA moieties toward the cytosol as carnitine esters. Excessive intracellular acylcarnitines are then cleared through the bloodstream and excreted in the urine (Chalmers et al, 1984). Therefore, the carnitine profile in plasma and tissues is characterized by abnormally low levels of free carnitine and increased levels of acylcarnitines, with inversion of the acyl/free carnitine ratio.

Evaluation of plasma carnitine levels and profiles was helpful in the identification of four children with small molecule disease, which was confirmed by urine organic acid GC/MS and enzymatic studies. As expected in these disorders, all patients had significantly reduced free carnitine together with increased acyl/free carnitine ratio in the blood.

Most CMP patients subjected to our screening protocol were classified as idiopathic, and showed significantly elevated plasma total carnitine levels. Skeletal muscle carnitine concentration was normal in five patients, indicating normal carnitine uptake in this tissue. In a single case, we observed low heart carnitine concentrations contrasting with high-normal plasma levels. Similar results have been reported in a series of 25 patients, including children and adults, with heterogeneous CMPs (Tripp and Shug, 1984). In 14 of these patients, plasma carnitine levels were above normal and skeletal muscle carnitine was normal in five of six patients. Myocardial carnitine was normal in two and low in one of three patients with high plasma carnitine.

Recently, low heart carnitine concentration has been observed in a family with X-linked dilated CMP, although carnitine concentration was normal in plasma, liver and muscle (Hug et al, 1990).

Taken together, these data suggest a primary defect of a specific carnitine carrier in cardiomyocytes. However, the reason for the increased concentration of carnitine in plasma remains elusive.

The Bio 14.6 hamster develops a CMP associated with progressive cardiac carnitine deficiency while maintaining normal or elevated plasma carnitine concentration (York et al, 1983). In this animal model, CMP seems to be due to a specific carnitine transport abnormality in the heart, related to a defective function of the cardiac carnitine-binding protein. However, it has been shown that non-specific membrane damage secondary to ischaemia or anoxia can also cause reduced myocardial and elevated plasma carnitine levels (Shug et al, 1978).

Similar secondary membrane damage with impairment of the carnitine carrier system has also been postulated to explain the low heart and elevated plasma carnitine levels found in a large series of 28 adult patients with mild, moderate or severe idiopathic dilated CMP, as well as in eight subjects with congestive heart failure of different origin (Regitz et al, 1990). The reduction in myocardial carnitine was proportional to the severity of the heart failure regardless of its origin.

Membrane damage can be excluded in our series of idiopathic CMP and in patients with CMP secondary to myocarditis because serum creatine kinase and lactate dehydrogenase were not elevated. Moreover, patients with myocarditis did not show significant elevation of plasma carnitine values.

Further studies are needed to confirm the postulated defect of a putative specific heart carnitine transport in humans.

In conclusion, plasma carnitine levels in children are useful biochemical markers for the diagnosis of CMP associated with primary or secondary carnitine deficiencies and help distinguish them from idiopathic forms. In selecting CMP patients for heart transplantation, it was possible to exclude children with treatable disease and to avoid surgery in fatal progressive disorders.

REFERENCES

Applegarth DA, Dimmick JE & Toone JR (1989) *Pediatr. Clin. North. Am.* 36: 49–65.

Burlina AB (1986) *Ital. J. Pediatr.* 12: 541–551.

Chalmers RA, Purkiss P, Watts RWE & Lawson AM (1980) *J. Inher. Metab. Dis.* 3: 27–43.

Chalmers RA, Roe CR, Stacey TE & Hoppel CL (1984) *Pediatr. Res.* 18: 1325–1328.

Dionisi Vici C, Bertini E, Bartuli A & Sabetta G (1988) *J. Pediatr.* 112: 678.

Dionisi Vici C, Garavaglia B, Burlina AB et al (1990) *Ann. Neurol.* 28: 278.

Dionisi Vici C, Burlina AB, Bertini E et al (1991) *J. Pediatr.* 118: 744–746.

Dubowitz V (1985) *Muscle Biopsy. A Practical Approach* pp 3–40. London: Baillière-Tindall.

Eriksson BO, Lindstedt S & Nordin I (1988) *Eur. J. Pediatr.* 147: 662–663.

Hug G, Schwartz DC, Tuuri D & Dillon T (1990) *Pediatr. Res.* 27 (part 2): 20A.

Kohlschutter A (1983) *Neuropediatrics* 14: 191–196.

Kohlschutter A & Hausdorf G (1986) *Eur. J. Pediatr.* 145: 454–459.

McGarry JD & Foster DW (1976) *J. Lipid Res.* 17: 277–281.

Nhyan WL (1988) *N. Engl. J. Med.* 319: 1344–1346.

Regitz V, Shug AL & Fleck E (1990) *Amer. J. Cardiol.* 65: 755–760.

Roe CR, Millington DS, Kahler SG et al (1990). In Coates PM & Tanaka K, *Fatty Acid Oxidation: Clinical, Biochemical and Molecular Aspects* pp 383–402. New York: Alan R. Liss.

Servidei S, Dionisi Vici C, Bertini E et al (1990) *Ital. J. Neurol. Sci.* 11: 194.

Shug AL, Thomsen JH, Folts JD et al (1978) *Arch. Biochem. Biophys.* 187: 25–33.

Siliprandi N, Sartorelli L, Ciman M & Di Lisa F (1989) *Clin. Chim. Acta.* 183: 3–12.

Tein I, De Vivo DC, Bierman F et al, (1990) *Pediatr. Res.* 28: 247–255.

Treem WR, Stanley CA, Hale DE & Coates PM (1988) *N. Engl. J. Med.* 319: 1331–1336.

Tripp ME & Shug AL (1984) *Biochem. Med.* 32: 199–206.

York CM, Cantrell CR & Borum PR (1983) *Arch. Biochem. Biophys.* 221: 526–533.

PART III

ADULT MEDICINE

Introduction: Carnitine in adults: an
overview
R. Ferrari

Carnitine concentration in the blood is 20 to 40 times less than that in tissue. Therefore, carnitine introduced with the diet or synthesized de novo in the liver or in the kidney, must be actively concentrated from the blood into fatty acid metabolizing organs, such as skeletal and, particularly, heart muscle. Therefore, in the last 20 years or so, there has been an expanding amount of research to clarify the role of carnitine in the pathogenesis and in the therapy of different cardiac conditions.

The finding in experimental animals and in humans that the ischaemic and failing myocardium has a low content of free carnitine has supported the concept that myocardial ischaemia and heart failure are conditions of relative carnitine insufficiency. It has been shown that exogenous administration of L-carnitine improves cardiac metabolism and function in different experimental models of ischaemia and failure. Professor Visioli offers an extensive overview of the existing data on the subject.

A possible anti-ischaemic effect of carnitine has been investigated

233

L-Carnitine and Its Role in Medicine:
From Function to Therapy. ISBN 0–12–253940–0

in CAD patients with typical effort angina and myocardial infarction. The evidence in favour, doubts and possible mechanisms of action are discussed in the chapters from our group and that of Professor Rizzon. Drs Regitz and Patel address issues pertaining to the role of carnitine in patients with heart failure and with low myocardial carnitine levels, where prognostic implications have been postulated. Finally, Professor Fernandez reviews data based on a large fourth-phase clinical trial conducted in Italy on coronary artery disease patients.

A new, interesting finding for a therapeutic use of L-carnitine was discovered in 1988 by Brevetti and colleagues. They showed that oral carnitine increases walking distance in patients with peripheral vascular disease without affecting general or regional haemodynamics. The same authors review the situation 3 years after their original findings, whilst Professor Hülsman provides an insight into the possible mechanism of action of L-carnitine at the smooth muscle level.

In 1978 Bohner et al (*Lancet* i: 126–128) reported a low muscle carnitine concentration in patients undergoing haemodialysis. Thereafter the effects of L-carnitine therapy were carefully examined. Dr Ahmad offers a critical and concise overview of the subject.

Only recently it has been recognized that carnitine plays a critical role not only in free fatty acid (FFA) metabolism, but also in that of carbohydrates. Quite correctly, in the 1990s, carnitine was recognized to act as a 'metabolic modulator', improving not only FFA, but also glucose utilization. This is discussed by Drs Lopascuk and Dhalla in the last two chapters.

Part IIIa

Cardiology

13

MOLECULAR MECHANISM OF ACTION OF L-CARNITINE IN TREATMENT OF MYOCARDIAL DISORDERS AT THE EXPERIMENTAL LEVEL

O. Visioli, E. Pasini, F. de Giuli and R. Ferrari

The purposes of this survey are: (i) to briefly consider some aspects of myocardial metabolism in aerobic conditions; (ii) to analyse the functional and molecular alterations caused by ischaemia and reperfusion with special attention to the pathways of lipid utilization and to the mechanism underlying the detrimental effects of free fatty acid

237

L-Carnitine and Its Role in Medicine:
From Function to Therapy. ISBN 0–12–253940–0

(FFA) during myocardial ischaemia and reperfusion; (iii) to discuss the role of L-carnitine in myocardial energy production and in reducing the damage mediated by ischaemia and reperfusion; (iv) to examine critically the experimental evidence suggesting that L-carnitine improves the adverse metabolic changes associated with myocardial ischaemia.

SUBSTRATE METABOLISM AND ENERGY PRODUCTION IN THE HEART

The energy needed for cardiac contraction comes from the breakdown of chemical substances or substrates. In the heart, this process occurs mainly aerobically, i.e. substrates are combined with oxygen to form water, carbon dioxide and energy (Figure 1). The amount of oxygen consumed is often used as a measure of the total energy available. The ultimate fate of the liberated energy is its conversion to heat. However, before this happens completely, part of the energy is used for contraction, a process during which the heart performs external work, as is usually the case in the intact body.

Knowledge of the fuels of the human heart started with the introduction of coronary sinus catheterization by Bing and his associates in 1954. The chemical composition of arterial blood entering the heart was compared with that of coronary sinus blood leaving the heart. From such studies it was established that glucose, lactate and FFA are the heart's major sources of energy (Bing et al, 1953). It has also been recognized that the myocardium is able to utilize such fuels as pyruvate, acetate, ketone bodies and amino acids, but the normal circulating levels are too low for them to be considered as major sources of energy, even when the external supply is increased (Drake, 1982). The heart can also use, under certain circumstances, its internal energy stores such as glycogen and lipid.

A cruder estimate of the type of substrate used by the heart can be achieved by the respiratory quotient, which is calculated by comparing the rate of oxygen uptake with the rate of carbon dioxide production. A respiratory quotient near to one implies oxidation of glucose and/or lactate, whereas a lower value implies fatty acid oxidation. Because the myocardial respiratory quotient was frequently low, early workers were alerted to the importance of lipids as the major myocardial fuel (Opie, 1969). However, there is still some controversy concerning the preferred myocardial substrate.

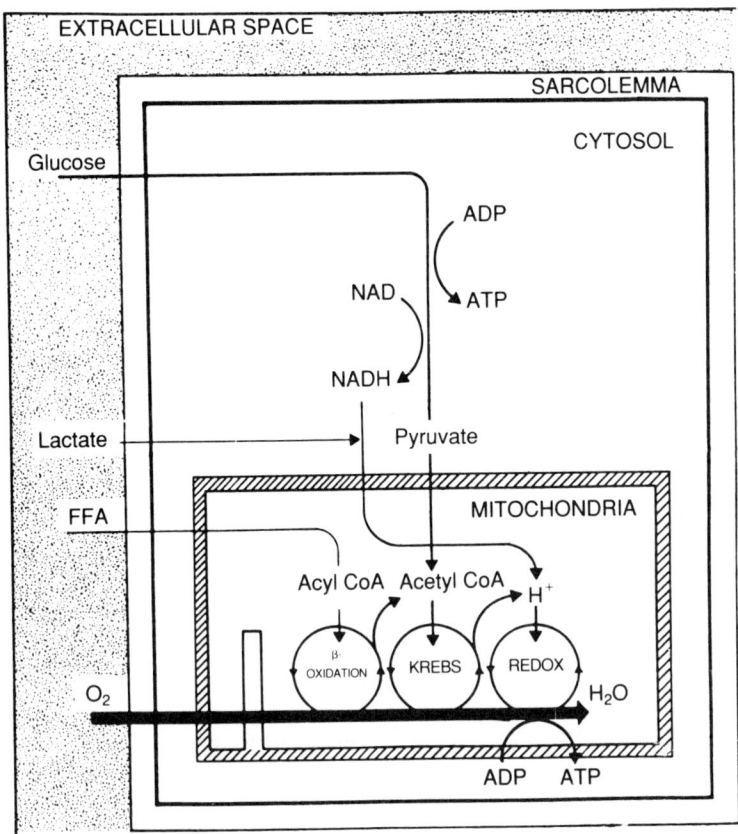

FIGURE 1. Schematic representation of aerobic metabolism in the myocardium.

The overall process of energy production involves the complete oxidation of substrates to carbon dioxide and water (Figure 1). Energy (as ATP) can be generated in the myocardium by two metabolic pathways, glycolysis (anaerobic) and oxidative phosphorylation (aerobic). Under normal conditions the majority (90%) of ATP is produced by the latter pathway (Kobayashi and Neely, 1979).

Before a carbohydrate (such as glucose) can enter the tricarboxylic acid cycle, it must be broken down via the glycolytic pathway. Therefore oxidation of glucose is dependent on the enzymes of anaerobic glycolysis. Lactate, the other major carbohydrate fuel, is dependent on the activity of the lactate dehydrogenase complex.

FREE FATTY ACID OXIDATION IN THE HEART

Although the heart is able to synthesize structural lipids for incorporation into the membranes, the most likely fate of a fatty acid molecule
taken up by the heart is oxidation. The first step in fatty acid oxidation
is their activation to form acyl CoA derivatives. Therefore the enzymes
initially concerned with fatty acids utilization are the acyl CoA
synthetases which exist in the heart with different fatty acid specificities
and locations. Short-chain fatty acids are oxidized by heart mitochondria in the absence of external CoA or of L-carnitine, the role of which
is discussed later in this chapter. This is because the relevant acyl
CoA synthetases are in the same compartment (mitochondrial matrix)
as the enzymes of β-oxidation and the citrate cycle. However, for the
oxidation of long-chain acids, this activation must be followed by the
transfer of long-chain acyl CoA into the interior of the mitochondria.

It is rather curious that the physiologically important long-chain
fatty acids are converted to their CoA derivatives on the wrong side
of the mitochondrial inner membrane, which is impermeable to
coenzyme A. This is particularly strange because the activation of fatty
acid is accomplished by two distinct enzymes that share the same
cytosolic coenzyme A pool, which is very small. One of these enzymes,
representing 80% of the total activity, is attached to the mitochondrial
outer membrane, and the other to the endoplasmic reticulum (De Jong
and Hulsman, 1970). Equally, ATP the product of fatty acid oxidation,
cannot freely reach the cytosol which is the site of its physiological
utilization. The transfer of ATP from the mitochondrial matrix to the
cytosol is, in fact, regulated by the enzyme adenine nucleotide
translocase (Figure 2). In this way, the entry of FFA into the
mitochondria, site of their oxidation to form ATP and the diffusion of
ATP out of the mitochondria is strictly dependent on and, therefore
regulated by, the function of the carnitine shuttle and adenine
nucleotide translocase activity.

Carnitine is synthesized almost exclusively in the liver, from lysine
and methionine (Bohmer, 1974). Bohmer et al (1977) found that heart
cells in culture possess a specific carnitine uptake mechanism. The
plasma concentration of carnitine is about 30 μM; in the heart the
concentration is about 100 times higher. More recently it has been
suggested (Hoppel, 1976) that: (i) L-carnitine, the naturally occurring
form, is able to stimulate fatty acid oxidation by tissue homogenates;
(ii) fatty acyl esters of carnitine are useful substrates for mitochondria;
(iii) these compounds are formed by enzyme-catalysed reversible acyl
transfer from CoA.

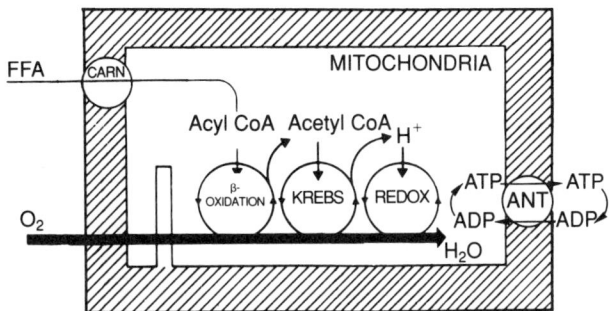

FIGURE 2. Schematic representation of free fatty acid oxidation. Role of carnitine shuttle (CARN) and of adenine nucleotide translocase (ANT).

Later it was recognized that two distinct classes of carnitine acyltransferases exist, normally referred to as carnitine acetyl- and palmitoyltransferases. Little is known about the heart carnitine palmitoyltransferase; however, inhibition experiments with purified liver enzymes have suggested that in mitochondria they exist in two forms with considerably different properties. One of these transferases, the outer or A enzyme, is accessible to extramitochondrial CoA, while the inner, or B enzyme, is within the inner membrane where it uses CoA of the matrix (Figure 3). The overall steps of free fatty acid oxidation can be summarized as follows:

1. extramitochondrial formation of acyl CoA;
2. transfer of the acyl group to carnitine by the outer transferase;
3. delivery of the carnitine ester to the inner transferase;
4. transfer of the acyl group to the matrix CoA;
5. β-oxidation;
6. transfer of intramitochondrial carnitine outside the mitochondria by a carnitine–acylcarnitine translocase system.

Experiments with heart mitochondria have demonstrated that penetration of the inner mitochondrial membrane by acylcarnitine occurs by the acylcarnitine–carnitine exchange or translocases. They are analogous to the ADP–ATP exchange (Figure 2).

The process exhibits 1:1 stoichiometry, so that the total carnitine content in mitochondria remains unchanged. This content is about 3 nmol mg^{-1} protein in isolated mitochondria, corresponding to a matrix concentration of 2–4 mM, similar to the concentration in the cytosol.

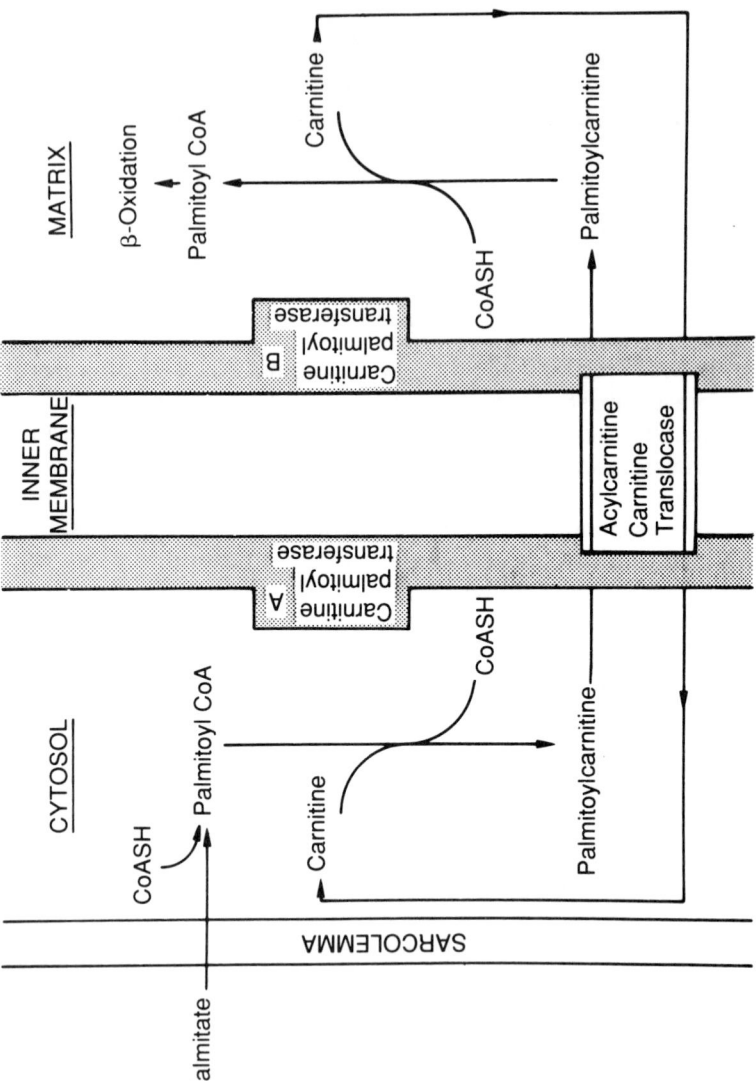

FIGURE 3. Schematic representation of the L-carnitine cycle in the heart.

ROLE OF L-CARNITINE IN THE HEART

The role of L-carnitine in energy production from fatty acid oxidation is obvious: L-carnitine takes part in the shuttle mechanism whereby long-chain fatty acids are transformed to acylcarnitine derivatives and transported across the inner mitochondrial membrane. This is impermeable to long-chain fatty acids and to their CoA esters. Once across the membrane, the acylcarnitine is reconverted to carnitine and to acyl CoA, which undergoes β-oxidation. This interesting action of L-carnitine is essential in heart free fatty acid metabolism.

L-carnitine has a role not only in energy production, but also, indirectly, in energy delivery from the mitochondria to the cytosol. In fact, long-chain acyl CoA is known to inhibit mitochondrial adenine-nucleotide translocase (Shug et al, 1975; Pande and Blanchaer, 1971), the enzyme responsible for the one-to-one exchange of ATP and ADP (Klingenberg et al, 1973). There is evidence that one of the most important effects of L-carnitine administration is the reduction of long-chain acyl CoA in heart tissue, resulting in a reduction of the inhibition of the adenine-nucleotide translocase. In this way, L-carnitine allows ATP to be formed from long-chain acyl CoA and transported from the mitochondria to the cytosol (Figure 2).

In the myocardium, L-carnitine has the important role of scavenging or buffering the toxic metabolites of FFA such as acyl CoA and acetyl CoA which in pathological conditions accumulate in the cytosol and/or in the mitochondria. These compounds are not able to cross heart membranes. L-Carnitine reacts with acyl and acetyl CoA to form acyl- and acetylcarnitines able to diffuse through the heart membranes. In this way they can be eliminated with the urine (Hulsman et al, 1960).

In addition, within the myocardium, L-carnitine is able positively to influence carbohydrate metabolism. It is known that an increased acyl CoA/CoA ratio inhibits the activity of pyruvate dehydrogenase, the key enzyme for the entry of pyruvate into the citric acid cycle. L-carnitine can either directly or indirectly activate pyruvate dehydrogenase. The indirect mechanism is related to a decrease in the acetyl CoA/CoA ratio as consequence of acetyl removal from CoA-mediated carnitine CoA acetyltransferase. It follows that the utilization of pyruvate, and consequently of glucose and lactate, under pathological conditions such as ischaemia (when the metabolism is predominantly anaerobic) increases after L-carnitine administration (Chapter 11 of this book).

It is often assumed that L-carnitine also has a role in permitting the import of acetylCoA by mitochondria, as it does with the long-chain derivatives. However, the doubts regarding this are threefold: (i) acetyl CoA is generated within the mitochondrial matrix; (ii) isolated mitochondria scarcely use external acetyl CoA, even in the presence of carnitine; (iii) isolated mitochondria apparently contain only one form of carnitine acetyltransferase (Edwards et al, 1974).

L-Carnitine is also able to improve the rate of anaerobic metabolism by a direct stimulation of phosphofructokinase.

MYOCARDIAL ISCHAEMIA

The term myocardial ischaemia describes a condition which exists when fractional uptake of oxygen in the heart is not sufficient to maintain the rate of cellular oxidation (Jennings, 1970). This leads to an extremely complex situation which has been studied extensively in recent years (Hillis and Braunwald, 1977; Nayler et al, 1979; Jennings and Reimer, 1981; Neely and Feuvray, 1981; Bourdillon and Poole-Wilson, 1982; Ferrari et al, 1986a).

A large amount of research has been directed to identify the time-course and the precise sequence of biochemical events leading to myocyte necrosis. It is obvious to intrinsic knowledge of this event could lead to rational treatments designed to delay myocardial death (Poole-Wilson, 1985).

At present there is no simple answer to what determines cell death and the lack of recovery of the ischaemic myocardium on reperfusion. Problems arise because:

1. ischaemic damage is not homogeneous and many factors may combine to cause cell death;
2. severity of biochemical changes and development of necrosis are usually associated (both processes being dependent on the duration of ischaemia) and the impossibility of establishing a causal relationship;
3. the inevitability of necrosis can only be assessed by reperfusion of the ischaemic myocardium. Restoration of flow, however, might result in numerous negative consequences, thus directly favouring the occurrence of cell death (Hearse, 1977; Nayler, 1981; Poole-Wilson, 1985; Ferrari et al, 1986a,b).

This latter concept has led to the idea that reperfusion may be deleterious, inducing further injury (Hearse, 1977; Nayler et al, 1980;

Braunwald and Kloner, 1985; Poole-Wilson, 1985). At the moment of reperfusion such phenomena may occur as intracardiac haemorrhage, 'no re-flow', loss of cell enzymes, morphological changes and deterioration of the ischaemic tissue (Braunwald and Kloner, 1985; Ferrari et al, 1986b; Hearse, 1990). The deleterious events associated with reperfusion cannot, however, be avoided by not reperfusing, or by prolonging the ischaemic period in the presence of protective agents. These agents, in the absence of reperfusion, do not restore normal contractile function and are only able to delay, but not avoid, the development of injury (Hearse, 1984; Hearse, 1990). It has been argued that, with the exception of the induction of arrhythmias (Manning and Hearse, 1984), it is difficult to believe that reperfusion causes further injury (Hearse, 1984).

FFAs might play an important detrimental role in the ischaemic and reperfusion-induced heart damage. Evidence that L-carnitine has a protective role in this regard is reviewed in the following discussion.

METABOLIC CHANGES DURING MYOCARDIAL ISCHAEMIA

Immediately after the onset of ischaemia, aerobic metabolism ceases, leaving anaerobic metabolism as the major source of energy production (Figure 4) (Neely et al, 1975). This has two important consequences: the intracellular pH drops (Cobbe and Poole-Wilson, 1980) and tissue content of ATP becomes severely reduced, generation of energy from the anaerobic myocardium being extremely inefficient and the cellular energy reserve in the form of creatine phosphate very limited (Ferrari et al, 1988). Intracellular acidosis inhibits calcium influx through the slow calcium channels and, therefore, reduces contractile activity of the ischaemic cell, which becomes quiescent. However, even when the myocardium is quiescent, energy, in the form of ATP, is required for maintenance of membrane integrity and ionic homeostasis, with extrusion of cytosolic calcium against the cellular and subcellular concentration gradients. The depletion of intracellular ATP results in an increase in the cytosolic calcium concentration, impairment of relaxation (Shen and Jennings, 1972; Nayler et al, 1980) and early activation of anaerobic glycolysis. Pyruvate cannot enter the mitochondria and is converted into lactate, allowing oxidation of NADH in the cytosol and consequently removing the inhibition on glyceraldehyde-

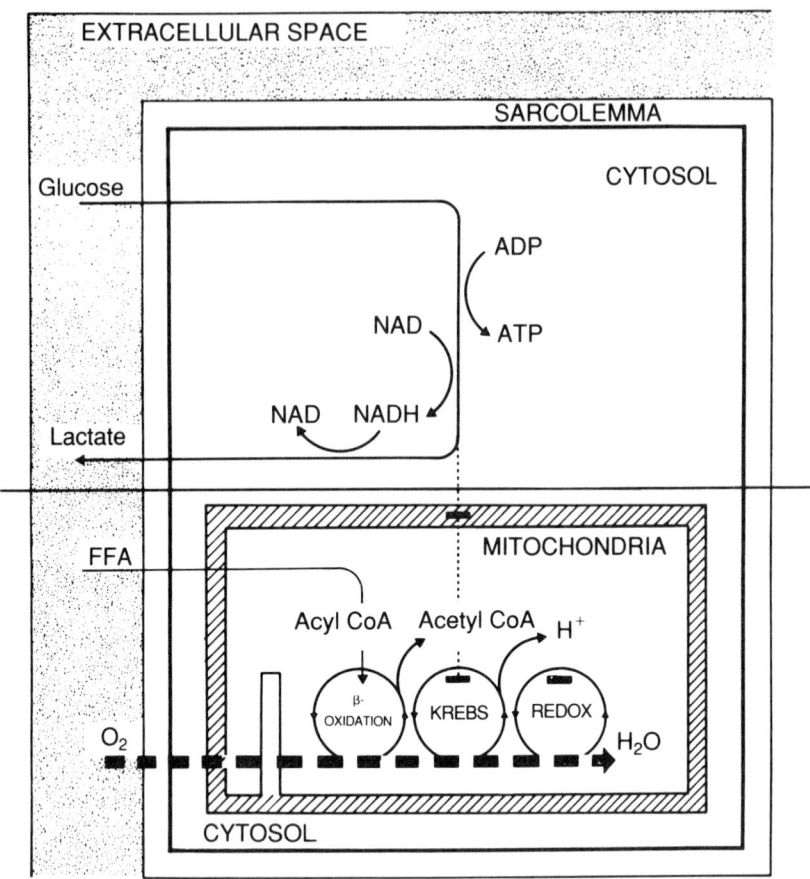

FIGURE 4. Schematic representation of the metabolism of the ischaemic heart.

3-phosphate dehydrogenase, the key enzyme of anaerobic glycolysis (Figure 5).

The clinically detectable signs of these metabolic changes have been demonstrated recently during balloon dilatation of a human coronary artery. They include loss of diastolic tone, regional areas of hypokinesia or akinesia, and increased myocardial content of potassium, lactate and hypoxanthine breakdown products of high-energy phosphate metabolism in the efflux of the coronary circulation (Hugenholtz et al, 1984, De Feyter et al, 1985). Interestingly, these abnormalities precede the other classical clinical signs of ischaemia such as ST segment elevation, chest pain and alterations in the systolic performance of the heart. This series of events is completely reversible: complete occlusion

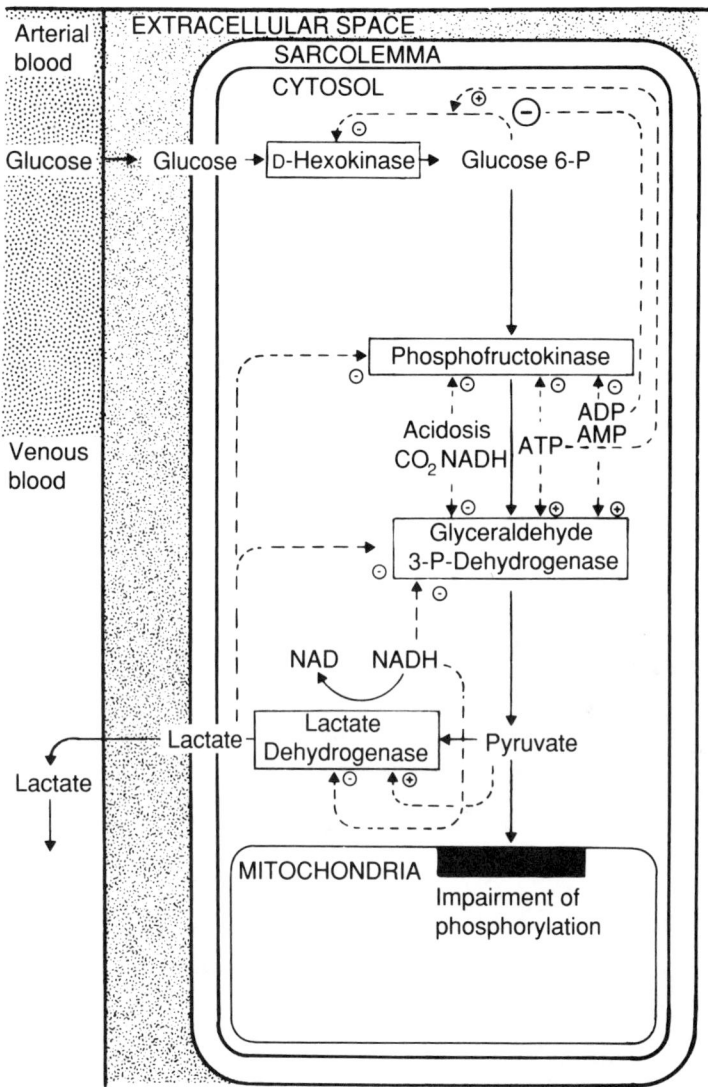

FIGURE 5. Schematic representation of the regulation of anaerobic glycolysis.

of a coronary artery for 5 to 10 minutes can be tolerated without any permanent defects. However, they denote an initial metabolic deterioration which heralds the onset of cellular disruption.

Prolongation of the ischaemic period beyond 10 to 30 minutes (depending on species and experimental models) results in greater changes in ionic homeostasis, an increase in tissue osmolality (Jennings et al, 1985), release of lysosomal enzymes (Ichihara et al, 1987), alteration of membrane phospholipids (Chien et al, 1981), complete depletion of both energy-rich phosphates and their adenine nucleotide precursors, mobilization of the endogenous stores of noradrenaline (norepinephrine) (Ferrari et al, 1989), reduction of L-carnitine content and accumulation of lipids.

These irreversible biochemical alterations produce swelling, disorganization of myofilaments and mitochondrial cristae, nuclear chromatin aggregations and cytoplasmic accumulation of free fatty acids, which are visible with the electron microscope (Figure 6) (Jennings and Ganote, 1976; Schwartz et al, 1984). They are associated with a limited degree of recovery of mechanical function during reperfusion, depending on the duration of the ischaemic episode (Ferrari et al, 1988).

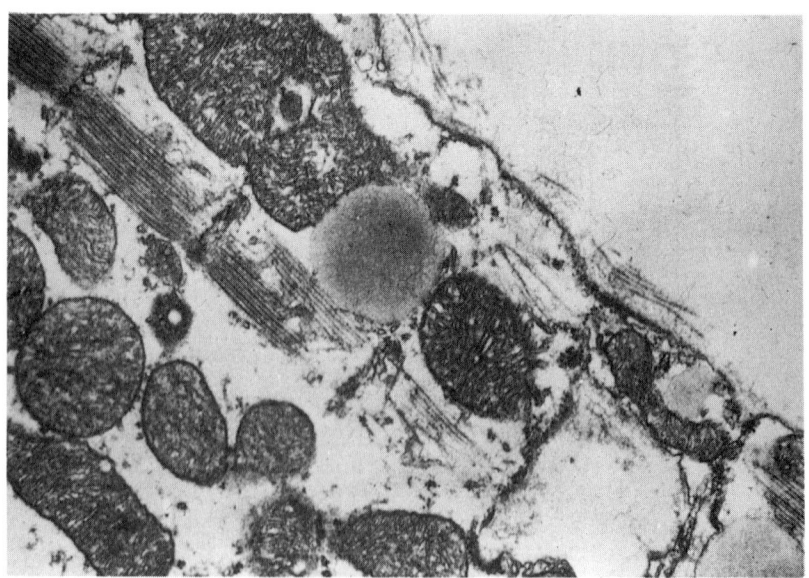

FIGURE 6. Electronmicrograph of longitudinal section of left ventricular free wall of rabbit hearts made ischaemic for 90 minutes. Note the presence of lipid droplets.

If the myocardium remains ischaemic for a longer period of time, the biochemical damage progresses further to involve structural disorganization and cell death. Reperfusion at this late state accelerates the progression towards necrosis.

Upon reperfusion, severely injured cells accumulate large amounts of calcium (Nayler, 1983; Ferrari et al, 1987), develop massive contracture bands and release intracellular macromolecules such as creatine phosphokinase into the extracellular space (Poole-Wilson et al, 1986). These events occur rapidly (within minutes) so that cells severely injured before reperfusion, rapidly become calcium overloaded and doomed to die.

It is relevant to recall here that the progression from reversible to irreversible damage is greatly accelerated by the presence of free fatty acids as myocardial substrate (Figure 7). Glucose or palmitate as myocardial substrates during the ischaemic period considerably accelerates irreversible damage, as indicated by the early increase of diastolic pressure, loss of mitochondrial ATP and accumulation of calcium.

Thus, ischaemia persisting for 60 or more minutes in man should herald the beginning of infarction, depending on the metabolic and mechanical state of the myocardium before the ischaemic episode. Hearts forced to beat at high rates, against a high preload (and therefore requiring higher degrees of oxygen delivery) with poorly developed collateral flow or exposure to higher concentrations of free fatty acids will have more extensive damage than those which are beating slowly, against reduced preload and have ample coronary collateral flow.

Evidence of such a series of events in man, in vivo, however, is more difficult to obtain. Our recent work on heart metabolism during intracoronary thrombolysis or during coronary artery bypass has shown that aerobic metabolism recovers only when coronary flow is reinstated within 60 minutes from the onset of symptoms (Ferrari et al, 1987). Later reperfusion is not associated with substrate utilization; oxygen wastage occurs and is coincident with a worsening of the mechanical performance of the ischaemic myocardium. Free fatty acids have deleterious consequences on this series of mechanisms.

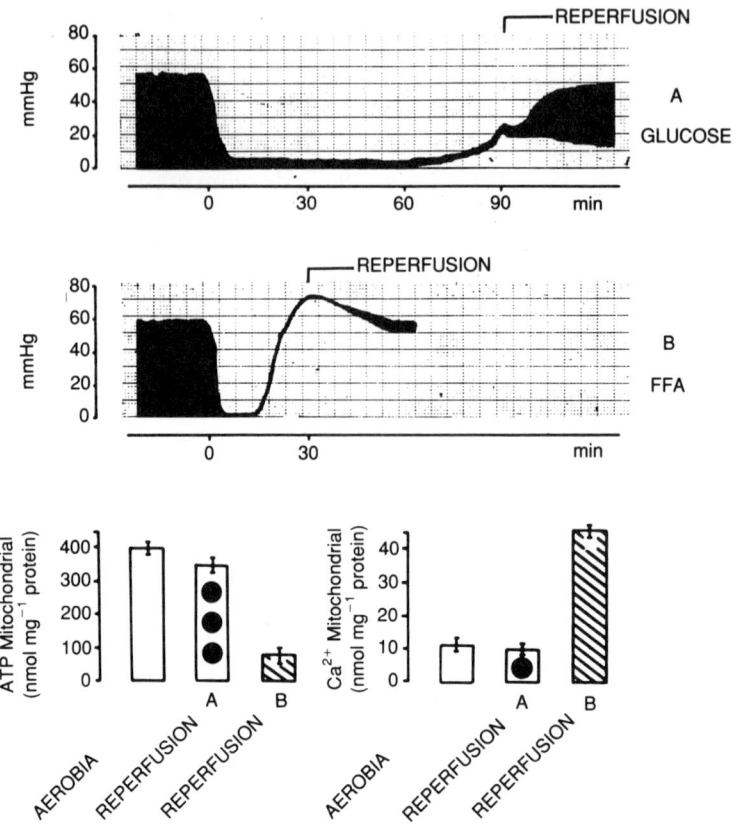

FIGURE 7. Importance of substrate in the development of ischaemic and reperfusion damage (top panels): typical tracing from isolated and perfused rabbit hearts.

DETRIMENTAL EFFECTS OF FATTY ACIDS AND THEIR DERIVATIVES IN ISCHAEMIC AND REPERFUSED HEART

It is well known that in ischaemic myocardial tissue, long-chain fatty acyl CoA and carnitine esters accumulate quickly, even in the absence of exogenous fatty acids (Idell-Wenger et al, 1978). Most of the accumulating long-chain acyl derivatives are hydrolysed from triglycerides and from membrane phospholipids. Exogenous fatty acids, being the main fuel for the myocardium under aerobic conditions, are disadvantageous under oxygen deprivation since their presence further augments the accumulation of long-chain acyl esters in the myocytes (Di Lisa et al, 1982). The accumulation of lipids as free amphiphiles and the degradation of lipids from cellular membranes may contribute to the progression of injury. Both the detergent effect of long-chain acyl compounds and the loss of constituent phospholipids can alter the barrier and transport function of cellular membranes and ultimately lead to their physical destruction (Katz and Messineo, 1981).

Oliver et al (1968) transferred these observations from the laboratory to the clinic. They documented a key association between severe myocardial complications and elevated levels of serum free fatty acids in patients suffering acute myocardial infarction. This association was confirmed, in part at least, in other clinical studies (Gupta et al, 1969; Rutenberg, 1969) and started the debate over the toxic role of fatty acids on cardiac function and structure which still continues.

Several studies have shown that raising the concentration of fatty acids in coronary artery perfusate promotes left ventricular dysfunction and heart failure in both aerobic and ischaemic myocardium (Severeid et al, 1969; Kjekshus and Mjos, 1972; Russo and Margolis, 1972). Conversely, lowering the fatty acid concentration appears to decrease the ischaemic injury, estimated in terms of surface ECG mapping (Kjekshus and Mjos, 1973; Mjos et al, 1974; Miller et al, 1976); mechanical function (Liedtke et al, 1984b; Miller et al, 1986) and biochemistry (Lochner et al, 1976; Katz, 1982). Drugs and strategies used to accomplish this effect include: lipid-free albumin (Kjekshus and Mjos, 1973); b-pyridylcarbinol to inhibit lipolysis (Kjekshus, 1974); p-chlorophenoxisobutarate, nicotinic acid and salicylates to depress free fatty acid extraction (Vik-mo et al, 1979); oxfenicine and 2-tetradecyblicidic acid to inhibit intracellular fatty acid transfer and activation (Liedtke et al, 1984a; Miller et al, 1986); and L-carnitine as will be discussed later.

MECHANISMS OF THE DETRIMENTAL EFFECTS OF FATTY ACIDS IN THE ISCHAEMIC AND REPERFUSED HEART

A variety of mechanisms have been suggested to explain the deleterious effects of fatty acids and their derivatives on cardiac structure and function in ischaemia and reperfusion. The old concept of fatty acids as non-specific detergents (Henderson et al, 1970) has been updated to include detailed considerations of phospholipid hydrolysis in membranes, enhanced activation of a variety of phospholipases which occurs in ischaemia and altered lipid-gel distributions in membrane biolipid, which in turn displace calcium and alter protein function (Katz and Messineo, 1981; Katz, 1982). The idea that fatty acids could act as antagonists to mitochondrial function and respiration have been recently expanded to include a number of sub-organelles, membrane and enzyme systems. In vitro, the uncoupling effects of fatty acids on mitochondrial oxidative phosphorylation is a well-known phenomenon (Borst et al, 1962; Hulsmann et al, 1960). The uncoupling ability is attributed to the stimulation of latent ATPase, ionophore and general detergent-like effects.

Fatty acids and their derivatives cause amphiphilic effects by their incorporation into membranes and consequent disruptions such as displacing calcium from negatively charged binding sites of phospholipids (Katz and Messineo, 1981). It has been proposed that the predominant requirement of a membrane perturbant is simply that the perturbing molecule reacts strongly within the membrane. The perturbation increases with increasing chain length of the amphiphile (Pressman and Hardy, 1956; Miller et al, 1972). It has been shown that amphiphile constituents further impair contractivity of the ischaemic myocardium (Liedtke et al, 1988), depress activity of ATP-dependent calcium transport in sarcoplasmic reticulum (Pitts et al, 1978; Lopaschuk et al, 1983), and Na^+,K^+-ATPase in sarcolemma, possibly through free radical-induced lipid peroxidation (Mak et al, 1986). Fatty acids and acyl CoA esters also have the ability to depress enzyme systems in mitochondria, sarcoplasma reticulum and sarcolemma (Liedtke, 1981) as well as generating free radicals (Liedtke et al, 1984b). In the cytosol, they have been found to inhibit triglyceride lipase (Severson and Hurley, 1982; McDonough and Neely, 1988). Lysophospholipids, breakdown products of phospholipids accumulating in membranes during ischaemia can cause arrhythmias, myocyte contracture and coronary artery constriction, even at subcritical micelle concentrations (Bergmann et al, 1981; Corr et al, 1984).

A site-specific interaction of long-chain acyl CoA esters with the mitochondrial ADP/ATP carrier has also been described (Shrago, 1978). Competitive inhibition with adenine nucleotides on the cytosolic side of the inner mitochondrial membrane and the reversal of this inhibition by removal of the acyl CoA by carnitine are properties which support the concept that long-chain acyl CoA esters modulate the carrier and influence the energetic state of the cell (Chua and Shrago, 1977; Ferrari, 1988).

Figure 8 is a scheme of the possible detrimental effects of fatty acids.

The literature incriminating fatty acids is not without criticism as some investigators have found no correlations between fatty acid excess and myocardial dysfunction. Most et al (1974) reported no further worsening of electrocardiographic (ST segment) changes on precordial mapping in a pig infarct model receiving lipid infusions.

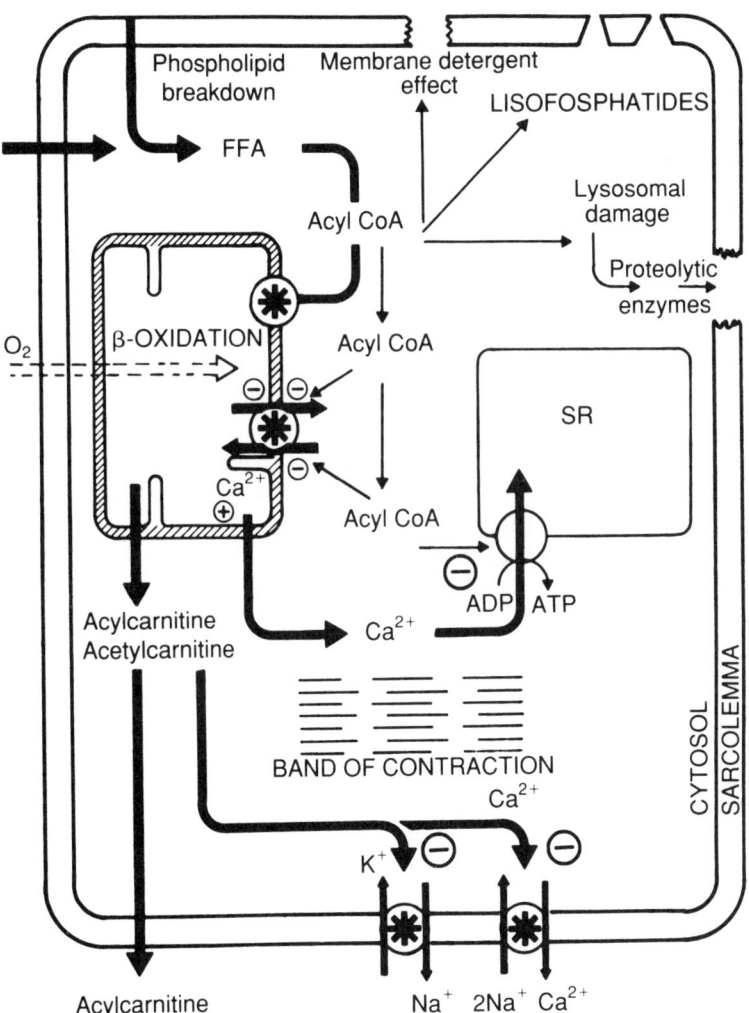

FIGURE 8. Schematic representation of free fatty acid toxicity in the ischaemic myocardium.

Others found only moderate changes in mechanical function associated with excess fatty acids during ischaemia (Shine and Douglas, 1988). Opie and colleagues (1971) noted in a series of dogs with coronary ligation that excess fatty acids exaggerated ectopic activity, but only in the presence of adrenaline infusions. Rutenberg et al (1969) in early clinical trials of arrhythmogenesis did note a correlation between cardiac complications and elevated plasma free fatty acids in infarcted patients, but cautioned that these effects were probably due to catecholamines.

EVALUATION OF THE CARDIAC PROTECTIVE EFFECTS OF L-CARNITINE IN LABORATORY ANIMALS

The finding that the ischaemic and failing heart is associated with a depauperation of carnitine (Whitmer et al, 1978; Shug et al, 1978; Idell-Wenger et al, 1978; Suzuki et al, 1981a, Borum et al, 1978; Hoppel et al, 1982; York, 1983; Yamashita et al, 1985, 1986; Whitmer, 1986, 1987), concomitant with intracellular accumulation of various components of free fatty acid metabolism known to be associated with tissue injury (Opie, 1979; Piper and Das, 1987), has stimulated a considerable amount of animal work on the possibility that L-carnitine may protect the ischaemic and failing heart.

Several different animal species, models as well as functional and metabolic parameters of injury have been utilized to test the possible beneficial effects of L-carnitine. We have, in the following survey, differentiated between the studies on ischaemia and those on heart failure.

PROTECTIVE EFFECTS OF L-CARNITINE AGAINST MYOCARDIAL ISCHAEMIA

Studies on mitochondrial function and on the energy status of the myocardium

In view of the essential role of L-carnitine in mitochondrial metabolism, the possibility that carnitine may protect the ischaemic reperfused heart through a mechanism involving the preservation of mitochondrial function and, consequently, of the myocardial energy stores has been considered. The studies which tested this hypothesis produced positive results (Imai et al, 1984; Branca et al, 1986; Bahl and Bressler, 1987; Duan and Karmazyn, 1990). It has been suggested that the beneficial effects of carnitine on mitochondrial function are due to its antagonists properties on lipid intermediates such as long-chain acyl CoA and acylcarnitine which alter mitochondrial function and reduce adenine nucleotide translocase activity (Pande and Blachaer, 1971; Chua and Shrago, 1977; Liedtke and Nellis, 1979; Katz and Messineo, 1981; Liedtke et al, 1981; Dipalma, 1986; Piper and Das, 1987; Van der Vusse et al, 1987). This hypothesis has been questioned by the fact that the concentration of lipid intermediates required to inhibit mitochondrial function in vitro is substantially higher than that achieved in vivo (La Nove et al, 1981) and other intracellular protective mechanisms against these compounds might be operating during ischaemia and reperfusion (Farnier and Rahim, 1985; de Villiers and Lochner, 1986).

Interestingly Duan and Karmazyn demonstrated that P_i induces mitochondrial dysfunction by inhibiting the electron transport chain system as well as ADP/ATP translocase activity. The former can be selectively prevented in a dose-dependent manner by carnitine. The P_i-induced dysfunction may be different from that produced by acyl CoA and its prevention may account for one of the important mechanisms of the protective effects of carnitine on the heart. Thus it is possible that carnitine exerts other intracellular functions in addition to its well-established role in fatty acid metabolism.

Interestingly, Imai et al (1984) suggested that the improvement of mitochondrial oxidative phosphorylation in dogs with coronary artery ligation is of central importance for the anti-arrhythmic effects of L-carnitine in the same experimental model. Furthermore Duan and Karmazyn (1989) were able to show that carnitine improves ventricular recovery after reperfusion in the ischaemic isolated rat heart through a mechanism mediated by improved mitochondrial respiratory activity. This study is particularly important as it shows that carnitine, through this mechanism, can protect the isolated rat heart in contrast to previous suggestions that the protective effects of carnitine could not be observed in this species due to the poor washout of cellular carnitine during the course of ischaemia (Neely et al, 1979; Hearse et al, 1980).

Studies with intact animals subjected to acute ischaemia

Indeed, the group at the University of Madison was the first to demonstrate the cardiac protective effect of carnitine in animal models with myocardial infarction (Folts et al, 1978; Liedtke et al, 1978, 1981; Shug et al, 1978; Liedtke and Nellis, 1979). These studies proved that L- or DL-carnitine, injected intravenously or directly into the coronary circulation of the open-chest, anaesthetized dog and/or swine prior to coronary artery ligation, attenuated the decrease in free carnitine, and the increase of both long-chain acylcarnitine and long-chain acyl CoA observed in the ischaemic area of heart from untreated animals. In addition, carnitine reduced the inhibition of myocardial adenine nucleotide translocase, improved adenosine triphosphate production, lessened electrocardiographic evidence of cell injury, improved the mechanical performance of the ischaemic and reperfused heart and protected the myocardial cell from subsequent episodes of ischaemia. These findings have been confirmed by Suzuki et al (1981b) who, in order to simulate the detrimental effects at high plasma FFA concentrations, treated their dogs with heparin and intralipid solution before and during coronary artery ligation. In this particular preparation, L-carnitine administration decreased plasma FFA levels reduced myocardial long-chain acyl CoA, improved tissue stores of high-energy phosphate and the mechanical performance of the hearts.

Interestingly these studies, together with those of Liedtke and Nellis (1979) using excess of free fatty acids, indirectly suggested a possible role of L-carnitine as a buffer or scavenger of their toxic metabolites; an effect which was later shown to be operating in patients with myocardial infarction. In 1982, Liedtke and colleagues, using a model of working swine heart, were able to demonstrate the superiority of L-carnitine over its racemate to protect the ischaemic heart.

Studies on ischaemic-induced arrhythmias

The accumulation of both acyl esters and lysophosphoglycerides has been suggested as an important factor in ischaemia and reperfusion-induced cardiac dysfunction, including the development of arrhythmias (Corr et al, 1979, 1981, 1984; Katz, 1982; Liedkte, 1988; Janse and Wit, 1989; Van der Vusse et al, 1989). Their amphiphilic properties may facilitate their incorporation into the sarcolemma with consequent perturbation of ion transport and electrophysiological derangements (Katz and Messineo, 1981; Corr et al, 1984).

Much attention has been focused on the loss of carnitine and accumulation of FFAs and related intermediates as the predisposing factor to malignant dysrhythmias during ischaemia. Consequently, several studies employing different experimental models have been conducted to test the possible antiarrhythmic effects of carnitine (Di Palma et al, 1975; Folts et al, 1978; Liedtke and Nellis, 1979; Suzuki et al, 1981; Hayashi et al, 1982, 1984; Kobayashi et al, 1983; Imai et al, 1984; Matusi et al, 1985; Nakaya and Tohse, 1986; Duan and Karmazyn, 1989; Yokota et al, 1989). All of them showed positive results, but the mechanism underlying the antiarrhythmic properties of L-carnitine is still poorly understood. Several studies demonstrated an association between preservation of mitochondrial function resulting in an improvement of mitochondrial oxidation of FFA intermediates such as long-chain acyl CoA and the antiarrhythmic effect of carnitine during both ischaemia and reperfusion (Liedtke and Nellis, 1979, Suzuki et al, 1981b; Imai et al, 1984; Duan and Karmazyn, 1989). Other studies reported beneficial effects of carnitine against electrophysiological derangements induced by hypoxia (Hayashi et al, 1982; Kobayashi et al, 1983; Hayashi et al, 1984), palmitoylcarnitine (Matsui et al, 1985; Yokota et al, 1989), lysophosphatidylcholine (Duan and Moffat, 1991) and reperfusion (Hayashi et al, 1984; Duan and Moffat, 1991). Furthermore, studies using excess free fatty acid have pointed out the possibility that carnitine may indirectly influence arrhythmias by reducing blood levels of FFAs and by buffering their toxic and arrhythmogenic metabolites (Folts et al, 1978; Liedtke and Nellis, 1979; Suzuki et al, 1981b).

Whatever the mechanism of action, there is clear evidence that carnitine can inhibit various cellular mechanisms of ischaemic and reperfusion arrhythmias, including abnormal automaticity and coupled beat, mainly by reducing the ischaemia-induced changes of the maximum diastolic potential.

PROTECTIVE EFFECTS OF L-CARNITINE AGAINST HEART HYPERTROPHY AND CARDIOMYOPATHIES

Studies on heart hypertrophy

Several workers have shown that cardiac hypertrophy induced by pressure-overload is associated with altered carnitine content. In this regard, rats (Riebel et al, 1983), rabbits (Levis and Cameron, 1979) and guinea-pigs (Wittels and Spann, 1968) subjected to surgically-induced pressure overload showed a reduced myocardial level of carnitine. On the contrary, hypertrophied hearts of spontaneously hypertensive rats (SHR) exhibited elevated levels of carnitine (Foster et al, 1985). Alterations in tissue carnitine content in cardiac hypertrophy may result from changes in the kinetics of the carrier-mediated transport process, changes in the diffusion component of uptake due to alterations in surface area for diffusion, and/or changes in carnitine efflux from the heart (Reibel et al, 1987). Alternatively, altered tissue carnitine may also result from changes in serum carnitine concentrations (Vary and Neely, 1982a, 1982b).

Interestingly Litwin et al (1990) have shown that inhibition of long-chain fatty acid oxidation with 2-tetradeglyclycidic acid, a compound that inhibits the activity of long-chain acyl CoA carnitine transferase induces cardiac hypertrophy and diastolic dysfunction. Exogenous administration of L-carnitine has been proved to reduce the degree of hypertrophy (Tripp and Shug, 1984; Yamashita et al, 1985, 1986; Whitmer, 1986; Whitmer, 1987).

Studies on cardiomyopathic striam hamsters

Carnitine stores are markedly reduced in striam hamsters with either the dilated or the hypertrophic forms of cardiomyopathy (Borum et al, 1978; Hoppel et al, 1982; York et al, 1983; Yamashita et al, 1985; Whitmer, 1986). A defect in the membrane transport of carnitine has been suggested to occur in these cardiomyopathic hamsters (York et al, 1983). High doses of L-carnitine have been shown to exert a beneficial effect on left ventricular contractility, rate of left ventricular relaxation; tissue content of high-energy stores and oxidative metabolism of animal models with two distinct forms of cardiomyopathy, i.e. dilated and hypertrophic. These effects occured with no resulting morbidity in the control or either group of cardiomyopathic hamsters throughout the treatment period. Total myocardial carnitine levels were restored to normal in the L-carnitine-treated dilated myopathic hearts, but no increase of total stores of carnitine was found in the hypertrophic hearts. Thus, the beneficial effects of L-carnitine on the myopathic hypertrophic heart cannot be explained by restoration of myocardial carnitine stores. L-Carnitine may have improved the use of other substrates such as glucose, resulting in increased energy metabolism and improved cardiac function (Borum et al, 1978; Hoppel et al, 1982; York et al, 1983; Yamashita et al, 1985; Whitmer, 1986).

Studies on other forms of cardiomyopathies

The effect of carnitine on free fatty acid, malondialdehyde, taurine and glutathione levels in myocardium was studied in rats administered isoproterenol to induce stress in the myocardium resulting in myocardial ischaemia. Carnitine decreased the levels of free fatty acid and malondialdehyde (an index of lipid peroxidation) when compared with control rats given isoproterenol alone. Taurine and glutathione also registered a fall in the carnitine-treated animals when compared with rats treated with isoproterenol alone. The results indicate that carnitine, by decreasing the levels of these parameters, helps the myocardium survive the stress induced by isoproterenol (Sushamakumari et al, 1989).

Carnitine has also been successfully used to prevent, in different animal species, adriamycin-induced cardiomyopathy, a condition associated with accumulation of FFAs and long-chain acyl CoA esters and disruption of intracellular calcium homeostasis. In addition, increasing myocardial carnitine content can increase heart function in cardiomyopathies associated with diabetes (Paulson et al, 1984, 1986b; Nicholls et al, 1991). The beneficial effect of L-carnitine in this condition can be explained by the effects of these agents on overcoming fatty acid inhibition of glucose oxidation.

CONCLUSION

In laboratory studies, L-carnitine has been shown to exert cardiac protection, particularly when used prophylactically and in conditions of clear carnitine deficiencies such as ischaemia and heart failure. The ultimate mechanism of action involves a reduction of the toxicity of long-chain CoAs and a consequent improvement of glucose oxidation suggesting that, in the heart, L-carnitine acts as a metabolic modulator.

REFERENCES

Bahl JJ & Bressler R (1987) *Annu. Rev. Pharmacol. Toxicol.* 27: 257–259.
Bergmann SR, Ferguson TB & Sobel BE (1981) *Am. J. Physiol.* 240: H229–H237.
Bing RJ (1954) *Harvey Lecture Series* 50: 27–70.
Bing RJ, Siegel A, Vitale A et al (1953) *Am. J. Med.* 15: 284–296.

Bohmer T (1974) *Biochim. Biophys. Acta* 343: 551–557.

Bohmer T, Eiklid K and Jonssen J (1977) *Biochim. Biophys. Acta* 465: 627–633.

Borst P, Loos JA, Christ EJ & Slater EC (1962) *Biochim. Biophys. Acta* 62: 509–518.

Borum PR, Park JH, Law PK & Roelofs RL (1978) *J. Neurol. Sci.* 38: 113–121.

Bourdillon PD & Poole-Wilson PA (1982) *Circ. Res.* 50: 360–368.

Branca D, Toninello A, Scutari, G et al (1986) *Biochem. Biophys. Res. Commun.* 139: 303–307.

Braunwald E & Kloner R (1985) *J. Clin. Invest.* 76: 1713–1719.

Chien KR, Reeves JP, Buia LM et al (1981) *Circ. Res* 48: 711–719.

Chua BH & Shrago E (1977) *J. Biol. Chem.* 252: 6711–6720.

Cobbe SM & Poole-Wilson A (1980) *J. Mol. Cell. Cardiol.* 12: 745–749.

Corr PB, Cain ME, Witkowski FX et al (1979) *Circ. Res.* 44: 822–832.

Corr PB, Snyder DW, Cain ME et al (1981) *Circ. Res.* 49: 354–363.

Corr PB, Gross RW & Sobel BE (1984) *Circ. Res.* 55: 135–154.

De Feyter PJ, Serryus PW, van der Brand M et al (1985) In Hungenholtz, PG & Goldman BS (eds) *Unstable Angina*, pp 229–237. Stuttgart: Schattauer.

De Jong JW & Hulsmann WC (1970) *Biochim. Biophys. Acta* 197: 127–135.

De Villiers M & Lochner A (1986) *Biochim. Biophys. Acta* 876: 309–312.

Di Lisa F, Raddino R, Bertorelli, D et al (1982). In Caldarera CM & Harris P (eds) *Advances in Studies on Heart Metabolism*, pp 269–274. Bologna. Clueb Publication.

Dipalma JR (1986) *Am. Fam. Physician.* 34: 127–129.

Dipalma JR, Ritchie DM & McMichael RF (1975) *Arch. Int. Pharmacodyn. Ther.* 217: 246–251.

Drake AJ (1982) *Basic Res. Cardiol.* 77: 1–11.

Duan J & Karmazyn M (1989) *Br. J. Pharmacol.* 98: 1319–1320.

Duan J & Karmazyn M (1990) *Eur. J. Pharmacol.* 189: 163–174.

Duan J & Moffat MP (1991) *Eur. J. Pharmacol.* 192: 355–363.

Edwards YH, Chase JFA, Edwards MR & Tubbs PK (1974) *Eur. J. Biochem.* 46: 209–215.

Farnier NC & Rahim M (1985) *Biochemistry* 24: 2387–2388.

Ferrari R, (1988) In de Jong (ed.) *Myocardial Energy Metabolism*, pp 35–43. Dordrecht-Boston-Lancaster: Martinus Nijhoff Publishing.

Ferrari R, Ceconi C, Curello S et al (1986a) *Eur. Heart J.* 7: 3–12.

Ferrari R, Albertini A, Curello S et al (1986b) *J. Mol. Cell. Cardiol.* 18: 484–498.

Ferrari R, Ceconi C, Curello S et al (1987) In Dhalla NS, Innes IR and Beamish RE (eds) *Myocardial Ischaemia*, pp 67–84. Boston, Martinus Nijhoff Publishing

Ferrari R, Curello S, Cargnoni A et al (1988) *J. Mol. Cell. Cardiol.* 20: 119–133.

Ferrari R, Boffa GM, Ceconi C et al (1989) *Bas. Res. Cardiol.* 84: 606–622.

Folts JD, Shug AL, Koke JR & Bittar P (1978) *Am. J. Cardiol.* 41: 1209–1214.

Foster KA, O'Rourke B & Reibel DK (1985) *Am. J. Physiol.* 249: E183–E186.

Gupta DK, Jewitt DE, Young R et al (1969) *Lancet* ii: 1209–1213.

Hayashi H, Suzuki Y, Masumura Y et al (1982) *Jpn. Heart J.* 23: 623–628.

Hayashi H, Suzuki Y, Abe M et al (1984) *J. Electrocardiol.* 17: 85–88.

Hearse DJ (1977) *J. Mol. Cell. Cardiol.* 9: 607–616.

Hearse DJ (1984) In Opie LH (ed.) *Calcium Antagonists and Cardiovascular Disease*, pp 129–135. New York: Raven Press.

Hearse DJ (1990) *Cardiovasc. Drugs Ther.* 4: 767–776.

Hearse DJ, Shattock MJ & Manning AS (1980) *Thorac. Cardiovasc. Surg.* 28: 253–258.
Henderson AC, Most AS, Parmely WW et al (1970) *Circ. Res.* 26: 439–449.
Hillis J & Braunwald E (1977) *New Engl. Med.* 17: 920–932.
Hoppel CL (1976) In Martonosi A (ed.) *The Enzymes of Biological Membranes*, pp 119–143. New York: Plenum Press.
Hoppel CL, Tandler B, Parland W et al (1982) *J. Biol. Chem.* 257: 1540–1548.
Hugenholtz PG, Deckers JW, van der Gieessen WJ et al (1984) *JUPHAR Proceedings*, pp 257–268: Macmillan.
Hulsmann, WC, Elliot WB & Slater EC (1960) *Biochem. Biophys. Acta* 39: 267–276.
Ichihara K, Haneda T, Ondera S & Abiko Y (1987) *J. Pharmacol. Exper. Ther.* 242: 1109–1113.
Idell-Wenger JA, Lee WG & Neely JR (1978) *J. Biol. Chem.* 253: 4310–4318.
Imai S, Matsui K, Nakazawa M et al (1984) *Br. J. Pharmacol.* 82: 533–542.
Janse MJ & Wit AL (1989) *Physiol. Rev.* 69: 1049–1051.
Jennings RB (1970) *J. Mol. Cell. Cardiol.* 1: 345–349.
Jennings RB & Ganote CE (1976) *Circ. Res.* 38: 180–190.
Jennings RB & Reimer KA (1981) *Am. J. Pathol.* 102: 241–255.
Jennings RB, Schaper J, Hill ML et al (1985) *Circ. Res.* 56: 262–278.
Katz AM (1982) *J. Mol. Cell. Cardiol.* 14: 627–631.
Katz AM & Messineo FC (1981) *Circ. Res.* 48: 1–13.
Kjekshus JK (1974) *Cardiovasc. Res.* 8: 73–80.
Kjekshus JK & Mjos OD (1972) *J. Clin. Invest.* 51: 1767–1776.
Kjekshus JK & Mjos OD (1973) *J. Clin. Invest.* 52: 1770–1778.
Kobayashi A & Neely JR (1979) *Circ. Res.* 44: 166–175.
Kobayashi A, Suzuki Y, Kamikawa T et al (1983) *Jpn. Circ. J.* 47: 536–541.
LaNove KF, Watts JA & Koch CD (1981) *Am. J. Physiol.* 241: H663–H666.
Levis NW & Cameron AJV (1979) *Metabol. Clin. Exp.* 28: 601–613.
Liedtke AJ (1981) *Prog. Cardiovasc. Dis.* 23: 321–336.
Liedtke AJ (1988) *J. Mol. Cell. Cardiol.* 20: 65–71.
Liedtke AJ & Nellis SH (1979) *J. Clin. Invest.* 64: 440–448.
Liedtke AJ, Nellis S & Neely JR (1978) *Circ Res.* 43: 652–661.
Liedtke AJ, Nellis SH & Whitesell LF (1981) *Circ. Res.* 48: 859–866.
Liedtke AJ, Nellis SH, Whitesell LF & Mahar CQ (1982) *Am. J. Physiol.* 243: H691–H697.
Liedtke AJ, Nellis SH & Mjos OD (1984a) *Am. J. Physiol.* 247: H378–H394.
Liedtke AJ, Mahar CQ, Ytrehus K & Mjos OD (1984b) *Basic. Res. Cardiol.* 79: 513–518.
Liedtke AJ, De Maison L, Eggleston AM et al (1988) *Circ. Res.* 62: 535–542.
Litwin SE, Raya TE, Gay RG et al (1990) *Am. J. Physiol.* 258: H51–H56.
Lochner A, Kotze JCN & Gevers W (1976) *J. Mol. Cell. Cardiol.* 8: 465–480.
Lopaschuk GD, Tahiliani AG, Vadlaumudi RVSV et al (1983) *Am. J. Physiol.* 245: H969–H976.
McDonough KH & Neely JR (1988) *J. Mol. Cell Cardiol.* 20: 31–39.
Mak IT, Kramer JH & Weglicki WB (1986) *J. Biol. Chem.* 261: 1153–1157.
Manning AS & Hearse DJ (1984) *J. Mol. Cell. Cardiol.* 16: 497–518.
Mathew S, Menon PVG & Kurup PA (1986) *Aust. J. Exp. Biol. Med. Sci.* 64: 79–87.

Matsui K, Nakazawa M, Takeda K & Imai S (1985) *Jap. J. Pharmacol.* 39: 263–271.

Miller KW, Paton WDM, Smith EB & Smith RA (1972) *Anesthesiology* 36: 339–351.

Miller NE, Mjos OD & Oliver MF (1976) *Clin. Sci. Mol. Med.* 51: 209–213.

Miller WP, Liedtke AJ & Nellis SH (1986) *Am. J. Physiol.* 251: H547–H553.

Mjos OD, Kjekshus JK & Lekven J (1974) *J. Clin. Invest.* 53: 1290–1299.

Most AS, Capone RJ, Szydlik P, Bruno CA & De Vona TS (1974) *Cardiology* 59: 201–212.

Nakaya H & Tohse N (1986) *Br. J. Pharmacol.* 89: 749–754.

Nayler WG, (1981) *Am. J. Pathol.* 102: 262–270.

Nayler WG, (1983) *Eur. Heart J.* 4: 33–41.

Nayler WG, Poole-Wilson PA & Williams A (1979) *J. Mol. Cell. Cardiol.* 11: 683–706.

Nayler WG, Ferrari R & Williams A (1980) *Am. J. Cardiol.* 46: 242–248.

Neely JR & Feuvray D (1981) *Am. J. Pathol.* 102: 282–291.

Neely JR, Whitmer JT & Rovetto MJ (1975) *Circ. Res.* 37: 733–741.

Neely JR, Garber D, McDonough K & Idell-Wenger J (1979) In Winbury MM & Abiko Y (eds), *Ischaemic Myocardium and Antianginal Drugs*, pp 225–234. New York: Raven Press.

Nicholls TA, Lopaschuk GD & McNeill JH (1991) *Am. J. Physiol.* (in press).

Oliver MF, Kurien VA & Greenwood TW (1968) *Lancet* i, 710–715.

Opie LH (1969) *Am. J. Cardiol.* 77: 100–122.

Opie LH (1979) *Am. Heart J.* 97: 375–380.

Opie LH, Thomas M, Owen P et al (1971) *Lancet* i, 818–822.

Pande SV & Blanchaer MC (1971) *J. Biol. Chem.* 246: 402–408.

Paulson DJ, Schmidt MJ, Traxler JS et al (1984) *Metabolism* 33: 358–363.

Paulson DJ, Traxler J, Schmidt MJ Noonan, J et al (1986) *Cardiovasc. Res.* 20: 536–541.

Piper HM, & Das A (1987) *Basic Res. Cardiol.* 82: 187–192.

Pitts BJR, Tate CA, Vanwinkle WB et al (1978) *Life Sci.* 23: 391–402.

Poole-Wilson PA (1985) In Parrat JR (ed.) *The Nature of Myocardial Damage Following Reoxygenation. Control and Manipulation of the Calcium Movement*, pp 99–108. New York: Raven Press.

Poole-Wilson PA, Harding DP, Bourdillon PDU & Tones MA (1986) *J. Mol. Cell. Cardiol.* 16: 175–187.

Pressman BC & Lardy HA (1956) *Biochim. Biphys. Acta* 21: 458–466.

Reibel DK, Uboh CE & Kent RL (1983) *Am. J. Physiol.* 244: H839–H843.

Reibel DK, O'Rourke, B & Foster KA (1987) *Am. J. Physiol.* 252: H561–H565.

Russo JV & Margolis S (1972) *Circulation* 215: 45–46.

Rutenberg HL, Pamintuan JC & Soloff LA (1969) *Lancet* ii, 559–564.

Schwartz P, Piper HM, Spahr R & Spieckermann PG (1984) *Am. J. Pathol.* 115: 359–361.

Severeid L, Connor WE & Long JP (1969) *Proc. Soc. Exp. Biol. Med.* 131: 1239–1243.

Severson DL & Hurley B (1982) *J. Mol. Cell. Cardiol.* 14: 467–474.

Shen AC & Jennings RB (1972) *Am. J. Pathol.* 67: 417–433.

Shine KI & Douglas AM (1988) *J. Mol. Cell. Cardiol.* 15: 251–260.

Shrago E (1978) *Life Sci.* 22: 1–6.

Shug AL, Shrago E, Bittar N et al (1975) *Am. J. Physiol.* 228: 689–692.

Shug AL, Thomsen JH, Folts JD et al (1978) *Arch. Biochem. Biophys.* 187: 25–33.
Sushamakumari S, Jayadeep A, Suresch Kumar JS & Menon VP (1989) *Ind. J. Exp. Biol.* 27: 134–137.
Suzuki Y, Kamikawa T, Kobayashi A et al (1981a) *Jpn. Circ. J.* 45: 687–694.
Suzuki Y, Kamikawa T & Yamazaki N (1981b) *Jpn. Circ. J.* 45: 552–555.
Tripp ME & Shug AL (1984) *Biochem. Med.* 32: 199–206.
Van der Vusse GJ, Prinzen FW, Van Bilsen M et al (1987) *Basic. Res. Cardiol.* 82: 157–162.
Van der Vusse GJ, Van Bilsen M & Reneman RS (1989) *News Physiol. Sci.* 4: 49–58.
Vary TC & Neely JR (1982a) *Am. J. Physiol.* 243: H154–H158.
Vary TC & Neely JR (1982b) *Am. J. Physiol.* 242: H585–H592.
Vik-mo H, Riemersma RA, Mjos OD & Oliver MF (1979) *Scand. J. Clin. Lab. Invest.* 39: 559–568.
Yamashita T, Hayashi H, Kaneko M et al (1985) *Jpn. Heart J.* 26: 833–844.
Yamashita T, Kobayashi A, Yamazaki N et al (1986) *Cardiovasc. Res.* 20: 614–620.
Yokota S, Hironaka Y & Ohara N (1989) *Res. Comm. Chem. Pathol. Pharmacol.* 66: 179–190.
York CM, Cantrell CR & Borum PR (1983) *Arch. Biochem. Biophys.* 221: 526–533.
Whitmer JT (1986) *J. Mol. Cell. Cardiol.* 18: 307–317.
Whitmer JT (1987) *Circ. Res.* 61: 396–408.
Whitmer JT, Idell-Wenger JA, Rovetto MJ & Neely JR (1978) *J. Biol. Chem.* 253: 4305–4315.
Wittels B & Spann JF (1968) *J. Clin. Invest.* 47: 1787–1793.

14

EFFECTS OF L-CARNITINE IN CORONARY ARTERY DISEASE PATIENTS

R. Ferrari and O. Visioli

Several reviews have been written regarding the action of endogenous carnitine in fatty acid metabolism in man (Bach, 1982; Borum, 1983; Bremer, 1983; Rebouche and Engel, 1983) and on its role in the metabolism of the ischaemic heart (Opie, 1979; Siliprandi et al, 1984; Logue, 1985a, 1985b, 1985c; Goa and Brodgen, 1987; Liedtke, 1987; Editorial, 1991).

Essentially, the rationale for the use of L-carnitine in patients with ischaemic heart disease relates to two major premises. Firstly, free carnitine concentrations in tissue from the infarcted area of patients who died of myocardial infarction is lower than that from heart tissues of patients who died from causes other than heart disease (Spagnoli et al, 1982; Suzuki et al, 1982a). Secondly, in patients suffering acute myocardial infarction there is a key association between severe

265

L-Carnitine and Its Role in Medicine:
From Function to Therapy. ISBN 0–12–253940–0

myocardial complications and elevated levels of serum free fatty acids (FFA), suggesting that accumulation of FFA is toxic to the heart (Oliver et al, 1968; Gupta et al, 1969; Rutenberg, 1969).

It has been demonstrated that the increase of long-chain coenzyme A (CoA) and acylcarnitine esters, consequent to the low myocardial free carnitine concentrations, inhibit adenyl-nucleotide translocase and ATP transport (Opie, 1979; Siliprandi et al, 1984) as well as the activity of pyruvic dehydrogenase which may result in increased lactic acid production (Ferrari et al, 1984a). Consequently, administration of exogenous L-carnitine reverses the inhibition of adenyl-nucleotide translocases and ameliorates pyruvate metabolism, reducing lactate production and acidosis (Thomsen et al, 1979; Ferrari et al, 1984a, 1984b; Reforzo et al, 1986).

Further, it has been postulated that L-carnitine has a scavenging or buffering action on toxic products of FFA which accumulate during ischaemia. L-Carnitine reacts with intracellular acyl CoA which cannot cross the heart membrane to form acylcarnitine, thus enabling diffusion of these deleterious compounds through the sarcolemma into blood and urine (Rizzon et al, 1989).

Recently, however, information has become available suggesting that L-carnitine may be advantageous not only for patients with myocardial infarction, but also for those with less severe coronary artery disease (CAD). L-Carnitine plays an important role not only in reducing FFA toxicity, but also in enhancing carbohydrate utilization, thus acting as a 'metabolic modulator' for the heart.

These new concepts have been generated by several studies. Bartles et al (1991) demonstrated that even after short periods of reversible ischaemia, as in the case of angina pectoris, there is a loss of L-carnitine from the heart. Capaldo et al (1991) and Lopaschuk (1991) showed that L-carnitine administration increases glucose utilization in patients with insulin-dependent diabetes as well as in the post-ischaemic reperfused hearts. Cederblad et al (1976) proved the existence of a close relationship between tissue carnitine levels and glycogen content.

These concepts form the basis of this chapter. Existing data on the role of L-carnitine in cardiovascular disorders are examined critically to assess its therapeutic potential and to define its novel mechanism of action. The effects of L-carnitine on patients with myocardial infarction are not considered, as they will be covered extensively in the next chapter.

EFFECTS OF L-CARNITINE IN PATIENTS WITH ISCHAEMIC HEART DISEASE

As mentioned in the previous chapter on the molecular mechanism of action of L-carnitine, administration of exogenous carnitine to laboratory animals prior to, or during, ischaemia increases tissue levels of free carnitine, decreases concentration of long-chain acyl CoA esters and affords cardiac protection (Folts et al, 1978; Shug et al, 1978; Liedtke and Nellis, 1979; Ferrari et al, 1984c; Bahl and Bressier, 1987; Bieber, 1988). These encouraging results have stimulated several studies on the effects of exogenously administered DL- or L-carnitine on haemodynamic and metabolic indices in coronary artery disease patients. In addition, the efficacy of therapy with L-carnitine in patients with chronic stable angina pectoris, ischaemic arrhythmias and heart failure has been investigated. All these aspects will now be examined separately.

EFFECTS OF L-CARNITINE ON HAEMODYNAMICS AT REST

The positive inotropic activity of L-carnitine observed in laboratory animals has also been detected in man. This effect, however, is more pronounced in patients with evidence of ischaemic heart disease who are subjected either to exercise or atrial pacing than in normal individuals.

An intravenous dose of L-carnitine (40 mg kg^{-1}) administered to healthy volunteers for 2 min produced modest variations in heart rate and arterial pressure (Schiavoni et al, 1983). We used the same intravenous dosage in patients with coronary artery disease (CAD) and normal left ventricular function (assessed in terms of regional ejection fraction and left ventricular end diastolic pressure, LVEDP) (Table 1). Acute administration of L-carnitine did not significantly change the parameters measured, including total coronary flow (Ferrari, 1988). Likewise, insignificant alterations in the pre-ejection period (PEP), left ventricular ejection time (LVET), the PEP/LVET ratio and in echocardiographic indices of cardiac performance were observed in CAD patients at rest (Schiavoni et al, 1983). On the contrary, Cherchi et al (1982) reported a reduced PEP/LVET ratio (relative to placebo) in CAD patients consequent to oral administration of 60 mg kg^{-1} of

TABLE I.

Effect of L-carnitine (40 mg kg^{-1}) on haemodynamic parameters at rest. Data represent the mean ± SE of 16 patients with coronary artery disease. No statistically significant (NS) differences were observed

	Before	After L-carnitine	
Heart rate (beats per min)	79 ± 4	76 ± 3	NS
Mean aortic systolic pressure (mmHg)	146 ± 4	144 ± 6	NS
Mean aortic diastolic pressure (mmHg)	76 ± 6	73 ± 2	NS
Pulmonary artery pressure (mmHg)	18 ± 1	18.2 ± 3	NS
Cardiac output (litres per min)	5.9 ± 0.7	5.9 ± 0.6	NS
Coronary sinus blood flow (ml per min)	127 ± 14	129 ± 12	NS
Heart rate × systolic blood pressure	11.53 ± 0.12	11.38 ± 0.14	NS

L-carnitine. Giordano et al (1983) found a similar beneficial effect on cardiac performance after a more prolonged period of carnitine (2 mg day^{-1}) administration. After 10 days of intravenous treatment, a significant increase in PEP, concomitant with a reduction in LVET was observed as compared with baseline values.

EFFECTS OF L-CARNITINE ON MYOCARDIAL METABOLISM AT REST

Although L-carnitine has little effect on heart function at rest, it should exert important changes on its metabolism. This information, however, is rare, mainly because measurements of heart metabolism in man is strictly dependent upon invasive methodology, i.e. catheterization of the coronary sinus (Bing, 1954).

We had the opportunity to investigate the effects of a central venous infusion of L-carnitine (40 mg kg^{-1}) on resting heart metabolism in 25 selected CAD patients without previous myocardial infarction and with normal myocardial function. Part of these data have been published before (Ferrari et al, 1984a, 1984b). Myocardial metabolism was measured in terms of arterial–coronary sinus difference, myocardial percentage of extraction and myocardial uptake of FFA, lactate and glucose (Ferrari, 1988).

In our patients there was a linear relationship between myocardial arterial–coronary sinus difference for the different substrates and their availability in the arterial blood (Ferrari et al, 1984a, 1984b). As expected, the two major substrates metabolized from the heart before administration of L-carnitine were glucose and FFA (Figure 1). The oxygen extraction ratio for carbohydrates in the form of glucose and lactate accounted for up to 11% of oxygen consumption and that of FFA for about 39% (Figure 2). Thus, the human heart, like that of the rat, prefers fatty acids as a respiratory fuel (Neely and Morgan, 1974; Zierler, 1976).

Administration of L-carnitine had several important effects:

1. a significant reduction in arterial concentration of FFA (Figure 3);
2. a significant increase in myocardial uptake of FFA (Figure 1);
3. a reduction in myocardial uptake of glucose (Figure 1);
4. no major changes in myocardial uptake of lactate (Figure 1);
5. no significant increase in the overall oxygen consumption of the heart (Figure 2).

The reduction of circulating FFA occurred in the absence of major

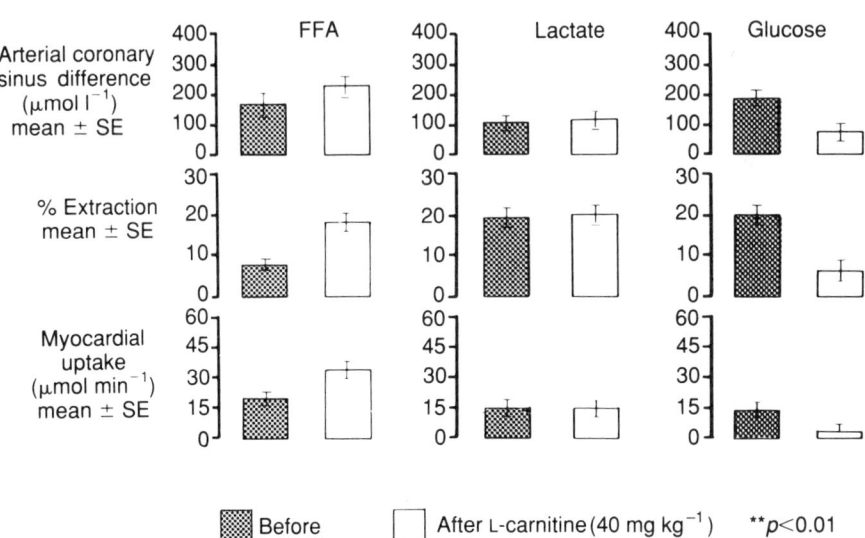

FIGURE 1. Effect of L-carnitine on arterial coronary-sinus difference, % extraction and myocardial uptake of FFA, lactate and glucose of 16 patients with coronary artery disease studied at rest. Data represent the mean ± SE. L-Carnitine significantly ($p < 0.05$, analysis of variance) increased myocardial uptake of FFA and reduced that of glucose.

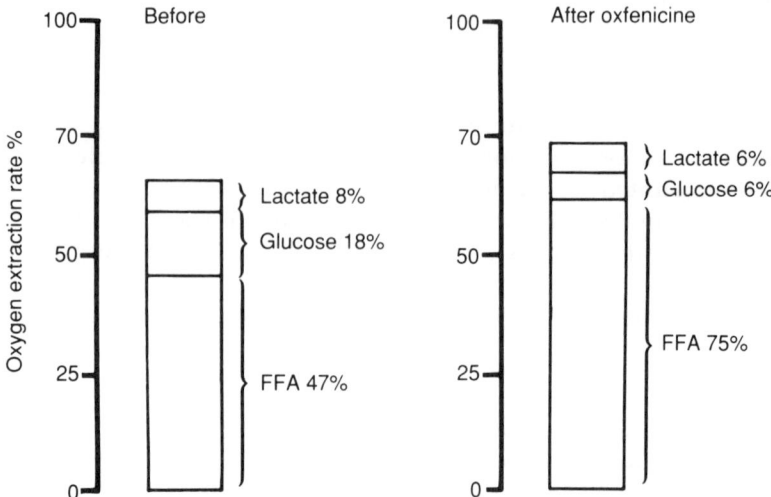

Figure 2. Effect of L-carnitine on myocardial oxygen consumption of 16 patients with coronary artery disease studied at rest. L-Carnitine did not significantly modify overall oxygen consumption, but increased the oxygen utilized for oxidation of FFA with respect to that used for carbohydrates.

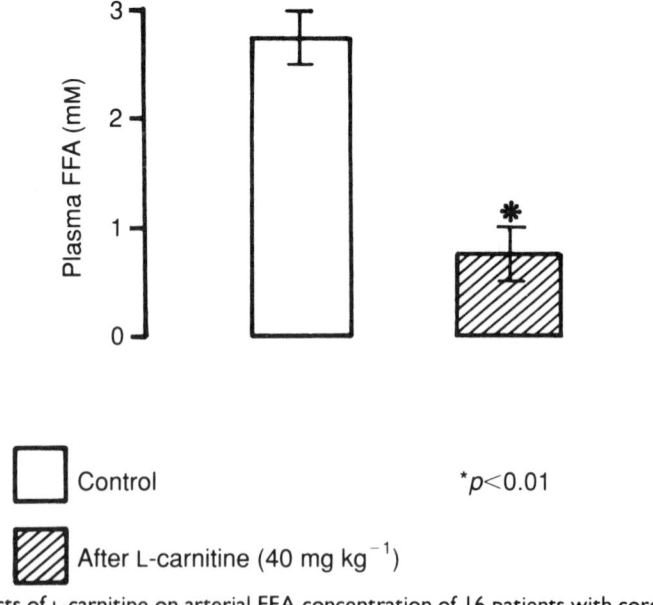

Figure 3. Effects of L-carnitine on arterial FFA concentration of 16 patients with coronary artery disease at rest. Data represent the mean ± SE L-carnitine significantly ($p < 0.001$, student's T-test) reduced circulating FFA.

systemic haemodynamic changes that could account for an increased utilization of these substrates. Thus, this effect appears to be primarily dependent on the metabolic and systemic action of L-carnitine. The stimulation of FFA oxidation by L-carnitine in all tissue is well known (Fritz, 1959; Opie, 1979). Since we measured only the myocardial uptake of FFA in our study, it is impossible to establish whether the effects of L-carnitine involved primarily the heart or other organs. Certainly administration of L-carnitine to our CAD patients stimulated myocardial FFA utilization.

These data indirectly suggest that the heart of CAD patients, even in the absence of previous myocardial infarction, lacks L-carnitine. The recent findings of Bartles et al (1991), showing that during each single attack of angina there is a release of L-carnitine from the heart into the coronary sinus, strongly support this hypothesis. It is probable that CAD patients exibit defects in carnitine uptake, which is energy-dependent (Bieber, 1988) and are not able to balance the loss of carnitine that occurs during acute ischaemia. The chronic perpetuation of this series of events leads to a condition of relative L-carnitine deficiency.

The reduction of circulating FFA and the stimulation of their myocardial uptake is clinically relevant for two main reasons: (i) high levels of FFA are arrhythmogenic and correlate with a poor prognosis (Oliver et al, 1968; Gupta et al, 1969; Rutenberg, 1969); (ii) the amount of heat, and consequently of energy, liberated per gram of fat oxidized is about 37.8 kJ g^{-1}, more than twice that per gram of carbohydrate, which is about 16.8 kJ g^{-1}. Interestingly, enthalpies are quite similar when calculated in terms of oxygen consumption (Fat: 20.5 kJ gO$_2$$^{-1}$; carbohydrates: 21.2 kJ gO$_2$$^{-1}$). This is in accordance with the finding that more oxygen is required to oxidize a gram of fat than a gram of carbohydrate.

Accordingly, in our CAD patients, after L-carnitine administration, overall myocardial oxygen consumption was unchanged. This is essential for patients with coronary artery disease who have a limited supply of oxygen and suggests that L-carnitine acts as 'metabolic modulator', influencing not only FFA metabolism but also that for carbohydrates with the final oxidation of the two substrates following the same step: reduction of acetyl CoA in the Krebs cycle (Ferrari, 1988).

The finding that acute administration of L-carnitine increases myocardial utilization of FFA at the expense of glucose is also a very important effect with clinical relevance, particularly in relation to chronic treatment with L-carnitine. Carbohydrates, especially those stored in the form of glycogen, represent a pool of emergency substrates utilized anaerobically by the myocardium under conditions of acute and severe energy need, like stress, exercise or, more relevant to this discussion, during acute ischaemia. The relatively high myocardial glucose utilization in CAD patients due to L-carnitine deficiency might lead to a depauperation of glycogen stores, thus reducing the myocardial metabolic defence against attacks of acute ischaemia. Conversely, administration of L-carnitine for prolonged periods of time improves FFA consumption and reduces myocardial glucose utilization, thus restoring glycogen stores. A clear relationship between carnitine concentration and enzyme activities representative of different metabolic pathways has been demonstrated in skeletal muscle of healthy volunteers (Cederblad et al, 1976). In particular, a highly significant correlation was found between carnitine concentration and muscle glycogen content as well as with the overall anaerobic glycolytic activity. We are at present investigating whether this correlation is also valid for heart muscle. If this turns out to be the case, chronic administration of L-carnitine to CAD patients will exert a favourable 'metabolic pre-conditioning', restoring the natural metabolic defence against ischaemia. It is also relevant to recall here that it has been suggested recently that shifting myocardial metabolism from lipids to carbohydrates induces cardiac hypertrophy and diastolic dysfunction (Litwin et al, 1990). L-Carnitine acting as a metabolic modulator restores a balanced myocardial metabolism and should avoid these negatives events.

EFFECTS OF L-CARNITINE ON HAEMODYNAMICS DURING EXERCISE OR INDUCED TACHYCARDIA

An improved cardiac performance during exercise has been demonstrated in healthy volunteers and athletes who received high doses of L-carnitine (Marconi et al, 1985; Angelini et al, 1986; Dal Negro et al, 1986; Vecchiet et al, 1990). Evaluations of the effect of carnitine on exercise tolerance in symptomatic CAD patients demonstrated improvements in exercise capacity (Kosolcharoen et al, 1981; Kamikawa et al, 1984; Cherchi et al, 1985; Canale et al, 1988). Increased in overall exercise time and in the time of onset of ischaemia were noted in all the studies. Echocardiographic evaluation suggests improvement in left ventricular function after 30 days of treatment with 2 g day^{-1} of L-carnitine (Cherchi et al, 1985).

Several studies have examined the effects of carnitine on the response to induced tachycardia in CAD patients (Thomsen et al, 1979; Ferrari et al, 1984a, 1984b; Reforzo et al, 1986). All report a reduction in the tachycardia-induced increase in LVEDP. In addition, Reforzo and coworkers (1986) and Thomsen and colleagues (1979) showed that either DL or L-carnitine diminished the magnitude of ischaemic-type ST-segment depression that occurred during atrial pacing and increased the maximal heart rate and rate-pressure product tolerated by the CAD patients. Carnitine also prolonged the time of onset of angina.

EFFECTS OF L-CARNITINE ON MYOCARDIAL METABOLISM DURING INDUCED TACHYCARDIA

Myocardial metabolism under stress conditions has been investigated in controlled studies in CAD patients subject to atrial pacing (Thomsen et al, 1979; Ferrari et al, 1984a, 1984b; Reforzo et al, 1986).

Single intravenous doses of L-carnitine 40 or 140 mg kg^{-1} or DL-carnitine 20 or 40 mg kg^{-1} decreased production of lactate from the myocardium or maintained a positive extraction of the substrate at peak sinus pacing relative to that seen in untreated or placebo-treated control groups. Moreover, the mean myocardial FFA extraction ratio increased significantly (Ferrari et al, 1984a, 1984b).

Figures 4 and 5 summarize our data. Figure 4 shows that in CAD patients a constant atrial stimulation at 140 beats per minute, prolonged enough to cause typical angina pain, causes no major change in myocardial uptake of FFA and a clear production of lactate and glucose in the coronary sinus, suggesting anaerobic metabolism and impairment of glucose utilization. Figure 5 shows that in the same patients pre-treatment with L-carnitine converted lactate production at peak pacing stress into extraction, thus preventing anaerobiosis. In addition, there was an increase in the uptake of FFA as well as in that of glucose, confirming the role of L-carnitine as a metabolic modulator, improving not only FFA, but also carbohydrate metabolism. The finding that glucose and lactate uptake were maintained confirms the data of Lopaschuk (1991) and supports the concept that L-carnitine is important in the critical condition of energy need. All these alterations are due to the metabolic properties of L-carnitine, since the increase in coronary flow induced by atrial pacing was not affected.

There is no simple explanation for these effects of L-carnitine. During ischaemia, the reduced oxygen availability leads to a decrease in

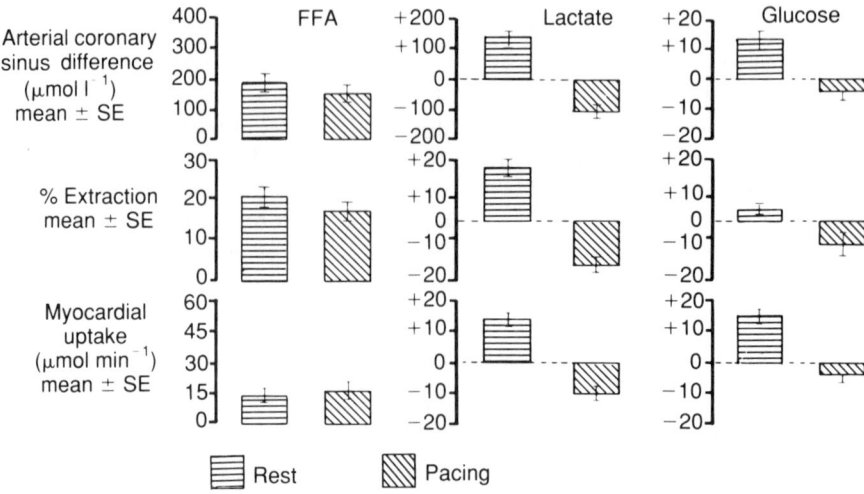

FIGURE 4. Effects of atrial pacing on arterial coronary sinus difference, % extraction and myocardial uptake of FFA, lactate and glucose of 25 patients with coronary artery disease. Data represent the mean ± SE. Atrial pacing caused a production of lactate into the coronary sinus and an impairment of glucose utilization.

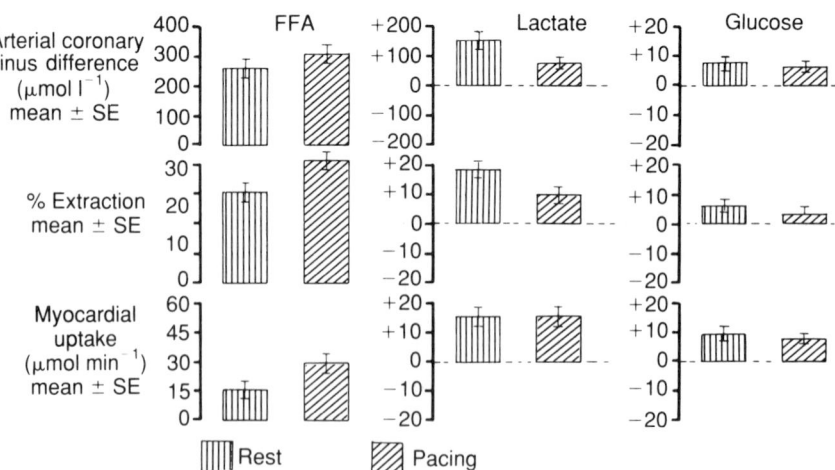

FIGURE 5. Effects of L-carnitine on arterial coronary sinus difference, % extraction and myocardial uptake of FFA, lactate and glucose of 25 patients with coronary artery disease subjected to atrial pacing. Data represent the mean ± SE. L-Carnitine converted lactate production (see Figure 4) to FFA and glucose.

mitochondrial electron transport, which, in turn, causes an accumulation of NADH and long-chain acyl CoA. An increased NADH/NAD ratio and acyl CoA/CoA ratio inhibits the activity of pyruvate dehydrogenase (PDH), the enzyme which regulates the entry of pyruvate into the citric acid cycle. Under these conditions pyruvate is preferentially converted to lactate with consequent lactate production.

L-Carnitine can reduce lactate production under ischaemic conditions either by activating PDH directly or by provoking a decrease in the acetyl CoA/CoA ratio, as a consequence of acetyl removal from CoA, mediated by carnitine CoA acetyltransferase. Therefore, the utilization of pyruvate and consequently of lactate in the oxidative pathway, induced by L-carnitine, may be attributed to enhanced PDH activity, rather than to an increase in oxygen availability induced by L-carnitine.

Another possible explanation for the effects of L-carnitine on lactate metabolism is an indirect effect on phosphofructokinase (PFK) activity, the enzyme regulating the rate of anaerobic glycolysis. The activity of this enzyme is inhibited by a high cytosolic ATP concentration, whilst it is stimulated by low cytosolic ATP concentration. Under ischaemic conditions the ATP concentration in the cytosol decreases either as a result of reduced oxidative metabolism or because the activity of adenine-nucleotide translocase is inhibited by long-chain acyl CoA. This causes sequestration of ATP into the mitochondrial matrix with a decrease of cytosolic ATP and a consequent stimulation of PFK. By removing long-chain acyl CoA, carnitine prevents its inhibitory action of adenosine-nucleotide translocase, thus improving the ATP transfer to the cytosolic compartment. The increased cytosolic ATP levels might decrease PFK activity and lactate production.

EFFECTS OF L-CARNITINE IN PATIENTS WITH STABLE ANGINA PECTORIS

The available short-term controlled studies in patients with stable angina pectoris indicate that orally administered L-carnitine 900–2000 mg daily improves exercise tolerance and increases the time of ST-segment depression (Garzya and Amico, 1980; Kosolcharoen et al, 1981; Kamikawa et al, 1984; Selveres, 1984; Cherchi et al, 1985; Canale et al, 1988). In the study of Garzya and Amico (1980) patients received isosorbide dinitrate together with either L-carnitine or DL-carnitine. L-Carnitine was significantly more effective than the racemate in reducing the frequency of angina attacks and glyceryl trinitrate consumption.

The clinical importance of these findings has been further evaluated in a large, open, multicentre study of more than 1000 patients with stable angina pectoris (Fernandez et al, 1985). L-Carnitine was administered at 2 g daily for 12 months. During the initial 6 months of therapy with L-carnitine, anginal attacks decreased in frequency by 60%. Similarly, 60% of the patients discontinued the use of glyceryl trinitrate. In addition, a significant reduction occurred in the need for traditional cardiovascular drugs, such as calcium antagonists, beta-blockers, diuretics and cardiac glycosides.

Symptomatic improvement has also been reported by Orlando and Rusconi (1986), who treated elderly patients with chronic, stable ischaemic heart disease. After 2 months of therapy with 4–6 mg daily of L-carnitine, these patients reported a decrease in palpitations, asthenia and precordial pain. The New York Heart Association (NYHA) functional class improved and there was an amelioration in the left ventricular shortening fraction, assessed by echocardiography.

Interestingly, the study of Fernandez et al (1985) also reports a reduction in the use of conventional antiarrhythmic drugs in patients with atherosclerotic disease or angina who received oral L-carnitine for 1 year. The antiarrhythmic potential of carnitine was further evaluated in a double-blind, parallel group trial examining the effects of L-carnitine on ventricular arrhythmias in patients with acute myocardial infarction (Rizzon et al, 1989); 56 subjects received infusion of 100 mg kg^{-1} of L-carnitine or placebo every 12 h for a total of 36 h. After 2 days of therapy, there was a significant decrease in hours of multiform preventricular contractions (PVC$_s$), number of PVC$_s$ per hour and number of episodes of ventricular tachycardia. These antiarrhythmic effects have been confirmed in a similar study by Martina et al (1991).

It is of interest to recall here that in the Rizzon et al (1989) study, the antiarrhythmic effect of L-carnitine was accompanied by a significant decrease of serum FFA concomitant with increases in serum and urinary levels of free carnitine and short- and long-chain carnitine esters during the first 48 hours after admission to the coronary unit. This suggests that L-carnitine acts by buffering myocardial toxic free fatty acid esters which may be arrhythmogenic. Suzuki et al (1982b) reported a reduction in the frequency of ventricular arrhythmias in haemodialysis patients treated with 2 mg day^{-1} of L-carnitine. This therapy resulted in an increase in plasma carnitine concentration, which was below normal levels before treatment, and in a reduction of plasma FFA concentration.

This potential antiarrhythmic effect of carnitine is particularly interesting in that it occurs in the absence of negative inotropism, which is often a limiting component for the utilization of traditional antiarrhythmic drugs.

EFFECTS OF L-CARNITINE IN PATIENTS SUBJECTED TO HEART SURGERY AND WITH CARDIOGENIC SHOCK

Pre-operative administration of L-carnitine has been attempted to improve the metabolic alteration caused by the total and global ischaemia imposed on CAD patients during aorto–coronary bypass surgery. The rationale for this use of carnitine is provided by the favourable results obtained in animal models with ischaemia (Folts et al, 1978; Shug et al, 1978; Suzuki et al, 1981; Ferrari et al, 1984c; Siliprandi et al, 1984; Liedtke, 1988) and in CAD patients exposed to tests aimed to induce ischaemia. Bohles et al (1986) studied 40 patients undergoing aorto–coronary bypass surgery who received either oral L-carnitine (1 g daily in 3 doses, for 2 days prior to surgery) plus 0.5 g intravenously immediately before surgery or no treatment. The concentration of myocardial free carnitine significantly increased, and that of long-chain acylcarnitine decreased in patients receiving carnitine therapy. Treated patients showed a reduced concentration of lactate in the myocardium correlated with significantly elevated concentrations of ATP, suggesting that metabolism of long-chain FFA was improved.

Corbucci and Peduto (1991), in an open study with a design similar to that of Bohles et al (1986), showed that administration of L-carnitine reduces the increase in plasma lactate concentration caused by heart surgery. Part of the data generated by this study are reported in Figure 6. These results indicate clearly that L-carnitine reduces the generalized cellular acidosis consequent to heart surgery, probably by reducing the inhibition of pyruvate dehydrogenase caused by accumulation of long-chain acyl CoA. Following this line of evidence, the same authors administered L-carnitine to 80 patients with cardiogenic shock in an open study randomized against bicarbonate. L-Carnitine significantly improved survival over bicarbonate (Corbucci et al, 1991).

Whilst these results are clearly of interest, particularly considering that mortality in cardiogenic shock is highly correlated to acidosis and to plasma lactate concentration (Cohen et al, 1983; Cooper et al, 1990; Kette et al, 1990), further evidence is needed before the role of

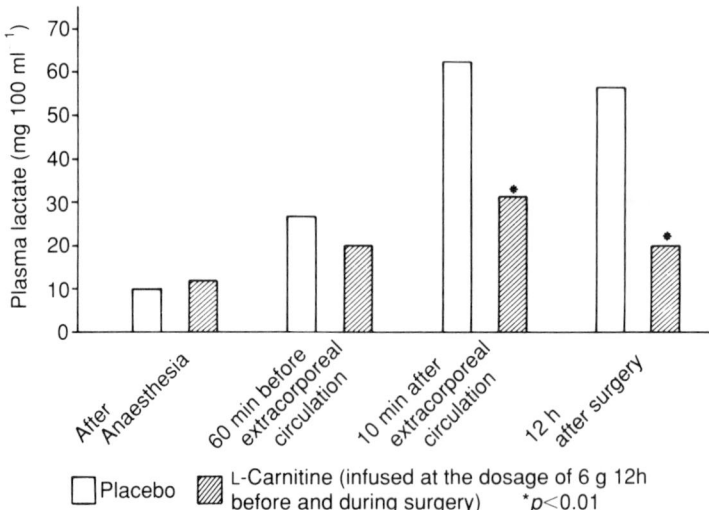

FIGURE 6. Effect of L-carnitine on venous lactate concentration of patients with ischaemic heart disease subjected to heart surgery. Data represent mean ± SE. L-Carnitine significantly reduced ($p < 0.01$, variance analysis) blood lactate concentration after surgery (Corbucci et al, 1991).

L-carnitine as an adjuvant in the treatment of cardiogenic shock is defined.

EFFECTS OF L-CARNITINE IN OTHER CARDIOVASCULAR DISORDERS

Heart failure and left ventricular dysfunction

A reduced carnitine concentration was found in the myocardium of patients undergoing cardiac transplant. Significant reduction in free carnitine concomitant with increases in short- and long-chain acylcarnitine has been detected in papillary muscle biopsy from patients with chronic heart failure undergoing valve replacement (Suzuki et al, 1982a). Similarly, a reduced carnitine concentration has been reported in patients with less severe congestive heart failure secondary either to dilated cardiomyopathy or to coronary artery, valvular or hypertensive heart disease (Regitz et al, 1990), suggesting a possible role of L-carnitine in heart failure. This possibility was evaluated by

Ghidini et al (1988) in a controlled study involving 38 patients treated with oral L-carnitine (1g, twice daily) for 45 days. They demonstrated improvement of NYHA functional class, echocardiographic measures of left ventricular wall motion and size, as well as a reduction in the incidence of cardiac arrhythmias. In addition, L-carnitine administration caused a marked decrease of digoxin requirements.

Cardiotoxicity induced by cytotoxic antibiotics

Development of cardiotoxicity has limited the long-term use of anthracycline antibiotics. The cardiotoxic effects of these agents include: tachycardia, coronary spasm, elevated serum levels of the MB-CPK isoenzyme, electrocardiographic abnormalities and congestive heart failure. These toxic effects might depend upon accumulation of FFA and long-chain acyl CoA esters (Pepine, 1991). In animals, L-carnitine protects cardiac myocytes from the deleterious effects of doxorubicin (Alberts et al, 1978; Maccari and Ramacci, 1981; Neri et al, 1986).

A few uncontrolled trials have investigated the effects of L-carnitine administration on different indices of cardiac performance in patients treated with a cumulative dose of anthracyclines, less than 500 mg m^{-2} (Furitano et al, 1984; De Leonardis et al, 1985, 1987; Neri et al, 1986). The expected increase in serum CPK-MB did not occur in patients receiving L-carnitine prior to administration of either doxorubicin or daunorubicin. A negative inotropic effect, evaluated by means of maximum velocity of circumferential fibre-shortening (VCF max) assessed by echocardiography, occurred in patients treated with doxorubicin alone, but not in those receiving concomitant L-carnitine 1 g intravenously.

These results are encouraging and, if confirmed by controlled studies, constitute a valid and innovative approach to reduce anthracycline-induced cardiotoxicity (Goa and Brogden, 1987; Pepine et al, 1991).

Hyperlipidaemia

Preliminary findings in open studies in patients with types II, IV or V hyperlipidaemia indicate that 3–4 g of L-carnitine daily significantly decrease serum concentrations of cholesterol, triglyceride or both and increase those of HDL-cholesterol (Pola et al, 1979, 1983; Rossi and Siliprandi, 1982, Adamo et al, 1986). In addition, it has been reported that plasma concentrations of FFA of patients with chronic hepatitis or cirrhosis decreased after a 14-day treatment of L-carnitine 1g daily (Goa and Brogden, 1987). These data need to be confirmed in much larger trials, but could be of clinical relevance for patients with ischaemic heart disease.

CONCLUSION

The role of L-carnitine as an exogenously administered therapeutic agent for treatment of ischaemic heart disease is becoming clearer. L-Carnitine has been found to improve tachycardia and exercise tolerance and to reduce signs and symptoms of ischaemia in patients with coronary artery disease. It improves myocardial function and clinical status of patients with stable angina pectoris and initial heart failure. In addition, it holds considerable potential as a therapeutic agent in difficult to manage conditions such as cardiogenic shock, cardiac arrhythmias and cardiotoxicity associated with anthracycline therapy.

These effects are achieved through a beneficial modulation of the disturbed cardiac metabolism and, therefore, differ in the intimate mechanism of action from the effects of compounds traditionally used for the management of ischaemia. L-Carnitine is virtually without side-effects. The novel mechanism of action and the excellent tolerance make carnitine a particularly attractive choice for adjunctive therapy in this condition.

REFERENCES

Adamo S, Tonon M, Carrara M et al (1986) In Borum P (ed.) *Clinical Aspects of Human Carnitine Deficiency*, p 244. New York: Pergamon Press.
Alberts DS, Peng YM & Moon TE (1978) *Biomedicine* 29: 265–267.
Angelini C, Vergani L, Costa L et al (1986) In Borum, P (ed.) *Clinical Aspects of Human Carnitine Deficiency*, p 38. New York: Pergamon Press.
Bach AC (1982) *Zeitschift für Ernahrungswissenschaft* 21: 257–265.
Bahl JJ & Bressler R (1987) *Annu. Rev. Pharmacol. Toxicol.* 27: 257–260.
Bartles GL, Remme WJ, Pillay M et al (1991) *J. Am. Coll. Cardiol.* (in press).
Bieber LL (1988) *Annu. Rev. Biochem.* 57: 261–283.
Bing RJ (1954) *Harvey Lecture Series* 50: 27–70.
Bohles H, Noppency T, Akcetin Z et al (1986) *Curr. Ther. Res.* 39: 429–435.
Borum PR (1983) *Annu. Rev. Nutr.* 3: 233–259.
Bremer J (1983) *Physiol. Res.* 63: 1420–1480.

Canale C, Terrachini V & Biagini A (1988) *Int. J. Clin. Pharmacol. Ther. Toxicol.* 26: 221–224.

Capaldo B, Napoli R, Di Bonito P et al (1991) *Diabetes Res. Clin. Pract.* (in press).

Cederblad G, Bylund AC, Holm, J & Schersten T (1976) *Scand. J. Clin. Lab. Invest.* 36: 547–552.

Cherchi A, Lai C, Gioglia G et al (1982) *IX World Congress of Cardiology, Moscow, Jun 20–26.*

Cherchi A, Lai C, Angolino F et al (1985) *Intern. J. Clin. Pharmacol. Ther. Toxic.* 23: 569–572.

Cohen RD & Woods HF (1983) *Diabetes* 32: 181–191.

Cooper DJ, Walley KR & Russell JA (1990) *Ann. Intern. Med.* 113(3): 256.

Corbucci CB & Peduto VA (1991) (in press).

Corbucci CB, Perduto VA, Lettieri B & Musu A (1991) (in press).

Dal Negro R, Zoccatelli O, Pomari G & Turco P (1986) *Clin. Trials J.* 23: 242–248.

De Leonardis V, Neri B, Bacalli S & Cinelli P (1985) *Int. J. Clin. Pharmacol. Res.* 5: 137–142.

De Leonardis V, De Scalzi M & Neri B (1987) *Int. J. Clin. Pharmacol. Res.* 7: 307–311.

Fernandez C, La Menza B & Pola P (1985) *Associazione Nazionale Cardiologi Extraospedalieri*, 29: 2–9.

Ferrari R (1988) In de Jong JW (ed.) *Myocardial Energy Metabolism*, pp 35–43. Dordrecht-Boston-Lancaster: Martinus Nijhoff Publishers.

Ferrari R, Cucchini F, Di Lisa F et al (1984a) *Clin. Trials J.* 21: 40–58.

Ferrari R, Cucchini F & Visioli O (1984b) *Int. J. Cardiol.* 5: 213–216.

Ferrari R, Di Lisa F, Raddino R et al (1984c) In Ferrari R, Katz A, Shug A & Visioli O (eds) *Myocardial Ischaemia and Lipid Metabolism*, pp 135–157. New York: Plenum Press.

Folts JD, Shug AL, Koke JR & Bittar N (1978) *Am. J. Cardiol.* 41: 1209–1214.

Fritz IB (1959) *Am. J. Physiol.* 197: 297–304.

Furitano G, Paterna S, Perricone R et al (1984) *Clin. Res.* 10: 107–111.

Garzya G & Amico RM (1980) *Int. J. Tissue React.* 2: 175–180.

Ghidini O, Azzurro M, Vita G & Sartori G (1988) *Int. J. Clin. Pharmacol. Ther. Toxic.* 26: 218–220.

Giordano MP, Corsi M, Roncarolo P et al (1983) *Curr. Ther. Res.* 33: 305–311.

Goa KL & Brogden RN (1987) *Drugs* 34: 1–24.

Gupta DK, Jewitt DE, Young R et al (1969) *Lancet* ii: 1209–1213.

Kamikawa T, Suzuki Y, Kobayashi A et al (1984) *Jpn Heart J.* 25: 587–597.

Kette F, Weil MH, von Planta M et al (1990) *Circulation* 5: 1660–1666.

Kosolcharoen P, Nappi J & Peduzzi P (1981) *Curr. Ther. Res.* 30: 753–764.

Liedtke AJ (1987) In Kaiser J (ed.) *Carnitine—its role in lung and heart disorders*, pp 100–111. Munich: Karger.

Liedtke AJ (1988) *J. Mol. Cell. Cardiol.* 20: 65–70.

Liedtke AJ & Nellis SH (1979) *J. Clin. Invest.* 64: 440–458.

Litwin SE, Raya TE, Gay RG et al (1990) *Am. J. Physiol.* 258: H51–H56.

Logue RB (1985a) In Logue RB (ed.) *The Heart* pp 81–94. New York: McGraw-Hill.

Logue RB (1985b) In Logue RB (ed.) *The Heart* pp 568–569. New York: McGraw-Hill.

Logue RB (1985c) *Metabolic Regulation and Myocardial Function*. In Logue RB (ed.) *The heart*, pp 653–654. New York: McGraw-Hill.
Lopaschuk GD (1991) In Lopaschuk GD (ed.) *Current Concepts in Carnitine Research*, pp. 1–5. Atlanta Georgia.
Maccari F & Ramacci MT (1981) *Biomedicine* 35: 65–67.
Marconi C, Sassi G, Carpinelli A & Cerretelli P (1985) *Eur. J. Appl. Physiol.* 54: 131–135.
Martina B, Zuber M, Weiss Ph et al (1991) *Lancet* (in press).
Neely JR & Morgan HE (1974) *Annu. Rev. Physiol.* 36: 413–459.
Neri B, Cini-Neri G, Bartalucci S & Bandinelli M (1986) *Anticancer Res.* 6: 659–662.
Oliver MF, Kurien VA & Greenwood TW (1968) *Lancet* i: 710–715.
Opie LH (1979) *Am. Heart J.* 97: 375–388.
Orlando G & Rusconi C (1986) *Clin. Trials J.* 23: 338–344.
Pepine CJ (1991) *Clin. Ther.* 13: 2–21.
Pola P, Savi L, Grilli M et al (1979) *Curr. Ther. Res.* 27: 208–216.
Pola P, Tondi P, Dal Lago A et al (1983) *Drugs under Exp. Clin. Res.* 12: 925–935.
Rebouche CJ & Engel AG (1983) *Mayo Clinic Proceedings* 58: 533–540.
Reforzo G, De Andreis Bessone PL, Rebaudo F & Tibaldi M (1986) *Curr. Ther. Res.* 40: 374–383.
Regitz V, Shug AL & Fleck E (1990) *Am. J. Cardiol.* 65: 755–760.
Rizzon P, Biasco G & Di Biase M (1989) *Eur. Heart J.* 10: 502–508.
Rossi CS & Siliprandi N (1982) *Johns Hopkins Med. J.* 150: 51–54.
Rumbak MJ (1990) *Ann. Int. Med.* 113(3): 254–255.
Rutenberg, HL, Pamintuan JC & Soloff LA (1969) *Circulation* II-215: 45–46.
Schiavoni G, Pennestri F, Monigiardo R et al (1983) *Drugs Under Exp. Clin. Res.* 9: 171–185.
Selveres G (1984) *Archivio di Medicina Interna* 36: 61–66.
Shug AL, Thomsen JH & Folts JD (1978) *Arch. Biochem. Biophys.* 187: 25–33.
Siliprandi N, Di Lisa F & Toninello A (1984) *G. Ital. Cardiol.* 14: 804–808.
Spagnoli LG, Corsi M, Villaschi S et al (1982) *Lancet* i: 1419–1420.
Suzuki Y, Kawikawa T & Kobayashi A (1981) *Jpn Circ. J.* 45: 687–694.
Suzuki Y, Masumura Y & Kobayashi A (1982a) *Lancet* i: 116.
Suzuki Y, Narita M & Yamazaki N (1982b) *Jpn. Heart J.* 23: 349–359.
Thomsen JH, Shug AL, Yap YU et al (1979) *Am. J. Cardiol.* 43: 300–306.
Vecchiet L, Di Lisa F, Pieralisi G et al (1990) *Eur. J. Appl. Physiol.* 61: 486–490.
Zierler KL (1976) *Circ. Res.* 38: 459–463.

15

TREATMENT OF ACUTE MYOCARDIAL INFARCTION WITH L-CARNITINE

P. Rizzon M. Di Biase and G. Biasco

Carnitine is a water-soluble, naturally-occurring amino acid. It plays an important role in fatty acid metabolism by promoting their transport into the mitochondria where the oxidation enzymes are located (Opie, 1979). The cardiac muscle has a carnitine content (1.5 μmol per g wet tissue) which is approximately twice that of the liver and 30 times higher than that of blood (Rebouche and Engel, 1983). The myocardium is unable to synthesize carnitine so it extracts this compound directly from the blood (Sartorelli et al, 1982).

Since, in the aerobic heart, the oxidation of fatty acids accounts for approximately 70% of the utilized substrates, primary or secondary carnitine deficiencies lead to a substantial reduction in energy production.

EXPERIMENTAL BACKGROUND FOR THE USE OF CARNITINE IN ACUTE MYOCARDIAL INFARCTION

Free carnitine loss from the myocardium

Free carnitine loss from the myocardium has been observed repeatedly in the experimental ischaemic heart as well as in the myocytes of

L-Carnitine and Its Role in Medicine:
From Function to Therapy. ISBN 0–12–253940–0

patients with myocardial infarction. Shug et al (1978) observed a loss of free carnitine in perfused anoxic rat heart of between 20 and 60% (mean 50%), while Suzuki et al (1981) demonstrated a significant decrease (40%) in tissue concentration of free carnitine after ischaemia induced by 15-min ligation of left descending coronary artery of dog hearts. A decrease in tissue levels of free carnitine both in infarcted and non-infarcted areas after coronary occlusion (15–120 min) was also observed in another experimental study (Suzuki et al, 1980). Spagnoli et al (1982) observed a myocardial carnitine deficiency in humans by measuring L-carnitine concentrations at necroscopy in infarcted and peri-infarcted areas. A loss of carnitine has also been demonstrated by Bartels and Remme (1990) after pacing-induced ischaemia in patients with coronary artery disease.

All these data suggest that ischaemia and anoxia induce a loss of free carnitine from the myocardium which determines a secondary carnitine deficiency.

Changes in fatty acid metabolism

During myocardial ischaemia the amount of oxygen to support oxidative phosphorylation is reduced and NADH accumulation occurs. Increased NADH/NAD ratio reduces the rate of β-oxidation of fatty acids and leads to a decrease in the levels of acetyl CoA and to an increase of acyl CoA and long-chain acylcarnitine (Liedtke et al, 1978). The associated depletion in free carnitine causes the accumulation of long-chain acyl CoA and free fatty acids in the cytosol (Pande, 1975). Because high concentrations of long-chain acyl CoA inhibit adenine nucleotide translocase activity (Shrago et al, 1976; Shug and Subramanian, 1987), ATP availability in ischaemic myocardium is impaired both by a reduced supply of oxygen and by the accumulation of long-chain acyl CoA. The accumulation of long-chain acyl carnitine and long-chain acyl CoA also leads to a disruption of the critical transport process across the mitochondrial membrane by inhibiting the membrane Na^+–K^+-stimulated ATPase (Wood et al, 1977). These data have been also confirmed by experimental studies in vivo demonstrating that after occlusion of coronary branches, long-chain acylcarnitine and long-chain acyl CoA concentrations increase while ATP levels significantly decrease (Liedtke et al, 1978; Suzuki et al, 1980, 1981).

The accumulation of free fatty acids or their derivatives induce changes in myocardial contractility and arrhythmias.

Liedtke et al (1978) demonstrate that both an excess in serum-free fatty acids and ischaemia cause the deterioration of haemodynamic parameters (aortic pressure, left ventricular systolic pressure, left ventricular work, epicardial motion and oxygen consumption), while their association induces an even greater deterioration of the same parameters. These changes were associated with a concomitant increase of long-chain acyl CoA and long-chain acylcarnitine levels.

Regarding the arrhythmic effects, after the report of Oliver et al (1968) suggesting that plasma free fatty acid (FFA) levels could be a predictive index of the vulnerability of patients with myocardial infarction to lethal arrhythmias, many experimental (Opie et al, 1971; Kostis et al, 1973; Kato et al, 1979) and clinical (Gupta et al, 1969; Nelson, 1970) research studies have demonstrated that FFA or their derivatives evoke arrhythmias. The threshold concentration of FFA at which arrhythmias occur in man is 1200 μmol l^{-1} (Oliver et al, 1968). In particular, conduction disturbances (Kurien and Yates, 1971), ventricular arrhythmias (Kurien and Oliver, 1970; Kurien and Yates, 1971; Katz and Messimes, 1982; Tausey and Opre, 1983) and a reduction of the ventricular fibrillation threshold (Kato et al, 1979) induced by fatty acids have been reported.

The mechanism involved in the arrhythmia induction is probably mainly due to a decreased mitochondrial Ca^{2+} binding activity (Sugiyama et al, 1982) which increases the intracellular Ca^{2+} concentration. These effects might cause changes in the action potential which has been demonstrated to be further shortened by fatty acids during ischaemia (Cowan and Vaughan-Williams, 1980). Other proposed mechanisms are a biotoxic detergent effect on membranes enhanced by high molar ratios of fatty acids/albumin (Willebrands et al, 1973), a non-specific detergent action on biomembranes which leads to a cation loss (Kurien and Oliver, 1970) and an interference by fats on glycolytically-derived ATP in the cytoplasm (Prasad and McLeod, 1969).

To summarize, ischaemia induces a loss of free carnitine from the myocardium and increases levels of free fatty acids and their derivatives which impair haemodynamic parameters and evoke arrhythmias.

Effects of exogenous carnitine supplement during myocardial ischaemia

Many experimental studies have demonstrated that the administration of carnitine, if supplied before or during ischaemia or anoxia:

1. increases free carnitine levels in infarcted and non-infarcted areas (Suzuki et al, 1980, 1981);

2. decreases levels of long-chain acyl CoA and long-chain acylcarnitine in ischaemic and infarcted areas (Shug et al, 1978; Suzuki et al, 1980, 1981);

3. increases ATP levels in infarcted and ischaemic areas (Suzuki et al, 1980, 1981);

4. decreases the adenine nucleotide translocase inhibition induced by long-chain acyl CoA (Shug and Subramanian, 1987);

5. improves the haemodynamic parameters impaired by anoxia or ipoxia (Neely et al, 1979; Liedtke and Nellis, 1979);

6. shows an anti-arrhythmic activity by preventing ventricular fibrillation induced by prolonged ischaemia or anoxia (Shug et al, 1975; Suzuki et al, 1981; Imai et al, 1984);

7. reduces ST-segment elevation during ischaemia (Shug et al, 1975; Thomsen et al, 1976);

8. improves the contractile recovery of myocardium and reduces the incidence of ventricular arrhythmias during reperfusion after a 30-min low-flow ischaemia (Duan and Karmazyn, 1989).

It may be concluded that exogenous administration of carnitine during ischaemia and anoxia has beneficial effects on haemodynamic parameters and ventricular arrhythmias and protects against haemodynamic and arrhythmic complications associated with reperfusion.

The mechanisms by which carnitine exerts its activity are probably linked to an improved mitochondrial function and to a reduction in the concentration of FFA and their derivatives which are transported by carnitine out of the mitochondria and out of the myocardial cells.

L-CARNITINE IN THE TREATMENT OF ACUTE MYOCARDIAL INFARCTION

Metabolic effects

The metabolic effects of L-carnitine administered during the acute phase of myocardial infarction were evaluated by Rizzon et al (1989).

Fifty-six patients with acute myocardial infarction were enrolled in the double-blind, parallel and placebo-controlled study. They had been admitted to the Coronary Care Unit between 3 and 12 h from the onset of pain and not submitted to thrombolytic treatment. Allocation of treatment to patients was random after stratification based on the time from onset of pain and site of infarction. The first group of 28 patients received intravenous L-carnitine at a dose of 100 mg kg body w^{-1} every 12 h for 36 h while the second group of 28 patients received placebo intravenously. Blood samples were taken at regular intervals and patients' urine was also collected over the same period of time. Concentration of free carnitine, short-chain acylcarnitine esters and long-chain acylcarnitine esters were measured in the serum and urine.

In the untreated group of patients serum free carnitine concentrations increased progressively from 38 ± μmol l^{-1} to 55 ± 17 μmol l^{-1} after 26 h, reaching a statistically significant difference (p <0.01) at 16 h after the beginning of the study (data compared with serum free carnitine levels observed in 11 healthy control subjects) (Figure 1). Urinary excretion of free carnitine also increased (Table 1).

These data show that ischaemia associated with acute myocardial infarction induces a similar loss of free carnitine from the myocardium in humans, as previously documented in experimental studies. The dramatic increase of free carnitine concentrations in serum and urine suggests that carnitine could also be released by skeletal muscle, as a result of stress; moreover, an increased carnitine synthesis in the liver and kidneys cannot be excluded.

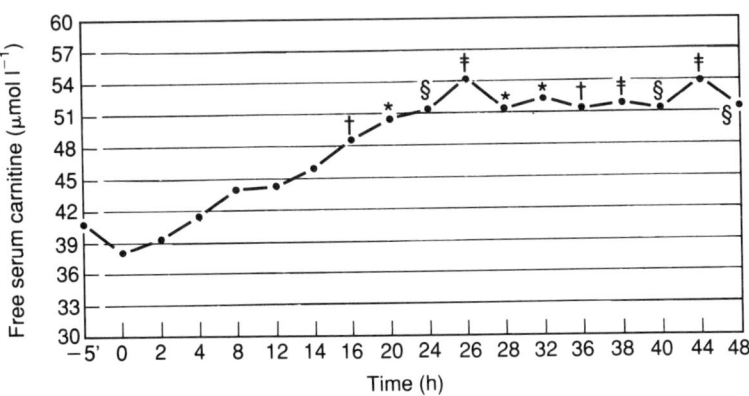

* = p<0.01; † = p<0.02;

§ = p<0.001; ‡ = p<0.002;

FIGURE I. Free serum carnitine concentration during the first 24 h after acute myocardial infarction in 28 patients receiving placebo (normal 43 ± 8 μmol l^{-1}).

TABLE I.

Urinary concentrations of free carnitine (FC), short- (SCACE) and long-chain acylcarnitine esters (LCACE) in 11 healthy subjects and in the group treated with L-carnitine and placebo during the first 48 h after acute myocardial infarction (AMI)

Urinary concentrations μ mol l^{-1}	Healthy subjects		AMI (placebo)		AMI (L-carnitine)	
	0–24 h	24–48 h	0–24 h	24–48 h	0–24 h	24–48 h
FC	126 ± 51	—	*547 ± 631	*576 ± 608	*30991 ± 18070†	26954 ± 11934
SCACE	146 ± 123	—	219 ± 257	154 ± 150	2676 ± 4224†	1818 ± 2151
LCACE	6.7 ± 4.3	—	8.2 ± 4.9	9.5 ± 8.2	230 ± 192†	†200 ± 142

* = $p < 0.05$;   † = $p < 0.001$.

In the carnitine-treated group of patients a significant increase ($p<0.01$) of serum (Figure 2) and urinary (Table 1) levels of short- and long-chain acylcarnitine esters were observed compared with the untreated group. This increase may be explained as a consequence of esterification between exogenous carnitine and the acyl groups within the cells catalysed by CoA: carnitine acyl transferase. This esterification, which is favoured by the increased availability of free carnitine which reacts with acyl CoA to form acylcarnitine, allows the washout of acyl compounds into the blood and, consequently, into the urine. By eliminating acyl compounds in excess, carnitine prevents their negative effects and exercises a protective function during ischaemia.

An increase of HDL-cholesterol with a reduction in total cholesterol/HDL ratio was also observed by De Ritis et al (1982).

Antiarrhythmic effects

The possibility that L-carnitine could have an anti-arrhythmic effect during acute myocardial infarction was suggested by De Ritis et al (1982).

The anti-arrhythmic effects of carnitine in acute myocardial infarction were evaluated by Rizzon et al (1989). Fifty-six patients with acute myocardial infarction were submitted to Holter monitoring during the first 48 h of admission to the Coronary Care Unit. Twenty-eight received intravenous L-carnitine at a dose of 100 mg kg body wt^{-1} every 12 h for 36 h while 28 patients received placebo.

Analysis of Holter tape records showed that during the second day following acute myocardial infarction in the carnitine-treated group there was a statistically-significant reduction in (Table 2): (i) the number of premature ventricular beats per hour; (ii) hours with multiform premature ventricular beats; (iii) hours with couplets; (iv) hours with non-sustained ventricular tachycardia; (v) the number of total non-sustained ventricular tachycardias. A significant difference in favour of the L-carnitine group was also observed on the second day of treatment when the number of patients with premature ventricular beats, greater or less than 10 per hour, was considered. Similar results, confirming anti-arrhythmic activity of L-carnitine during the second day after acute myocardial infarction, were reported by Martine et al (1990) in 12 patients treated with L-carnitine i.v., when compared with eight patients receiving placebo.

These data favour the conclusion that L-carnitine possesses some anti-arrhythmic effects in humans during myocardial infarction, thus confirming previous experimental observations.

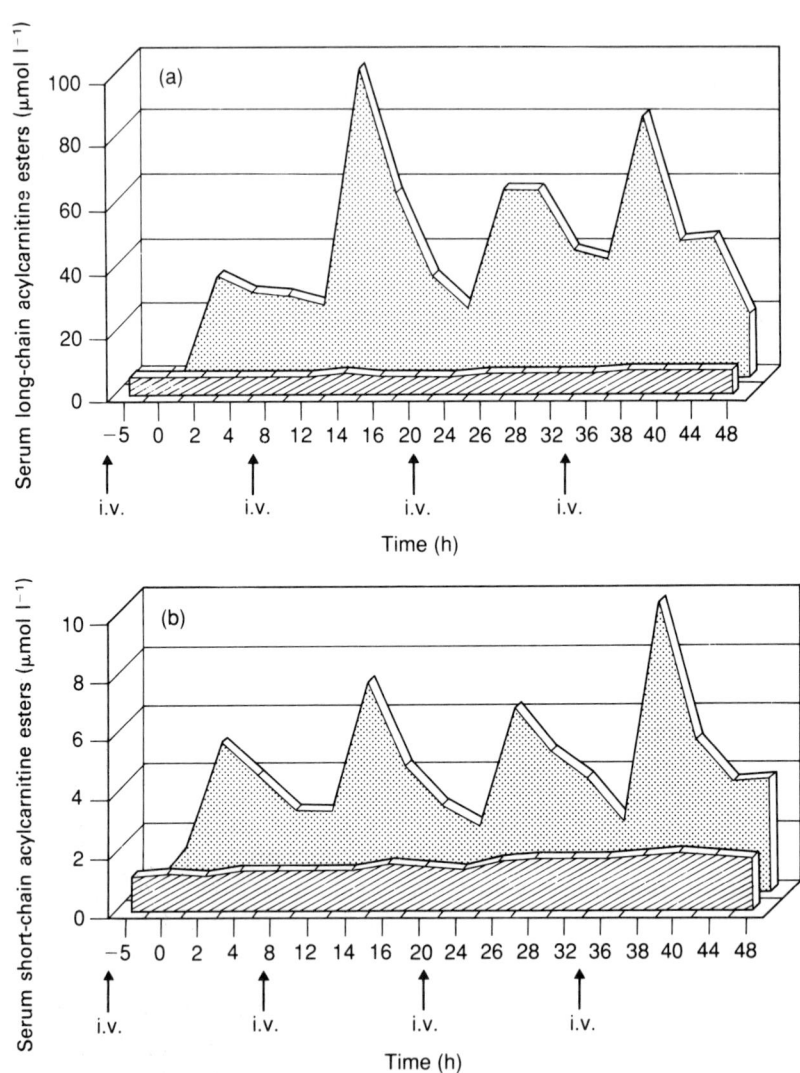

FIGURE 2. Serum short-chain (a) and long-chain (b) acylcarnitine ester concentrations during the first 48 h after admission to the Coronary Care Unit in the L-carnitine-treated group ▦ and in the placebo group ▨. The treated group shows a significant increase in acylcarnitine concentrations compared with the placebo group.

TABLE 2.

Ventricular arrhythmias in the L-carnitine-treated group and in the placebo group (first 48 h after acute myocardial infarction)

Measurements	1st day		2nd day	
	Placebo	L-Carnitine	Placebo	L-Carnitine
Recording time (h)	22.4 ± 3.4	22.5 ± 5	20.4 ± 7.2	20.4 ± 7.6
PVBs/h	93 ± 272	60 ± 115	20 ± 36*	4 ± 7
Time with multiform PVBs (h)	11.1 ± 9	8.9 ± 8	7.3 ± 8*	2.9 ± 4
Time with paired PVBs (h)	6.6 ± 7.6	5.6 ± 6.8	2.8 ± 4.4†	0.6 ± 1.2
Number of paired PVBs (24 h)	23 ± 54	23 ± 46	7 ± 16	0.7 ± 1.5
Time with VT (h)	4.1 ± 5.9	3 ± 4	0.7 ± 1.1*	0.2 ± 0.4
Number of VT episodes	17 ± 43	23 ± 97	1 ± 2*	0.2 ± 0.5

* = $p < 0.05$; † = $p < 0.02$.
PVBs, premature ventricular beats; VT, non-sustained ventricular tachycardia.

These effects could be explained by the detoxifying effects of L-carnitine in ischaemic myocardium exerted by reducing fatty acid metabolite levels in ischaemic cells which are transported out of the mitochondria and out of the cells by L-carnitine. This hypothesis is supported by the statistically-significant increased concentrations of short- and long-chain acyl-carnitine esters in serum and urine, observed in the group of patients treated with intravenous L-carnitine compared with patients receiving placebo.

Effects on the reduction of the necrotic area

The capability of L-carnitine to reduce the extent of the necrotic area in acute myocardial infarction was assessed by Rebuzzi et al (1984) utilizing the measurement of CPK and MB-CPK plasma levels and by Chiariello et al (1986) utilizing electrocardiographic parameters.

In the study of Rebuzzi et al (1984), where 12 patients with acute myocardial infarction were treated with 40 mg kg^{-1} day^{-1} of L-carnitine, there was a significantly-reduced release of MB-CPK and a minor CPK maximum value compared with the control group. In the randomized study of Chiariello et al (1986), L-carnitine was administered to 177 patients with acute myocardial infarction at a dosage of 3 g every 8 h for 48 h. The treated patients showed a statistically-significant reduction in the decline in R-wave compared with the 174 untreated patients. Comparing only patients with anterior myocardial infarction, a 26% decline in R-wave in favour of the treated patients was observed.

These data, obtained in two studies which used two different methods, seem to confirm that L-carnitine has a beneficial effect in reducing the extent of the necrotic area during myocardial infarction. The mechanism by which L-carnitine favours myocardial survival is probably due to the improvement of mitochondrial function which, in turn, is due to the reduction of acyl CoA ester concentrations in ischaemic cells not yet irreversibly affected.

REFERENCES

Bartels GL & Remme WJ (1990) *Eur. Heart J.* 11 (abstract supplement): 41.
Chiariello M, Brevetti G, Policicchio A et al (1986) In Borum PR (ed.) *Clinical Aspects of Human Carnitine Deficiency*, pp 242–243. New York: Pergamon Press.

Cowan JC & Vaughan-Williams EM (1980) *J. Mol. Cell. Cardiol.* 12: 347–369.
De Ritis G, Pietropaoli P, Milletti M et al (1982) *Eur. Rev. Med. Pharmacol. Sci.* 4: 477–484.
Duan J & Karmazyn M (1989) *Br. J. Pharmacol.* 98, 1319–1327.
Gupta DK, Young R, Jewitt DE et al (1969) *Lancet* ii, 1209–1213.
Imai S, Matsui K & Nakazawa M (1984) *Br. J. Pharmacol.* 82: 533–542.
Kato T, Suzuki S, Kamme T et al (1979) *J. Appl. Biochem.* 1: 139–146.
Katz AM & Messineo FC (1982) *J. Mol. Cell. Cardiol.* 14(3): 119–122.
Kostis JB, Mavrogeorgis EA, Horstmann E & Gotzoyannis S (1973) *Cardiology* 58: 89–95.
Kurien VA & Oliver MF (1970) *Lancet* i: 813–815.
Kurien VA & Yates PA (1971) *Eur. J. Clin. Invest.* 1: 225–241.
Liedtke AJ & Nellis SH (1979) *J. Clin. Invest.* 64: 440–447.
Liedtke AJ, Nellis SH & Neely JR (1978) *Circ. Res.* 43: 652–661.
Martine B, Zuber M, Burkert F et al (1990) *Schweiz. Med. Wochenschr.* 32 (supplement II): 8.
Nelson PG (1970) *Br. Med. J.* 3: 735–737.
Neely JR, Garber D, McDonough K & Idell-Wenger J (1979) In Winbury MM & Abiko Y (eds) *Perspectives in Cardiovascular Researches*, pp 225–234. New York: Raven Press.
Oliver MF, Kurien VA & Greenwood TW (1968) *Lancet* i, 710–714.
Opie LH (1979) *Am. Heart J.* 97: 375–388.
Opie LH, Norris RM, Thomas M et al (1971) *Lancet* i, 818–822.
Pande SV (1975) *Proc. Natl Acad. Sci. USA* 72: 883–887.
Prasad K & McLeod DP (1969) *Circ. Res.* 24: 939–950.
Rebouche CJ & Engel AG (1983) *Arch. Biochem. Biophys.* 220: 60–70.
Rebuzzi AG, Schiavoni G, Amico CM et al (1984) *Drugs Exp. Clin. Res.* 10 (4): 219–223.
Rizzon P, Biasco G, Di Biase M et al (1989) *Eur. Heart J.* 10: 502–508.
Sartorelli M, Ciman M, Rizzoli V & Siliprandi N (1982) *Ital. J. Biochem.* 31: 261–268.
Shrago E, Shug AL, Sul H et al (1976) *Circ. Res.* 38 (supplement I): 75–78.
Shug AL & Subramanian R (1987) *Z. Kardiol.* 76 (supplement 5): 26–33.
Shug AL, Shrago E, Bittar N et al (1975) *Am. J. Physiol.* 228: 689–692.
Shug AL, Thomsen JH, Folts JD et al (1978) *Arch. Biochem. Biophys.* 187: 25–33.
Spagnoli LG, Corsi M, Villaschi S et al (1982) *Lancet* i, 1419–1420.
Sugiyama S, Miyazaki Y, Kotaka K et al (1982) *J. Electrocardiol.* 15 (3): 227–232.
Suzuki Y, Kamikawa T & Yamazaki N (1980) In Frenkel RA & McGarry JD (eds) *Carnitine Biosynthesis, Metabolism and Functions*, pp 341–352. New York: Academic Press.
Suzuki Y, Kamikawa T, Kobayashi A et al (1981) *Jpn. Circ. J.* 45: 687–694.
Tansey MJB & Opie LH (1983) *Lancet* ii, 419–422.
Thomsen JH, Shug AL, Yap VU et al (1976) *Am. J. Cardiol.* 43: 300–306.
Willebrands AF, Ter Welle HF & Tasseron SJA (1973) *J. Mol. Cell. Cardiol.* 5: 259–273.
Wood JM, Bush B, Pitts BJR & Schwartz A (1977) *Biochem. Biophys. Res. Commun.* 74: 677–684.

16

ROLE OF CARNITINE IN HEART FAILURE

V. Regitz and E. Fleck

DIAGNOSTIC AND PROGNOSTIC FEATURES IN HEART FAILURE

Heart failure is one of the leading causes of death in western societies, causing 7.8% of deaths (52 189/687 516) in the Federal Republic of Germany in 1988 (Statistisches Bundesamt, unpublished data). The most frequent cause of heart failure is coronary heart disease, followed by hypertensive and valvular heart disease and cardiomyopathy. Recent findings emphasize that the clinical features of heart failure are independent from the underlying aetiology.

The clinical syndrome of heart failure is characterized by a reduced cardiac index, elevated filling pressures as well as the activation of neurohumoral compensatory mechanisms (Francis, 1985). However, the prognosis and clinical course of heart failure are not determined

295

L-Carnitine and Its Role in Medicine:
From Function to Therapy. ISBN 0–12–253940–0

by these peripheral changes but by the function of the myocardium itself (Katz, 1970, 1988; Levine et al, 1982). Heart failure alters the myocardium in several animal models, and also in humans in a comparable way. Initial damage to the myocardium is followed by a period of myocardial hyperfunction that is associated with qualitative and quantitative alterations of the metabolism and composition of the myocardium (Rabinowitz, 1973; Meerson, 1983). This state can only be tolerated for a limited time, progressive deterioration of function leading ultimately to end-stage heart failure (Meerson, 1983; Pfeffer et al, 1988).

The most attractive hypotheses to explain myocardial dysfunction in heart failure postulates biochemical defects in the myocardium other than the alteration in loading conditions or ischaemic damage as a cause for the functional deficits. These biochemical causes of contractile dysfunction have not yet been conclusively described. The assessment of changes in the complex metabolism of the myocardium may improve the understanding of both the underlying biochemical defects and also the role of exogenous factors in a multifactorial system. It may also contribute to the development of therapeutic strategies.

Carnitine, a small amino acid derivative plays a major role in fatty acid oxidation as well as in other central metabolic pathways. Fatty acid oxidation is the major energy-providing pathway of the myocardium; its inhibition has been shown to impair myocardial function (Neely and Morgan, 1974; Rebouche and Engel, 1983; Bressler et al, 1990). The hypothesis that myocardial carnitine deficiency may cause malfunction of the heart has been confirmed in several animal models and in humans (Engel and Angelini, 1973; Chapoy et al, 1980; Paulsen and Shug, 1981; Waber et al, 1982; Paulson et al, 1984; Whitmer, 1987). Systemic carnitine deficiency has been shown to lead to dilated or hypertrophic cardiomyopathy (Engel and Angelini, 1973; Regitz et al, 1982; Shug and Paulson, 1984; Ino et al, 1988).

This article discusses animal models with spontaneous and induced alterations of carnitine metabolism, with reduced myocardial carnitine levels and impaired cardiac function. Further, human cardiac diseases associated with myocardial carnitine loss will be described. The role of myocardial carnitine deficiency and its consequences for myocardial metabolism and myocardial function will be discussed.

LOSS OF CARNITINE IN ANIMAL MODELS OF DILATED CARDIOMYOPATHY—FUNCTIONAL CONSEQUENCES OF CARNITINE LOSS

Myocardial carnitine deficiency in dog cardiomyopathy

Spontaneous dilated cardiomyopathy in a family of dogs has been reported recently (Keene et al, 1986 and unpublished data). Two of the six members of the family were affected with severe congestive heart failure: peripheral and pulmonary oedema, atrial fibrillation and a reduced fractional shortening in echocardiography. These dogs showed severely depressed myocardial L-carnitine concentrations compared with normal control animals. In the two dogs, treatment with high doses of L-carnitine was instituted and was associated with increased myocardial L-carnitine concentrations. There was a simultaneous improvement in clinical status and myocardial function. Withdrawal of L-carnitine from these animals caused myocardial dysfunction and clinical signs of heart failure to recur. This study was interpreted as evidence that myocardial L-carnitine deficiency played a central role in the pathogenesis of heart failure in these animals.

Syrian hamsters with myocardial carnitine deficiency

Syrian hamsters with inborn hypertrophic and dilated cardiomyopathy develop myocardial carnitine deficiency during the first months of life (Shug and Paulson, 1984; Whitmer, 1987). Carnitine deficiency in these animals is associated with significant alterations in myocardial energy metabolism. Carnitine substitution restored myocardial carnitine concentrations to normal, improved myocardial function and restored myocardial ATP concentrations in the isolated heart model (Whitmer, 1987).

Myocardial carnitine deficiency in streptozotocin-treated diabetic rats

It is well known that streptozotocin-treated diabetic rats develop myocardial carnitine deficiency (Paulson et al, 1984). Myocardial carnitine deficiency in diabetic rats is associated with functional impairment if the animal hearts are studied in an isolated heart model. Parallel to functional impairment and the carnitine loss there is a significant increase of long-chain acyl CoA esters in the myocardium. When myocardial carnitine levels were reduced to only about 74% of normal, long-chain acyl CoA esters rose to 150% of controls (Paulson et al, 1984). Thus, small changes in myocardial carnitine concentrations are associated with other significant biochemical defects in this model. Substitution of carnitine improved myocardial function as well as tolerance to ischaemia. The concentration of long-chain acylcarnitine increased, whereas that of long-chain acyl CoA decreased, with carnitine treatment (Paulson et al, 1984).

Common features of myocardial carnitine loss in animal models

An association between myocardial carnitine loss and functional defects of the myocardium has been established in the three quoted animal models. However, other metabolic defects in addition to carnitine deficiency may also be present.

In diabetic rats the primary defect is not carnitine deficiency but the diabetic state. There is some evidence of mitochondrial loading with acetyl CoA which is probably prevented from being used for energy production by a lack of pyruvate entering the citric acid cycle. One of the major metabolic roles of carnitine is to protect the acetyl CoA/free CoA pool and to maintain sufficient amounts of free CoA for mitochondrial function (Tubbs et al, 1980). This sensitive equilibrium seems changed in diabetics. It remains to be determined if altered acetyl CoA/free CoA ratios are causally linked to reduced carnitine content or functional impairment. In the dog model no parameters of myocardial metabolism aside from carnitine have been measured (Keene et al, 1986, and unpublished data). Thus, more complex metabolic defects cannot be excluded. In the Syrian hamster it is well known that several morphological and biochemical defects coexist with the disease (Whitmer, 1987).

In summary, myocardial carnitine deficiency is associated with functional impairment in several animal models of heart failure that are caused by completely different mechanisms. Thus, carnitine deficiency seems to represent a non-specific indicator of metabolic stress on the myocardium. Explaining the biochemical mechanism leading to the carnitine loss in these models may improve our understanding of metabolic changes in heart failure. The crucial experiment in all models is to show that carnitine substitution restores normal cardiac function. A few experiments indicate such a possibility (Choi et al, 1977; Paulson et al, 1984; Whitmer, 1987). Thus, the correction of secondary metabolic changes may improve cardiac function. Perhaps the myocardial carnitine loss induces harmful metabolic effects, which may be suppressed by carnitine substitution, independent from the primary metabolic defect.

MYOCARDIAL CARNITINE LOSS IN END-STAGE HEART FAILURE

Studies in end-stage heart failure have been greatly facilitated by the development of transplant programmes, with the consequent opportunity for using the explanted hearts for metabolic studies. Because all hearts investigated are in the same 'end'-stage of heart failure, there is only one point of the regression line function/biochemical changes available. Thus, possible relations between biochemical changes and function cannot be assessed in these hearts. However, explanted hearts can be used to describe an end-point and offer the opportunity for methodological studies because there is enough material available. So far, three working groups have studied alterations of carnitine metabolism in explanted hearts with end-stage heart failure (Regitz et al, 1988a; Pierpont et al, 1989; Bressler et al, 1990).

The Deutsches Herzzentrum Berlin (DHZB)-study

Myocardial carnitine content in dilated cardiomyopathy was investigated in explanted hearts from 39 patients with end-stage heart failure. These explanted hearts were compared with 10 left-ventricular and 14 right-atrial biopsies that were taken from donor hearts during heart transplantation. To assess whether myocardial carnitine deficiency is specific for dilated cardiomyopathy or if it also occurs in heart failure of different origin, myocardial carnitine levels were also determined in 27 patients with coronary or valvular heart disease. The 66 patients with heart failure were characterized by reduced cardiac index, by reduced left-ventricular ejection fraction and by elevated left-ventricular end-diastolic pressure (Table 1). Samples for carnitine determinations

TABLE I.

Haemodynamic parameters of patients with end-stage heart failure due to dilated cardiomyopathy (DCM) of different origins.

	DCM n = 39	HF n = 27
LVEF (%)	25 ± 9	23 ± 9
LVEDP (mmHg)	20 ± 10	25 ± 12
CI (l min^{-1} × m^2)	2.4 ± 0.9	2.3 ± 0.6

were taken from the base of the left ventricle in all 66 patients and from the free wall of the right ventricle in 63 of 66 patients. In addition, the mid area (38/66) and the apex (41/66) of the left ventricle were investigated as well as the interventricular septum (32/66) and right atrium (43/66).

Carnitine concentrations were determined using the radioenzymatic assay of Parvin and Pandee (1977). The regular assay with a standard curve of 0.2–5.0 nmol was used for large samples from explanted hearts and the microassay with a standard curve from 20–500 pmol was used for endomyocardial biopsies. The two assays correlated with $r = 0.95$. (Figure 1). Carnitine concentrations were related to non-collagen protein as described by Lilienthal and Bradford (Lilienthal et al, 1949; Bradford, 1976).

Regional distribution of myocardial carnitine in explanted hearts

To assess the distribution of carnitine independent of the absolute values a rank-analysis was conducted in 25 patients with dilated cardiomyopathy ($n = 15$) and with heart failure of different origins ($n = 10$) in whom samples were obtained from all six areas of the heart. Samples were ranked according to carnitine concentrations in every heart: the area with the highest carnitine concentration was given 6 points, the sample with the lowest content, 1 point. For each area, mean ranks for 25 patients were calculated. The highest ranks were obtained in the left ventricle, the lowest values in the right atrium. This is in agreement with the distribution of the absolute carnitine concentrations in these hearts (Figure 2).

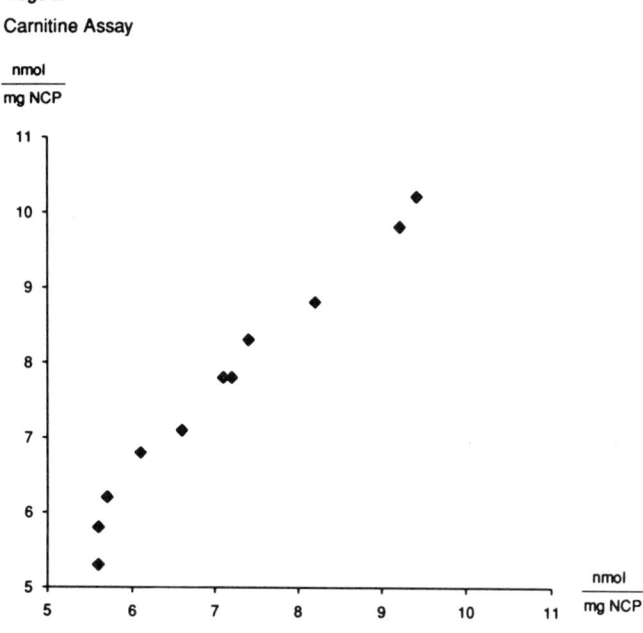

Regular

Carnitine Assay

FIGURE 1. Correlation between microassay and regular carnitine assay. In tissue samples from 11 patients carnitine concentrations were determined using the regular assay and, after adequate dilution of the tissue homogenate, using the microassay. All samples were determined in triplicate. The assays correlated with $r = 0.95$; $p < 0.0001$.

Myocardial carnitine loss in explanted hearts

The patients with heart failure due to dilated cardiomyopathy showed significantly reduced myocardial carnitine levels in all areas of the explanted hearts. Figure 3 depicts total myocardial carnitine levels in three areas of the left ventricle, in the right ventricle septum and right atrium of all the explanted hearts, compared with 10 left-ventricular and 14 right-atrial controls. As in patients with dilated cardiomyopathy, myocardial carnitine content was significantly reduced in the explanted hearts of patients with coronary heart disease. Carnitine levels in hearts from patients with dilated cardiomyopathy and coronary heart disease were not different from each other (Figure 4).

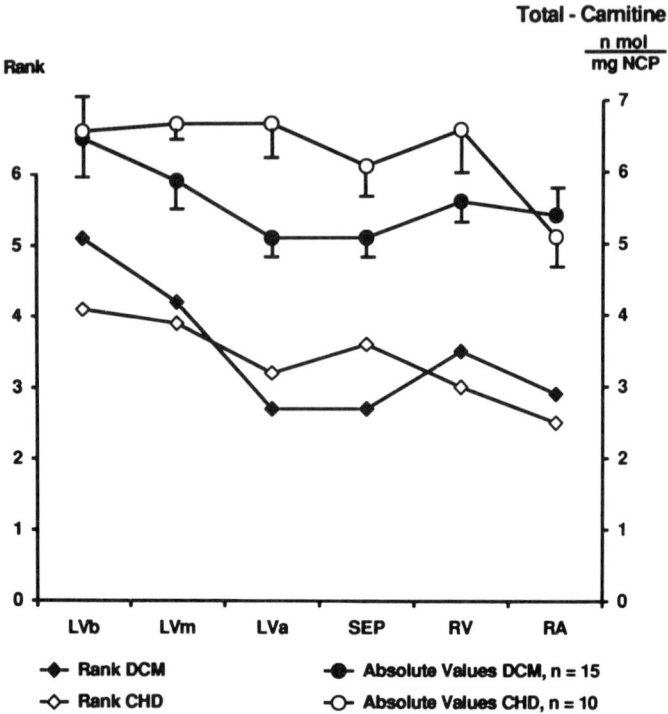

FIGURE 2. Regional distribution of carnitine in end-stage heart failure. Rank statistical and absolute values for carnitine concentrations in six areas from explanted hearts with dilated cardiomyopathy ($n = 15$) and coronary heart disease ($n = 10$). To determine the carnitine content in different areas of the explanted hearts independent from the absolute values, we attributed rank numbers to the different areas in one heart. The area with the highest carnitine concentration obtained 6 points (rank 6); 1 point was attributed to the area with the lowest carnitine content. For each area the mean rank and mean carnitine concentration for 25 hearts was calculated. LVB, LVM, LVA, left ventricle basis, mid area and apex; SEP, interventricular septum; RV, right ventricle; RA, right atrium.

Literature review

After our first publication of reduced myocardial carnitine levels in explanted hearts (Regitz et al, 1988a) two more studies reported comparable data for hearts obtained at cardiac transplantation (Pierpont et al, 1989; Bressler et al, 1990). Bressler (1990) reaches the same conclusions of reduced carnitine levels in heart failure, but in the study of Pierpont et al (1989) the difference between controls and heart

Total-Carnitine

$$\frac{n\ mol}{mg\ NCP}$$

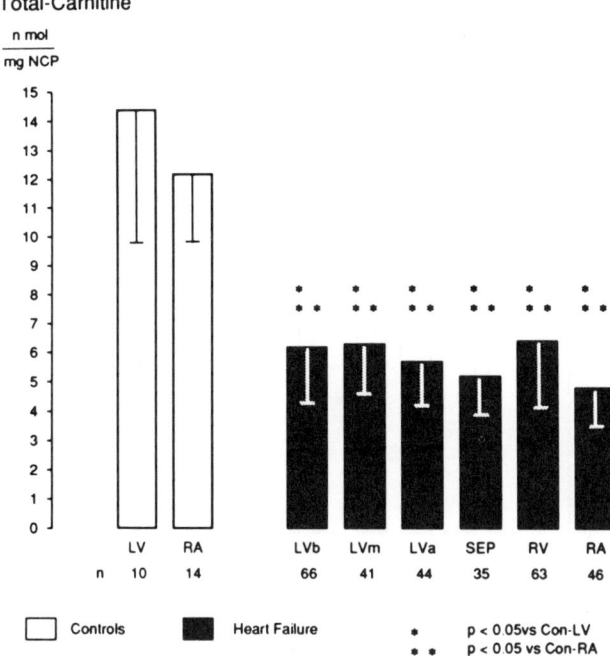

FIGURE 3. Myocardial carnitine loss in end-stage heart failure: Carnitine concentrations in explanted hearts from patients in end-stage heart failure in comparison with controls from left ventricle ($n = 10$) and right atrium ($n = 14$) from healthy donor hearts. In the explanted hearts a significant loss of myocardial carnitine was found in comparison with controls.

failure was only significant in 7 of 51 patients. The reason for this is that control carnitine values were rather low (left ventricle 5.7 ± 1.0, right ventricle 6.2 ± 1.8 μmol mg^{-1} non-collagen protein). This is significantly lower than the control values obtained by Patel et al (1991) or in our group; it is also lower than myocardial carnitine levels in normal rats or dogs (Borun, 1978; Keene et al, unpublished data). Control values in Pierspont's paper have been obtained at autopsy; neither the underlying disease leading to autopsy nor the interval between death and autopsy are mentioned. There are several systemic diseases—liver diseases, kidney diseases, catabolic states or just old age—that are associated with altered carnitine metabolism (Shug and Paulson, 1984). As these diseases are common in patients who have died, it is not sufficient to simply select autopsy cases without cardiac disease to obtain normal cardiac carnitine levels. In addition to in vivo myocardial carnitine loss, breakdown of myocardial membrane and

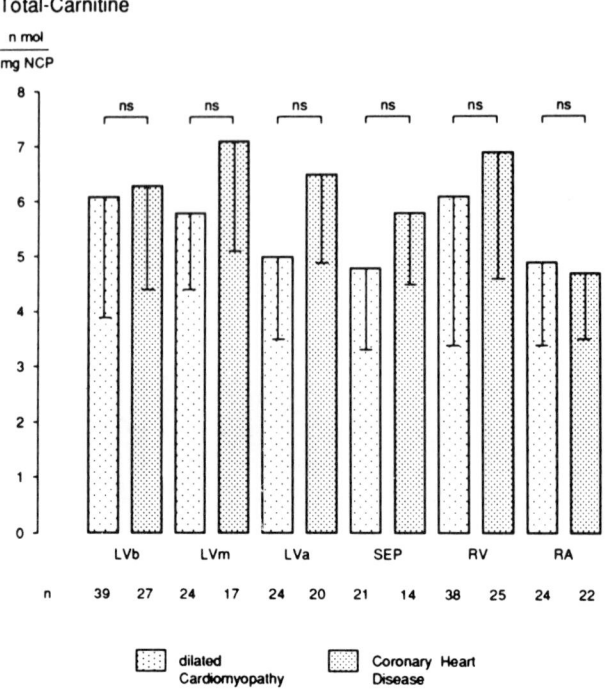

Total-Carnitine

FIGURE 4. Myocardial carnitine loss in end-stage heart failure, comparison between carnitine concentrations in dilated cardiomyopathy and coronary heart disease. No significant difference exists between the two groups.

leakage of carnitine from the cells may occur if the time interval between death and autopsy is relatively long, although carnitine is not broken down enzymatically. For these reasons, the use of autopsy hearts to obtain normal values should be restricted. Endomyocardial biopsies or biopsies from healthy donor hearts are probably more representative of in vivo carnitine levels.

CHARACTERISTIC FEATURES OF MYOCARDIAL CARNITINE LOSS IN END-STAGE HEART FAILURE

Lack of correlation between carnitine loss and aetiology of heart failure

There is often no correlation between myocardial carnitine loss and the aetiology of end-stage heart failure. Patients with dilated cardiomyopathy and heart failure due to coronary or valvular heart disease do show a comparable loss of myocardial carnitine in several studies (Regitz et al, 1988a, 1990; Bressler et al, 1990; A. Patel et al, unpublished data). Individual patients with myocarditis and valvular disease were also studied, and in these there were no differences in comparison with the groups already mentioned (Regitz et al, 1988b). Thus, the myocardial carnitine loss in heart failure is not a primary, disease-specific finding. It probably represents a secondary phenomenon following pressure or volume load, or a response to increased wall stress or filling pressures or a compensatory metabolic mechanism.

High inter-individual variability of myocardial carnitine content

Patients with end-stage heart failure and the same aetiology (such as dilated cardiomyopathy) show great differences in myocardial carnitine content (Regitz et al, 1988a; Bressler et al, 1990), although their functional deficits are comparable. Thus, decreased myocardial carnitine is not simply an answer to haemodynamic changes. Different compensatory mechanisms may be effective in different patients and may lead to differing responses to metabolic stress.

Homogeneous distribution of myocardial carnitine loss in heart failure

We found a homogeneous distribution of carnitine in the right ventricle, in the septum and in the base and mid area of the left ventricle. This was true for all control groups in this and in other studies as well as for all patient groups evaluated. Carnitine concentrations in the septum and right ventricle were not significantly different from the left ventricle; however, there was a tendency to a lower carnitine content in the atria. Possibly the ventricle, with a higher mechanical load, utilizes the more efficient fatty acid oxidation to a greater extent than the atrial myocardium. Direct measurements of substrate utilization are needed to substantiate this hypothesis.

Because of the homogeneous distribution of carnitine in the myocardia of failing hearts, biopsies from the right ventricular septum may be used to estimate metabolite content in the heart and to use it for functional correlations.

MYOCARDIAL CARNITINE LOSS IN MILD TO SEVERE HEART FAILURE—MEASUREMENTS IN ENDOMYOCARDIAL BIOPSIES

In contrast to studies in explanted hearts, measurements in endomyocardial biopsies enable changes in the early stages of the disease to be monitored, to investigate possible correlations between metabolic changes and function and to obtain normal tissue for comparisons. Methodological problems inherent to the material available must however be solved before measurements can be accepted. So far two groups have reported reduced myocardial carnitine in endomyocardial biopsies from patients with mild to severe heart failure and have discussed functional consequences (Regitz et al, 1990; A. Patel et al, unpublished data).

Prerequisites for metabolic determinations in endomyocardial biopsies

Metabolic determinations in endomyocardial biopsies are only possible if suitable micromethods are available to measure samples of about 1–3 mg with sufficient sensitivity and reproducibility. A suitable reference system is also required. Wet weight measurements give rise to the greatest mistakes in small and bloody samples and are therefore not suitable. If carnitine determinations related to non-collagen protein and to wet weight are compared, the advantages of non-collagen protein become evident (Figure 5), with variances of about 30% in a group of healthy controls.

Knowing the regional distribution of metabolic changes in the failing heart is essential for the correct interpretation of measurements in endomyocardial biopsies (see above). As there is a relatively homogeneous distribution of carnitine in failing hearts with either coronary heart disease or cardiomyopathy, right-ventricular samples may be used to estimate carnitine content of the heart.

Finally determination of normal values is crucial. Nearly normal values can only be approached in endomyocardial biopsies without postmortem changes, the influence of premortal disease or the influence of anaesthesia. We therefore used endomyocardial biopsies of patients in whom coronary, valvular or pulmonary heart disease was excluded after complete invasive diagnosis including ventriculography, coronary

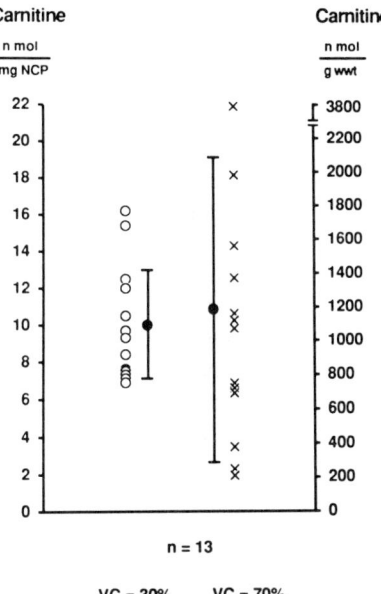

FIGURE 5. Importance of the reference system for metabolic determinations in endomyocardial biopsies. Myocardial carnitine levels in 13 controls related to non-collagen protein (left) and related to wet weight (right) are shown. The coefficient of variance was lower for the non-collagen protein-related values.

angiography and endomyocardial biopsy for the determination of normal values.

The DHZB study

Carnitine concentrations were determined in right-ventricular endomyocardial biopsies from 28 patients with dilated cardiomyopathy and eight patients with heart failure with different causes, and compared with 13 normal controls. Haemodynamic features of these patients are depicted in Table 2. In controls coronary, valvular, hypertensive or pulmonary heart disease was excluded after complete invasive diagnosis including right- and left-ventricular angiography, coronary angiography and endomyocardial biopsy (Table 2).

In 28 patients with dilated cardiomyopathy and mild to severe, but not yet end-stage, heart failure, myocardial carnitine was significantly reduced compared with 13 normal controls. Total (Figure 6a) as well

TABLE 2.

Haemodynamic parameters of patients with mild to severe heart failure due to dilated cardiomyopathy (DCM) or to heart failure of different origins (HF) and controls (Con).

	DCM $n = 28$	HF $n = 8$	Con $n = 13$
LVEF (%)	31 ± 11	34 ± 11	65 ± 5
LVEDVI (ml qm^{-1})	181 ± 57	192 ± 70	91 ± 11
LVESVI (ml qm^{-1})	125 ± 54	122 ± 58	32 ± 12
LVEDP (mmHg)	19 ± 10	15 ± 5	11 ± 3
CI (l min$^{-1} \times$ qm)	3.4 ± 1.1	4.2 ± 1.1	3.8 ± 0.9
RVEF (%)	39 ± 12	52 ± 10	57 ± 5

as free myocardial carnitine concentration were affected (Figure 6b). The extent of the reduction in free and total myocardial carnitine in the patients with coronary heart disease was not significantly different from the carnitine loss in patients with dilated cardiomyopathy.

In patients with left-ventricular ejection fractions below 30% the loss of total (Figure 7a) and free (Figure 7b) myocardial carnitine was more pronounced than in patients with ejection fractions between 30 and 50%. A significant non-linear relationship was found between free myocardial carnitine concentration and left-ventricular ejection fraction in the patients with dilated cardiomyopathy and controls (Figure 8).

Literature review

Carnitine levels in endomyocardial biopsies from human hearts have also been determined by A.L. Shug's group (A. Patel et al, unpublished data). Of 40 patients with dilated cardiomyopathy, hypertensive, coronary or valvular heart disease, 18 had myocardial carnitine concentrations below 5 nmol mg^{-1} non-collagen protein (NCP) (normal: 9 ± 2 nmol mg^{-1} NCP). This group also found no differences between the different aetiologies of heart failure. Patients were followed for more than 1 year and a significant association between myocardial carnitine levels and survival was documented.

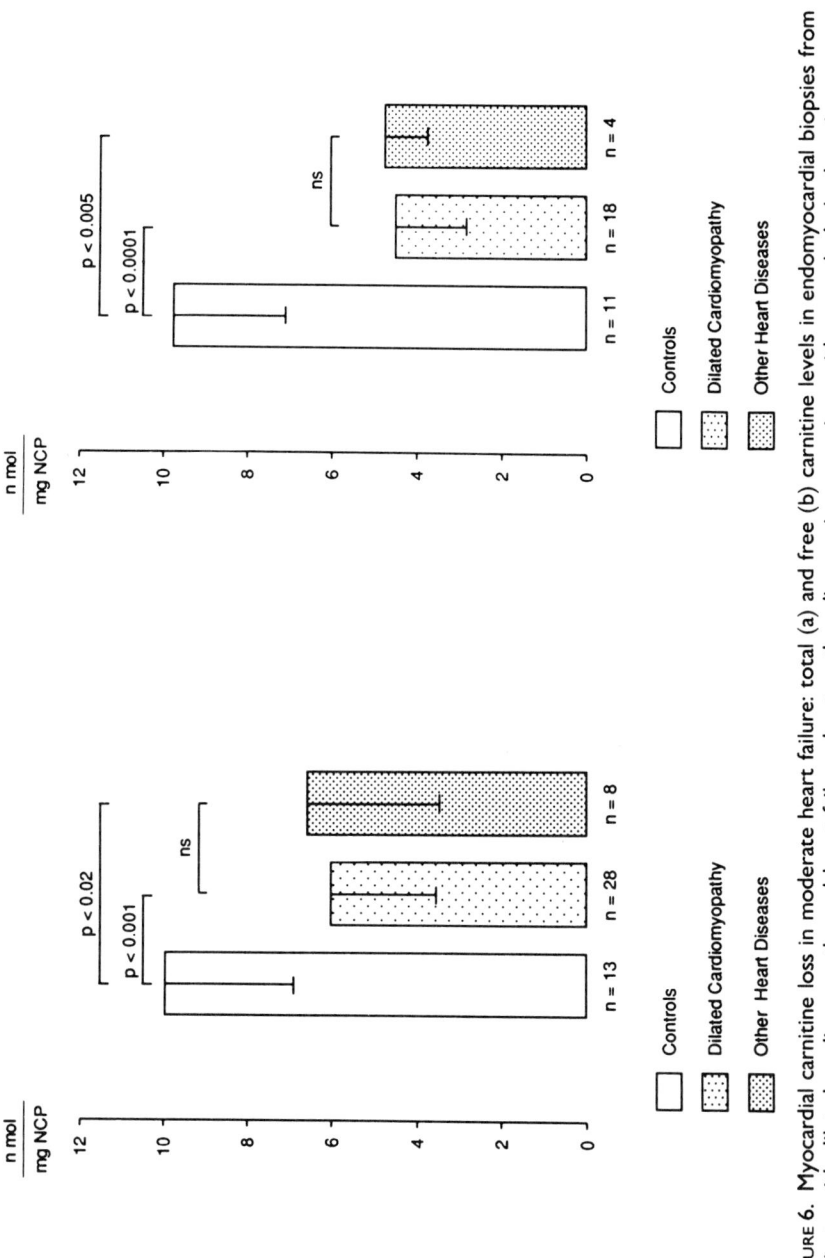

FIGURE 6. Myocardial carnitine loss in moderate heart failure: total (a) and free (b) carnitine levels in endomyocardial biopsies from patients with dilated cardiomyopathy and heart failure due to other diseases in comparison with controls. In both patient groups there was a significant loss of total and free myocardial carnitine in comparison with controls. No difference was found between the two patient groups.

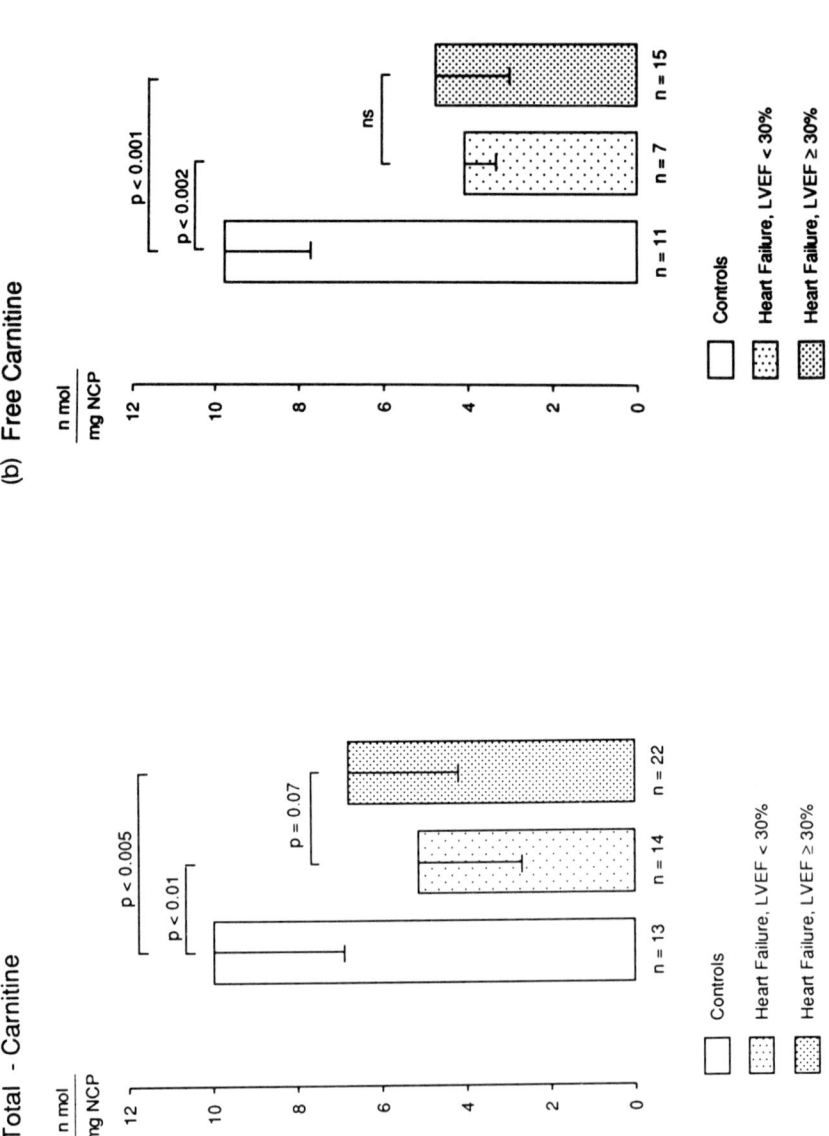

FIGURE 7. Myocardial carnitine loss in mild to severe heart failure: total (a) and free (b) carnitine levels in endomyocardial biopsies from patients with left-ventricular ejection fractions below 30% and with ejection fractions from 30–55% are shown. Both patient groups were significantly different from control. Patients with left-ventricular ejection fractions from 30–55% had higher myocardial

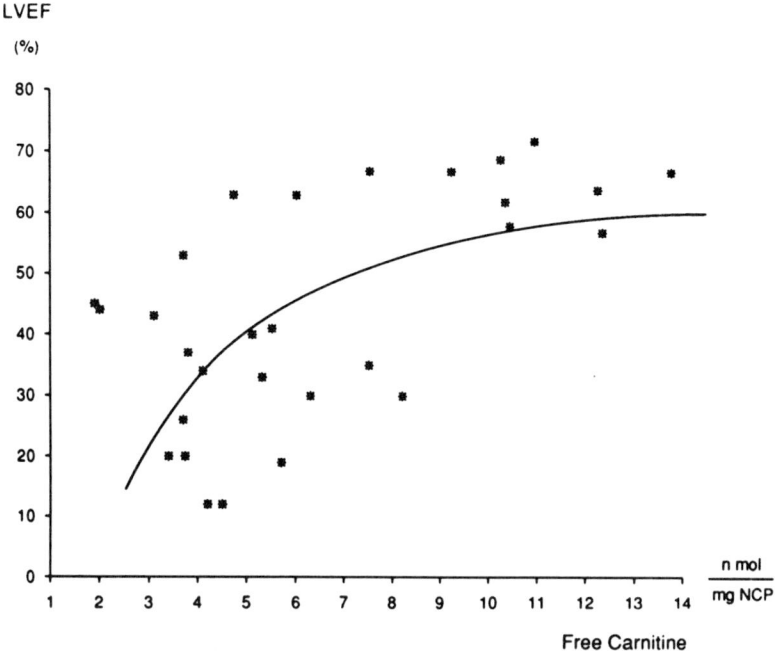

FIGURE 8. Non-linear relationship between myocardial carnitine and left-ventricular ejection fraction in patients with dilated cardiomyopathy and controls ($n = 29$). Using a non-linear fitting model the relationship LVEF $= (74.58 - 167.92) \div$ free carnitine is found. Transforming the equation with 1/free carnitine as new independent variable results in a linear correlation coefficient of $r = 0.76$; $p < 0.01$.

Characteristic features of myocardial carnitine loss in mild to severe heart failure

Association between myocardial carnitine loss, underlying cardiac diseases and cardiac function

We are able to compare the myocardial carnitine metabolism of patients with dilated cardiomyopathy and coronary heart disease, and to monitor it in individual patients with myocarditis and valvular heart disease (Regitz et al, 1988a, 1988b, 1990). In all patients the loss of carnitine was comparable; in agreement with other authors, no differences could be established between heart failure with different causes (Pierpont et al, 1989; Bressler et al, 1990; Patel, unpublished data). Therefore, carnitine deficiency is probably a secondary metabolic defect following pressure or volume load or a compensatory metabolic mechanism, and not a primary, disease-specific feature. Patients with the severest decrease of ejection fraction showed the most pronounced myocardial carnitine loss. A correlation between biochemical defects and decrease of myocardial function could be established. The correlation was closest in patients with cardiomyopathy, probably because in these patients the depressed ejection fraction corresponds to the impairment of myocardial function. In contrast, in coronary or valvular heart disease, regional wall motion disturbances, or unphysiological loading conditions caused by altered valve function, affect global cardiac function as a whole, including left-ventricular ejection fraction.

Although correlations between myocardial carnitine and left-ventricular ejection fraction can be established in dilated cardiomyopathy, there is a high inter-individual variability. Thus, carnitine levels do not only reflect functional impairment but, as already stated, probably also represent the metabolic response of the myocardium to stress. This response, however, may vary in different patients depending on duration of the disease, genetic disposition, nutritional status, availability of substrates, hormonal regulations and the availability of other compensatory mechanisms.

Carnitine loss in early heart failure

Patients with mild impairment of left-ventricular function, with ejection fractions from 30–55%, already have significant reductions in myocardial carnitine content as well as increased lactate dehydrogenase (LDH) activity (Regitz et al, 1988a). Thus, metabolic alterations may have been made in an effort to stabilize the metabolism and function of the myocardium before pronounced clinical manifestations or functional disturbances can be seen. In these cases there will be a discrepancy between pronounced metabolic alterations and less severe functional impairment. This does not limit the value of biochemical investigations in the myocardium; assessment of metabolic alterations may offer a second way of assessing myocardial damage in addition to changes in pumping function.

Prognostic significance of myocardial carnitine loss

A relationship between myocardial carnitine concentration and prognosis has been postulated (A. Patel et al, unpublished data). The same group reject a relationship between myocardial carnitine content and ejection fraction. However, this study did not analyse the relationship between survival and ejection fraction and there was no multivariate analysis to search for prognostic parameters. We speculate that relationships between survival and both carnitine and ejection fraction will be found and that carnitine and ejection fraction will not turn out to be independent prognostic parameters if large numbers of patients, or a more homogeneous group, is studied and if adequate multivariate analysis is done.

PLASMA CARNITINE IN HEART FAILURE

Rise of plasma carnitine in end-stage and less severe heart failure—the DHZB experience

Plasma carnitine concentrations were determined in patients with dilated cardiomyopathy (n = 38) and coronary heart disease (n = 22) and end-stage heart failure, in 16 patients with mild to severe heart failure and 15 controls. The haemodynamic parameters of patients whose plasma carnitine levels were determined were not different from the corresponding groups in whom myocardial carnitine determinations were performed. Plasma for the determination of free and total carnitine, as well as of creatinine, was taken just before transplantation or during a pre-operative ambulatory control or on the day of cardiac catheterization. Controls for plasma carnitine determinations were 15 patients with normal left-ventricular ejection fraction without significant cardiac or metabolic diseases (for example, diabetes mellitus).

Plasma carnitine levels in 16 patients with mild to severe heart failure and 60 patients with end-stage heart failure were significantly elevated compared with normal controls. This affected both total (Figure 9a) and free carnitine levels (Figure 9b). The ratio free/total plasma carnitine was 0.71 ± 0.03 in heart failure and 0.81 ± 0.05 in normal controls. No significant differences were found between the patients with dilated cardiomyopathy and coronary heart disease. Although the highest plasma carnitine concentrations were found in end-stage heart failure, the correlation between plasma carnitine and left-ventricular ejection fraction was not significant ($p < 0.07$, $r = 0.47$). No significant correlation was found between the concentration of carnitine in plasma and the myocardium.

As carnitine is eliminated by the kidney and plasma carnitine is increased in renal failure, we measured serum creatinine and correlated it with plasma carnitine to determine if the impairment of kidney function was linked to the rise in plasma carnitine in our patients. No significant correlation was established (Figure 10).

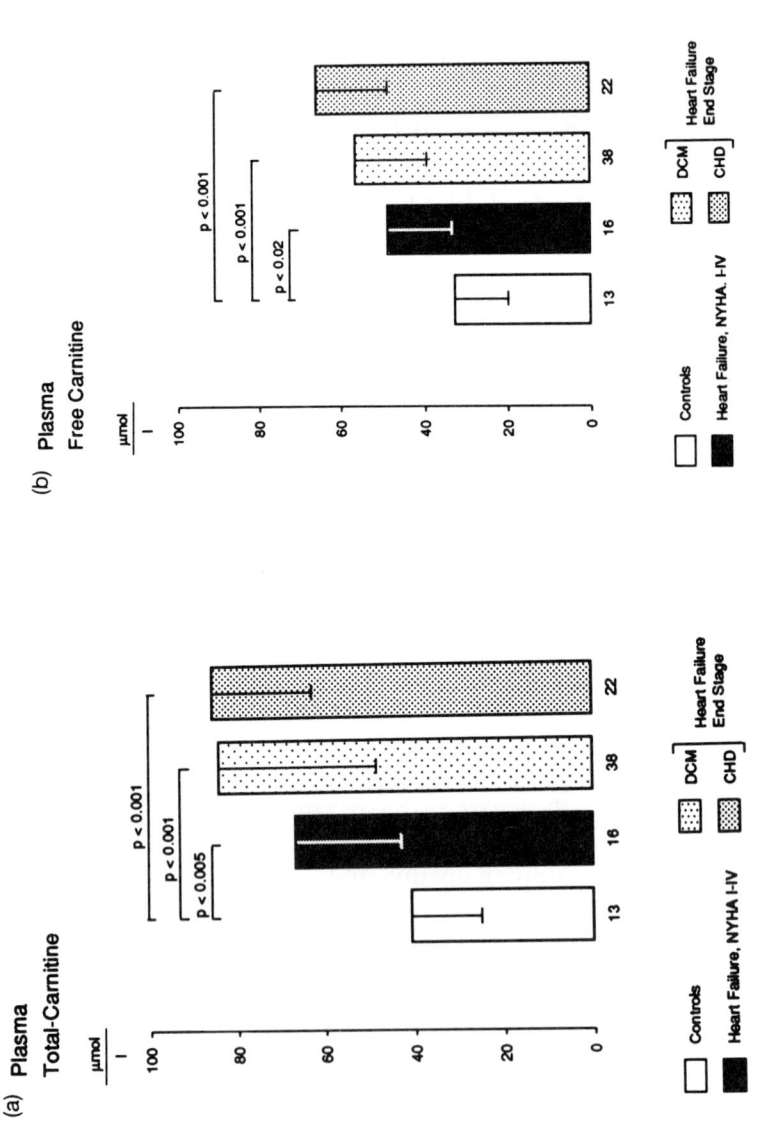

FIGURE 9. Total (a) and free (b) plasma carnitine in patients with end-stage heart failure, in patients with moderate to severe depression of left-ventricular function and in controls. There is a significant rise of plasma carnitine in all patient groups which is most pronounced in the patients with end-stage heart failure.

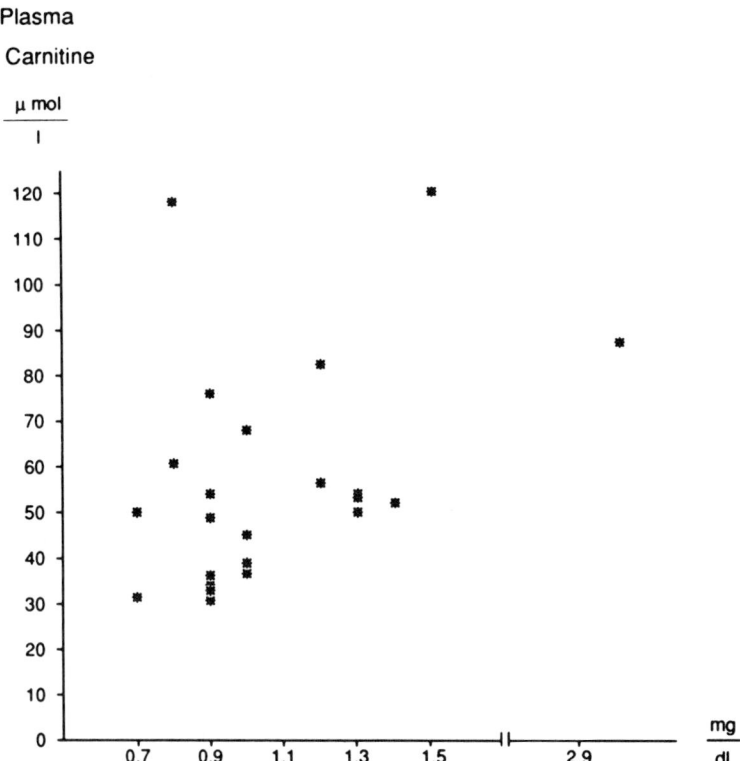

FIGURE 10. Relationship between plasma carnitine and serum creatinine in heart failure: no significant correlation was found.

Literature review

The rise in plasma carnitine concentration in heart failure has been described by several groups (Tripp and Shug, 1984; Conte et al, 1987; Pierpont et al, 1989; Regitz et al, 1990). Although the highest plasma carnitine levels have been described in patients undergoing heart transplantation, no significant correlation between plasma carnitine and myocardial function was established in the groups studied. This may be due partially to the small number and non-homogeneity of the patients investigated. Further, plasma carnitine levels are not only determined by myocardial function but also by several independent parameters such as regulation by hormones, or liver and kidney function (Boehmer et al, 1974; Chen and Lincoln, 1977; Shug and Paulson, 1984). They are certainly less closely linked to myocardial function than myocardial carnitine levels. Thus, an association between plasma carnitine concentrations and prognosis can probably be established if large numbers of patients in all disease states can be included. However, the correlation will be less close than the correlation between myocardial carnitine content and prognosis.

CARNITINE PALMITOYL TRANSFERASE ACTIVITY IN HUMAN HEART FAILURE

Carnitine palmitoyl transferase (CPT, EC 2.3.1.21) represents the rate-limiting step of fatty acid oxidation. It is responsible for the trans-esterification of cytoplasmic long-chain acyl CoA esters with free carnitine to long-chain acylcarnitine esters. In contrast to long-chain acyl CoA esters these carnitine esters are transported into the mitochondrial matrix where they undergo β-oxidation. It has been speculated that limited availability of free carnitine for the carnitine palmitoyl transferase reaction limits the uptake of long-chain fatty acid derivatives into the mitochondria. The determination of the Michaelis constant of CPT versus free carnitine may indicate whether, under physiological or pathological conditions, free carnitine concentrations can limit the transferase reaction.

CPT activity and the Michaelis constant of CPT versus free carnitine in explanted human hearts

We determined the carnitine palmitoyl transferase activity using the forward reaction (McGarry et al, 1978). We measured the radioactively-labelled palmitoyl carnitine that was formed from palmitoyl CoA and radioactively-marked free carnitine. Reaction velocity was determined with varying free carnitine concentrations to calculate the K_m (substrate concentrations at half maximal reaction velocity). Carnitine concentrations between 25 μM and 800 μM were used.

The total carnitine palmitoyl transferase activity was measured in the left ventricle and in the right atrium from 25 explanted hearts from patients with end-stage dilated cardiomyopathy or coronary heart disease. Functional parameters of these hearts were not different from hearts used for carnitine determinations. Six of the explanted hearts were randomly chosen for kinetic studies.

The activity of carnitine palmitoyl transferase in the right atrium from 25 explanted hearts was 960 ± 299 mU mg^{-1} NCP. This was significantly lower than the CPT activity in left-ventricular samples from the same 25 patients: 1199 ± 237 mU mg^{-1} NCP ($p < 0.05$).

The Michaelis constant of CPT versus free carnitine in six explanted hearts was about 300 mM. This corresponds to tissue concentrations of about 300 nmol carnitine per g wet weight, corresponding to between one quarter and one third of the physiological carnitine concentrations of about 1000 nmol per g wet weight (Figure 11).

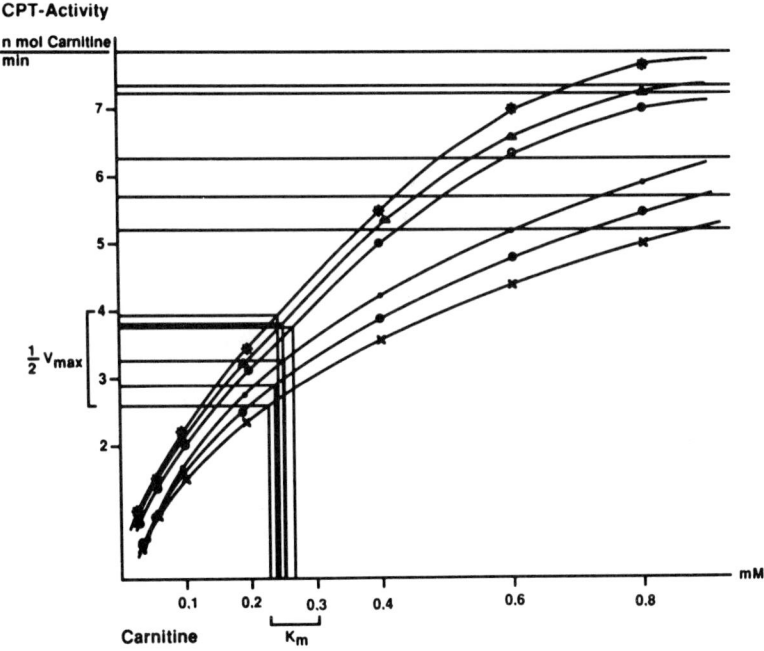

FIGURE 11. K_m of carnitine palmitoyl transferase (CPT) versus free carnitine in explanted human hearts. The reaction velocities (v) for carnitine concentrations from 25 to 800 μm in six experiments are shown as well as the calculated substrate concentration at half-maximal reaction velocity (K_m).

Consequences of experimental CPT inhibition

Bressler investigated the effects of CPT inhibition with tetradecylgly-cidic acid (TDGA) in normal rats and diabetic mice (Bressler et al, 1990). Both animal groups developed myocardial hypertrophy and increased glucose utilization. Systolic function was unchanged but diastolic stiffness was significantly increased in TDGA treated animals. It was concluded that a chronic decrease in long-chain fatty acid oxidation and the consequent increase in glucose utilization was detrimental to cardiac structure and function (Bressler et al, 1990).

Role of CPT in human heart failure

The regulation of the carnitine palmitoyl transferase is done by several allosteric inhibitors or activators. An important inhibitor is malonyl CoA, the first committed metabolite of fatty acid synthesis from glucose. Free carnitine does not limit the activity of carnitine palmitoyl transferase in the myocardium in vivo under physiological conditions. Investigations in rat myocardium have shown that the normal free carnitine concentrations in tissue are several times higher than the Michaelis constant of carnitine palmitoyl transferase for free carnitine. Only if carnitine concentrations fall below the Michaelis constant, i.e. the substrate concentration needed for half-maximal reaction velocity, may the concentration of free carnitine limit reaction velocity.

In the human myocardium we found a distribution of activities of carnitine palmitoyl transferase that are comparable to these described (Choi et al, 1977) for rat myocardium: higher CPT activities in the ventricle in comparison to the atria are confirmed by our data. In the explanted hearts we calculated a Michaelis-constant (K_m) of carnitine palmitoyl transferase against free carnitine of about 300 μM. Comparable to animal experiments, the K_m of carnitine palmitoyl transferase versus free carnitine under physiological concentrations was clearly below the tissue concentrations for free carnitine. As in patients with heart failure, a reduction of myocardial carnitine content to between one quarter and one third of physiological levels can occur. The velocity of carnitine palmitoyl transferase reaction and therefore the availability of fatty acids for oxidation in the mitochondria may well be controlled by the availability of free carnitine.

PATHOPHYSIOLOGY OF CARNITINE IN HEART FAILURE

Relationship between free and total carnitine

Tissue carnitine is present as free carnitine that is available for trans-esterifications with long-chain acyl CoA esters and as esterified carnitine, mainly acetylcarnitine and acylcarnitine. The distribution found by us with 80% of plasma and about 90% of tissue carnitine being present as free carnitine is in agreement with plasma levels that have been obtained in humans and tissue values from the rat heart (Boehmer et al, 1974; Borum, 1978; Tripp and Shug, 1984). The ratio of free to total carnitine in the plasma and in the tissue is not significantly changed in heart failure. Thus, a relative rise of carnitine esters in heart failure is not evident from our data. To document such a rise will be difficult as, according to previous findings, the increase of carnitine esters in the tissues will not exceed 10–30% of total carnitine (Folts et al, 1978). This, however, is in the range of the variability of the carnitine determination in endomyocardial biopsies. A supposed rise of carnitine esters cannot be documented in samples from explanted hearts as even unavoidable delays of a few minutes between taking out the heart and freezing the tissue lead to a rise of carnitine esters due to ischaemia.

Compartmentalization of myocardial carnitine

Measuring the loss of carnitine in tissue homogenates gives no information as to which compartments—cytosol, membranes or mitochondria are mainly concerned. As, however, more than about 90% of total carnitine in the non-ischaemic heart is stored in the cytosol and only about 10% in the mitochondria (Idell-Wenger et al, 1978), the loss of carnitine in heart failure will mainly affect the cytosol. It cannot be based on the reduction of the volume fraction of mitochondria that occurs in heart failure (Katz, 1988). Thus in patients with heart failure a reduction of effective carnitine concentrations that are available in the cytoplasm occurs.

Reasons for increased plasma and decreased myocardial carnitine concentrations in heart failure

Several metabolic alterations are associated with reduced tissue carnitine. Primary systemic carnitine deficiency is a rare inborn disease where carnitine biosynthesis is probably affected (Treem et al, 1988). Secondary carnitine deficiency syndromes are associated with defects in fatty acid oxidation and amino acid metabolism (Chapay et al, 1970; Chalmers et al, 1984; Roe et al, 1984). In both patient groups, the continuous elimination of toxic metabolites as carnitine esters leads to a depletion of the body in carnitine. Patients with primary and secondary carnitine deficiency differ from the heart failure patients studied by us in their low plasma carnitine levels.

Physiologically, carnitine is synthesized in the liver, and is accumulated in the myocytes to concentrations 20–50 times greater than the plasma levels (Molstadt et al, 1977; Siliprandi et al, 1987). High myocardial carnitine levels are maintained by the action of a specific carnitine carrier together with relative impermeability of the myocyte membrane for carnitine. Defects in the carrier system (as occurs in diphtheria), as well as non-specific membrane damage (as found in ischaemia) may lead to reduced myocardial carnitine concentrations (Bressler and Wittels, 1965; Folts et al, 1978; Shug et al, 1978; Thomson et al, 1979). Both mechanisms would be consistent with a rise in plasma carnitine levels as documented in our patients. Other possible mechanisms that may lead to an elevation of plasma carnitine, for example impaired kidney function, are not important in our patients with mainly normal or only moderately impaired kidney function (Chen and Lincoln, 1977).

Consequences of reduced myocardial carnitine content in heart failure; possible compensation by increased glucose utilization

Free carnitine levels in heart failure fall into the range of the K_m of CPT and thus the availability of free carnitine may limit fatty acid oxidation. Studies with CPT inhibition in animal models have shown that reduced fatty acid oxidation is not necessarily accompanied by accumulation of lipid droplets in the myocardium (Bressler et al, 1990) as it occurs in severe carnitine deficiency with myocardial carnitine levels falling below 5% of controls (Regitz et al, 1982).

Parallel to the myocardial carnitine loss and increase in plasma carnitine, alterations of glucose and/or lactate metabolism occur in heart failure (Regitz et al, 1988a). Patients with dilated cardiomyopathy have two-fold greater activity of myocardial lactate dehydrogenase (LDH) and hydroxybutyrate dehydrogenase (HBDH) (Figure 12a and b), indicating increased glucose or lactate utilization for energy production. As lactate production at rest does not usually occur in dilated cardiomyopathy (Pasternac et al, 1982), this probably corresponds to increased carbohydrate metabolism. We hypothesize that the combination of reduced myocardial carnitine levels and activation of LDH and HBDH indicate a switch of myocardial metabolism from preferred fatty acid utilization to preferred glucose or lactate utilization. The rise in glucose of lactase utilization could correspond to a metabolic compensation for limited fatty acid utilization. There is experimental evidence that such a shift is harmful in a *chronic* animal model (Bressler et al, 1990); however, no data are available for humans so far.

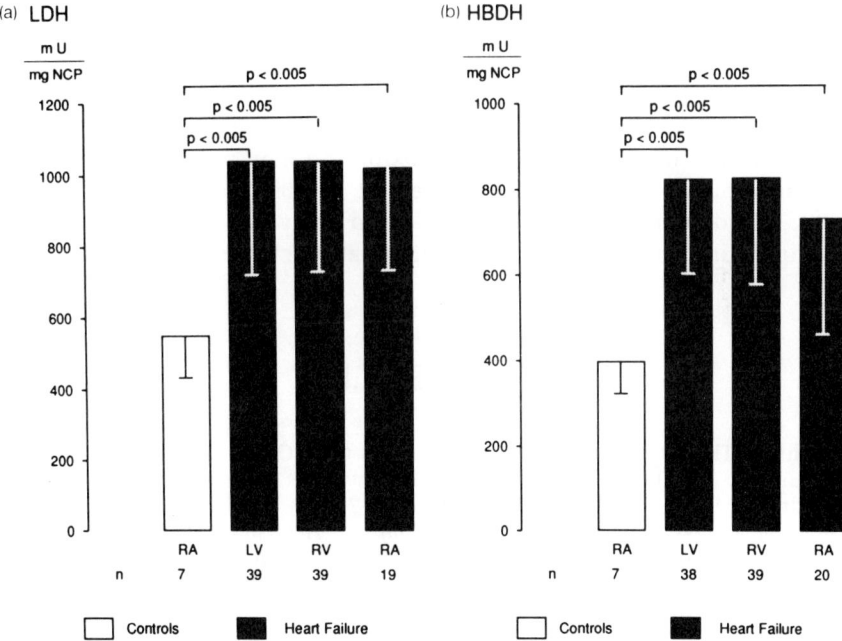

FIGURE 12. Rise of lactate dehydrogenase (LDH) and hydroxybutyrate dehydrogenase (HBDH) in end-stage human heart failure. LDH and HBDH activities are shown in explanted hearts from patients with end-stage heart failure in comparison with healthy donor hearts (right atrium, $n = 7$). In comparison with controls a significant rise of both LDH and HBDH was found in heart failure.

SUMMARY

In explanted hearts from patients with end-stage heart failure a significant myocardial carnitine loss occurs independently of the pathogenic origin. The myocardial carnitine loss affects all areas of the explanted hearts; the distribution of cartinine in end-stage heart failure is relatively homogeneous. In endomyocardial biopsies from patients with early mild to severe, but not yet end-stage, heart failure, a comparable loss of myocardial carnitine is found. In this group, the myocardial carnitine decrease is more pronounced in patients with more severe heart failure than in patients with less severe reduction of ejection fraction. Also patients with only moderately impaired left-ventricular ejection fraction (LVEF 30–55%) exhibit a significant decrease in myocardial carnitine content. Possible reasons include defects in the carnitine transport system of myocytes or non-specific membrane damage. In animal experiments, reduced myocardial carnitine concentrations were associated with impaired myocardial function. The decrease of myocardial carnitine in heart failure in some patients reaches levels of about one third of the physiological concentrations. In this range, the availability of free carnitine may limit the activity of carnitine palmitoyl transferase. Therefore, a limitation of myocardial fatty acid oxidation may occur in some heart failure patients. Indicators of increased glucose or lactate utilization can be demonstrated in parallel and may be interpreted as a compensatory mechanism for reduced fatty acid oxidation.

REFERENCES

Boehmer Th, Rydning A, Solberg HE (1974) Clin. Chim. Acta 57: 55–61.
Borum PR (1978) Biochem. J. 176: 677–681.
Bradford MM (1976) Anal. Biochem. 72: 248–254.
Bressler R & Wittels B (1965) Biochim. Biophys. Acta 104: 39–45.
Bressler R, Gay R, Copeland JG et al (1990) Life Sciences 44: 1897–1906.
Chalmers RA, Roe CR, Stacey JE et al (1984) Pediatr. Res. 12: 1325–1326.
Chapoy PR, Angelini C, Brown WJ et al (1980) N Engl. J. Med. 303: 1389–1393.
Chen S-H & Lincoln SD (1977) Clin. Chem. 23: 278–280.
Choi YR, Fogle PJ, Clarke PRH & Bieber LL (1977) J. Biol. Chem. 252: 7930–7931.
Conte A, Hess OM, Maire R et al (1987) Z. Kardiol. 76: 15–24.
Engel AG & Angelini C (1973) Science 179: 899–902.
Folts JD, Shug AL, Koke JR & Bittar N (1978) Am. J. Cardiol. 41: 1209–1214.
Francis GS (1985) Am. J . Cardiol. 55: 17A–21A.

Idell-Wenger JA, Grotyohann LW & Neely JR (1978) *J. Biol. Chem.* 12: 4310–4318.
Ino T, Sherwood WG, Benson LN et al (1988) *J. Am. Coll. Cardiol.* 11 (6): 1301–1308.
Katz AM (1970) *Physiol. Rev.* 50: 63–158.
Katz AM (1988) *Am. J. Cardiol.* 62: 3A–8A.
Keene B, Panciera DL, Regitz V et al (1986) *Scientific Proceedings of the Am. Coll. Vet. Intern. Med.* 2: 14.
Levine TB, Francis GS, Simon SR & Cohn JN (1982) *Am. J. Cardiol.* 49: 1659–1666.
Lilienthal JL, Zierler KL, Folk BP et al (1949) *J. Biol. Chem.* 182: 501–508.
McGarry JD, Leatherman GF & Foster DW (1978) *J. Biol. Chem.* 253: 4128–4136.
Meerson FZ (1983) In *The Failing Heart: Adaptation and Deadaptation* pp 128–179. New York: Raven Press.
Molstadt P, Bohmer T & Eiklid K (1977) *Biochim. Biophys. Acta* 471: 296–304.
Neely JR & Morgan HE (1974) *Annu. Rev. Physiol.* 36: 413–459.
Parvin R & Pande SV (1977) *Anal. Biochem.* 79: 190–201.
Pasternac A, Noble J, Streulens Y et al (1982) *Circulation* 65: 778–789.
Paulson DJ & Shug AL (1981) *Life Sci.* 28: 2931–2938.
Paulson DJ, Schmidt MJ, Traxler JS et al (1984) *Metabolism* 33: 358–363.
Pfeffer MA, Lamas GA, Vaughan DE et al (1988) *N Engl. J. Med.* 319: 80–86.
Pierpont MEM, Judd D, Goldenberg IF et al (1989) *Am. J. Cardiol.* 64: 56–60.
Rabinowitz M (1973) *Am. J. Cardiol.* 31: 202–210.
Rebouche CJ and Engel AG (1983) *Mayo Clin. Proc.* 58: 533–540.
Regitz V, Hodach RJ & Shug AL (1982) *Klin. Wochenschr.* 60: 393–399.
Regitz V, Shug AL, Shüler S et al (1988a) *Deutsche Medizinische Wochenschrift* 113: 718–786.
Regitz V, Strasser R, Chmielewski G et al (1988b) In H.P. Schultheiss (ed.) *New Concepts in Viral Heart Disease.* Berlin, Heidelberg: Springer-Verlag.
Regitz V, Shug AL & Fleck E (1990) *Am. J. Cardiol.* 65: 755–760.
Roe CR, Millington SD, Maltby DA et al (1984) *J. Clin. Invest.* 74: 2290–2295.
Shug AL & Paulson DJ (1984) In Ferrari A, Katz A, Shug S & Visioli O (eds), *Myocardial Ischemia and Lipid Metabolism* pp 203–224. New York: Plenum Press.
Shug AL, Thomsen JH, Folts JD et al (1978) *Arch. Biochem. Biophys.* 187: 25–33.
Siliprandi N, Di Lisa F, Pivetta A et al (1987) *Z. Kardiol.* 76 (Supplement 5): 34–40.
Thomson JH, Shug AL, Yap VU et al (1979) *Am. J. Cardiol.* 43: 300–306.
Treem WR, Stanley CA, Finegold DN et al (1988) *N. Engl. J. Med.* 319: 1331–1336.
Tripp ME & Shug AL (1984) *Biochem. Medic.* 32: 199–206.
Tubbs PK, Ramsay RR & Edwards RR (1980) In Frenkel RA & McGarry JD (eds) *Carnitine, Biosynthesis, Metabolism and Functions* pp 207–216. New York: Academic Press.
Waber LJ, Valle D, Neill C et al (1982) *Am. J. Pediatr.* 101: 700–705.
Whitmer JT (1987) *Circ. Res.* 61: 396–408.

17

MYOCARDIAL CARNITINE STATUS: CLINICAL, PROGNOSTIC AND THERAPEUTIC SIGNIFICANCE

A.K. Patel, J.H. Thomsen, P.K. Kosolcharoen and A.L. Shug

Carnitine (3-hydroxy-4N-trimethylaminobutyric acid) facilitates transport of long-chain fatty acids across the inner mitochondrial membrane (Bremer, 1983). Since long-chain fatty acids are the predominant energy-yielding substrate for oxidative metabolism by cardiac cells, carnitine deficiency may be associated with cardiac dysfunction. This chapter will review studies dealing with myocardial carnitine status in children, adults and various animal models, its association with cardiac disease, its prognostic significance and response to carnitine therapy.

L-Carnitine and Its Role in Medicine:
From Function to Therapy. ISBN 0–12–253940–0

CARNITINE DEFICIENCY IN CHILDREN

Clinical presentation, cardiac disease, response to therapy

The predominant clinical presentation in children with systemic carnitine deficiency is multisystem manifestation, mainly skeletal muscle weakness in myopathic cardiac deficiency or clinical features related to enzyme defects of fatty acid metabolism. Cardiac disease is manifest as either dilated or hypertrophic cardiomyopathy and endocardial fibroelastosis with congestive heart failure (Table 1).

Total plasma and skeletal muscle carnitine levels are low in systemic carnitine deficiency. Total plasma levels were normal and skeletal muscle carnitine low in myopathic carnitine deficiency. Myocardial histology in five patients showed lipid deposits consistent with a defect in fatty acid metabolism (Tripp et al, 1981; Matsuishi et al, 1985; Ino et al, 1988). The cardiac response to therapy with DL- or L-carnitine is usually good, despite only partial normalization of plasma or skeletal muscle carnitine concentration (Chapoy et al, 1980; Tripp et al, 1981; Waber et al, 1982; Matsuishi et al, 1985; Eriksson et al, 1988; Tein et al, 1990).

Myocardial carnitine status

Myocardial carnitine concentrations were documented in only three patients. In one autopsy patient, the level was in the low–normal range despite DL-carnitine therapy (Hart et al, 1978). In another autopsy patient, who did not receive carnitine therapy, the levels were markedly reduced (Tripp et al, 1981). In one case of documented primary systemic carnitine deficiency, myocardial carnitine concentrations were less than 1% of controls (Eriksson et al, 1988). Therefore, although response to therapy is usually good in children with carnitine deficiency and cardiac dysfunction, there is a paucity of information on myocardial carnitine concentrations in these patients.

TABLE I.

Plasma and skeletal muscle carnitine deficiency, cardiac disease, and response to therapy in children

Reference	Age	Clinical presentation		Carnitine				Response	Comments
		General	Cardiac	Pre-treatment		Post-treatment			
				Plasma	Muscle	Plasma	Muscle		
Hart et al (1978)	23 months	MCD *1*	DCM	Low	Low	—	—	DL-Car: died	Borderline LMC at autopsy
Chapoy et al (1980)	3.5 yr	SCD *1*	DCM	Low (<5%)	Low (<5%)	Low-N	Low-N	DL- & L-Car: good	?Family history of SCD
Tripp et al (1981)	15 months –9 yr	SD *3* Cardiomegaly *1*	EFE *3* DCM *1*	Low *3*	Low *2*	Low-N *1*	Low *1*	L-Car: good *1*	Familial cardiomyopathy; LMC in 1 autopsy patient
Waber et al (1982)	3.5 yr	Hypotonia *1*	DCM	Low (<2%)	Low (<10%)	Low-N	—	L-Car: good	Brother died of DCM
Matsuishi et al (1985)	5 yr 7 yr	Hypotonia *2*	HCM	Low *2*	Low *2* (<10%)	Low-N *2*	Low *2*	DL-Car: good	Myocardial biopsy: increased lipids, 1 patient
Eriksson et al (1988)	4 yr	Primary SCD	DCM	Low (<3%)	Low (<1%)		Low	L-Car: good	Myocardial carnitine concentration <1%
Ino et al (1988)	1 day– 11 months	Secondary SCD *11*	HCM *6* DCM *5*	Low (Free)	—	—	—	L-Car *8*: good *6*	Total plasma carnitine normal; NC 1, died 1
Tein et al (1990)	4.5–10 yr	Primary SCD *4*	DCM *4*	Low *4* (<15%)	Low *3*	Low *2*	Low *1*	L-Car: good *4*	Improved motor function in all

Numbers in italics are number of patients. MCD, myopathic carnitine deficiency; DCM, dilated cardiomyopathy; car, carnitine; LMC, low myocardial carnitine; SCD, systemic carnitine deficiency; N, normal; SD, sudden death; EFE, endocardial fibroelastosis; HCM, hypertrophic cardiomyopathy; NC, no change.

MYOCARDIAL CARNITINE DEFICIENCY: ANIMAL STUDIES

Relevance to human myocardial deficiency

A number of experimental studies in animals have shown myocardial carnitine deficiency with metabolic abnormalities in long-chain fatty acid utilization. This has relevance to clinical manifestations and therapy in people (Table 2). York et al (1983) studied cardiomyopathic hamsters (Bio 14.6) that have myocardial carnitine deficiency throughout their life. This is due to a defective carnitine transport mechanism, probably mediated by an abnormality in cardiac carnitine-binding protein. Plasma concentrations of carnitine were normal or increased. Oral carnitine therapy resulted in only partial repletion of myocardial carnitine. This animal model has some similarity to primary systemic carnitine deficiency with cardiac dysfunction in children.

Myocardial carnitine deficiency is also documented in experimentally-induced right- or left-ventricular hypertrophy (Wittels et al, 1968; Revis and Cameron, 1979; Reibel et al, 1982). This is associated with reduced total coenzyme A (CoA), reduced oxidation of long-chain fatty acids, increased incorporation of palmitate into triglyceride and lecithin, and increased lipid deposit in the heart. Carnitine treatment corrected abnormal palmitate metabolism (Wittels et al, 1968). Left-ventricular hypertrophy secondary to cardiomyopathy, hypertension, and valvular heart disease is common in people. It is not surprising, therefore, that myocardial carnitine deficiency is documented in human studies of left-ventricular hypertrophy (Patel et al, 1990; Regitz et al, 1990).

In an experimental model of ischaemia created by coronary artery ligation or anoxia in an isolated rat-heart preparation, abnormalities in carnitine concentrations have been documented, with levels increasing after carnitine therapy and reversal of the metabolic abnormality (Shug et al, 1978; Suzuki et al, 1980). Coronary artery disease is a leading cause of myocardial dysfunction and end-stage cardiac disease, which frequently lead to cardiac transplantation. Myocardial carnitine deficiency has been documented in this group of patients (Pierpont et al, 1989; Regitz et al, 1990).

TABLE 2.
Animal models of myocardial carnitine deficiency

Reference	Model	Method	Total carnitine level			Effect of carnitine treatment	Other findings
			Myo-cardium	Plasma	Skeletal muscle		
York et al (1983)	Hamster Bio 14.6	Congenital carnitine deficiency	Low	Normal or ↑	Normal or ↑	—	Defective carnitine transport mechanism; partial repletion of myocardial carnitine with treatment
Reibel et al (1983)	Rat	Aortic banding	Low (20%)	Normal	—	—	Total CoA ↓; no ↑ in long-chain acyl esters
Wittels & Spann (1968)	Guinea-pig	Aortic constriction	Low (50%)	—	—	Corrected palmitate metabolism	Oxidation of LCFA ↓; palmitate incorporation into triglyceride and lecithin ↑
Revis & Cameron (1979)	Rabbit	Aortic coarctation	Low (>50%)	—	—	—	Lipid deposit in heart ↑
Shug et al (1978)	Dog	Ischaemia (coronary ligation)	Low (free)	—	—	Reversed metabolic abnormality	Ischaemia < 10 min: total carnitine unchanged, free carnitine ↓, acetyl and LC acyl carnitine ↑, acetyl CoA, CoA, ATP, CP ↓; ischaemia 30 min: total carnitine ↓ due to loss of acetylcarnitine
	Rat	Anoxia (isolated heart)	—	—	—		
Suzuki et al (1980)	Dog	Coronary ligation	Low (free)	—	—	Reversed metabolic abnormality	Ischaemia 10–15 min: free carnitine ↓, ATP ↓, FFA ↑; ischaemia 60–120 min: ATP ↓ ↓, free carnitine > early phase

↑, increased; ↓, decreased; LCFA, long-chain fatty acids; LC, long-chain; CP, creatine phosphokinase; FFA, free fatty acids.

MYOCARDIAL CARNITINE DEFICIENCY: STUDIES IN ADULT HUMANS

Clinical studies

Low total and free myocardial carnitine concentrations have been documented in tissues obtained at autopsy, cardiac surgery, and right ventricular endomyocardial biopsy in patients with various types of underlying heart disease (Table 3) (Spagnoli et al, 1982; Suzuki et al, 1982; Pierpont et al, 1989; Patel et al, 1990; Regitz et al, 1990). Although there is a tendency for lower myocardial carnitine concentrations to be associated with more severe left-ventricular dysfunction and haemodynamic abnormality (Regitz et al, 1990), the statistical correlation is weak (Pierpont et al, 1989; Patel et al, 1990). In an autopsy study of myocardial infarction, low myocardial carnitine levels were found in the infarct zone, intermediate levels in the border zone, and normal levels in the healthy tissue (Suzuki et al, 1982). Therefore, right-ventricular biopsy in some patients with coronary artery disease and left-ventricular dysfunction may show normal myocardial concentrations, whereas low levels may be present in the ischaemic or infarcted zone.

Plasma concentrations of carnitine are usually elevated in patients with cardiomyopathy, end-stage coronary artery disease, valvular heart disease, or cardiac failure from other aetiological factors (Tripp and Shug, 1984; Pierpont et al, 1989; Patel et al, 1990; Regitz et al, 1990). This is in sharp contrast to carnitine deficiency and cardiac disease in children, whose plasma concentrations are either normal, as in myopathic carnitine deficiency, or reduced, as in systemic carnitine deficiency.

Mechanism of low myocardial carnitine

In humans, carnitine is synthesized from methionine and lysine in liver, kidneys and brain (Wolf and Berger, 1961; Tanphaichitr and Broquist, 1973). Since it is not synthesized in the myocyte, the myocardium is dependent on plasma carnitine for maintenance of an adequate carnitine concentration. The cardiac intracellular concentration of carnitine is approximately 40 times higher than the plasma concentration, which suggests an active transport system capable of transporting carnitine into myocytes against a concentration gradient (Table 4).

TABLE 3.

Human studies of myocardial carnitine deficiency

Reference	Cardiac abnormality	Source and type of tissue	Carnitine status			Other findings
			Myocardium		Plasma	
			Total	Free		
Suzuki et al (1982)	Mitral valve disease *16*; CHF	Surgery; papillary muscle	Normal	Low	—	Short- and long-chain acylcarnitine ↑
Spangioli et al (1982)	Myocardial infarction *7*	Autopsy; left ventricle	—	Low	—	Intermediate carnitine levels in border zone, normal levels in healthy tissue
Pierpont et al (1989)	DCM *31*; CAD *13*; Myocarditis *5*; RHD *2*	Cardiac transplant	Low ?	—	↑	Left ventricle carnitine > right ventricle; no correlation with haemodynamics
Regitz et al (1990)	DCM *28*; CAD *3*; valvular HD *3*; HTN *3*	Endomyocardial biopsy; right ventricle	Low	Low	↑	LMC correlated with severity of left-ventricular dysfunction
Patel et al (1990)	CM *10*; amyloid *2*; valvular HD *4*; CP *1*; VT *1*	Endomyocardial biopsy; right ventricle	Low	Low	↑	No correlation of myocardial carnitine with haemodynamics or degree of myocardial dysfunction

Numbers in italics indicate number of patients. CHF, congestive heart failure; DCM, dilated cardiomyopathy; CAD, coronary artery disease; RHD, rheumatic heart disease; HD, heart disease; HTN, hypertension; CM, cardiomyopathy; CP, constrictive pericarditis; VT, ventricular tachycardia.

In vitro studies in cultured skin fibroblasts have shown a defect in the specific, high-affinity, low-concentration, carrier-mediated carnitine uptake mechanism in primary systemic carnitine deficiency (Treem et al, 1988; Eriksson et al, 1989; Tein et al, 1990). A similar defect in myocardial carnitine uptake probably results in cardiomyopathy associated with primary systemic carnitine deficiency. Beneficial therapeutic response and partial repletion of tissue carnitine concentrations are likely a result of passive diffusion (Eriksson et al, 1989). In various types of acquired heart disease and low myocardial carnitine, it is postulated that a functional or structural defect in myocardial membrane transport results in an inability to maintain adequate myocardial concentrations. The exact nature of this defect has not been defined.

Prognostic implications

Early studies in patients with end-stage cardiac disease undergoing cardiac transplantation showed low myocardial carnitine concentrations (Regitz et al, 1990). There was a trend toward lower myocardial carnitine concentrations with more severe left-ventricular dysfunction and haemodynamic abnormalities. This would imply a worse prognosis in these patients. We evaluated 40 consecutive patients with various types of acquired heart disease to assess the impact of myocardial carnitine concentrations on prognosis (Patel et al, 1990).

Myocardial carnitine concentration was normal in 22 patients and low in 18. Three patients in the normal myocardial carnitine group

TABLE 4.
Mechanism of myocardial carnitine transport

Reference	Model	Postulated mechanism
Molstad et al (1977)	Cultured human heart cells (CCL 27)	Carnitine transport dependent on free sulfhydryl group
Vary & Neely (1983)	Isolated rat myocytes	Carrier-mediated transport system dependent on extracellular sodium
Siliprandi et al (1989)	Isolated rat myocytes	Exchange-diffusion transport: γ-butyrobetaine exchanged with plasma carnitine

died; one of these was a cardiac death. In the low myocardial carnitine concentration group seven patients died, six of them from cardiac causes. The log-rank test comparing survival distributions of patients with normal myocardial carnitine concentration to patients with low myocardial carnitine concentrations showed a p value of 0.02, a statistically significant difference in the two survival curves. Therefore myocardial carnitine levels may have significant prognostic implications.

Therapeutic implications

Administration of carnitine to patients with ischaemic heart disease and angina is associated with increased exercise tolerance and reduced ST depression (Thomsen et al, 1979; Kosolcharoen et al, 1981; Kamikawa et al, 1984; Cherchi et al, 1985). In myocardial infarction, administration of carnitine may limit infarct size (Chiariello et al, 1986) and protect against arrhythmias (Rizzon et al, 1989). However, this has not been compared with standard treatment. In elderly patients with congestive heart failure secondary to ischaemic or hypertensive heart disease, treatment with L-carnitine resulted in reduced heart rate, oedema, and dyspnoea, increased diuresis, and reduced digitalis consumption compared with the group not treated with carnitine (Ghidini et al, 1988). Objective improvements in exercise tolerance test or left-ventricular ejection fraction were not documented in this study and myocardial carnitine concentrations were not known. Since low concentrations of myocardial carnitine have been demonstrated in various types of acquired heart disease in adults, it is likely that some of these patients may respond favourably to L-carnitine therapy. Clinical trials are underway to define this role of L-carnitine therapy.

SUMMARY

Cardiomyopathy with associated congestive heart failure is common in children with primary or systemic carnitine deficiency. However, there are only three patients in whom documented low myocardial carnitine concentrations have been reported. In other patients, myocardial concentrations are presumed to be low based on low levels in the plasma and skeletal muscle and favourable cardiac response to therapy. In adult patients with various types of acquired heart disease, documented myocardial carnitine deficiency is often accompanied by normal or elevated plasma levels. Therapy with L-carnitine has been reported to produce subjective improvement in cardiac failure, decreased arrhythmia and improved exercise tolerance, and limitation of infarct size in ischaemic heart disease. However, these observations need to be confirmed by carefully controlled studies in which carnitine therapy is compared with conventional therapy in patients whose cardiac carnitine status is known. Low myocardial carnitine concentrations appear to have adverse prognostic implications. Further clinical trials are underway to define the role of carnitine therapy in this group of patients with low myocardial carnitine concentrations.

REFERENCES

Bremer J (1983) *Physiol. Rev.* 63: 1420–1480.
Chapoy PR, Angelini C, Brown WJ et al (1980) *N. Engl. J. Med.* 303: 1389–1394.
Cherchi A, Lai C, Angelino F et al (1985) *Int. J. Clin. Pharmacol. Ther. Toxicol.* 23: 569–572.
Chiariello M, Brevetti G, Policicchio A et al (1986) In Borum PR (ed.) *Clinical Aspects of Human Carnitine Deficiency*, pp 242–243. New York: Pergamon Press.
Eriksson BO, Lindstedt S & Nordin I (1988) Hereditary defect in carnitine membrane transport is expressed in skin fibroblasts. *Eur. J. Pediatr.* 147: 662–663.
Eriksson BO, Gustafson B, Lindstedt S & Nordin I (1989) *J. Inher. Metab. Dis.* 12: 108–111.
Ghidini O, Azzurro M, Vita G & Sartori G (1988) *Int. J. Clin. Pharmacol. Ther. Toxicol.* 26: 217–220.
Hart ZH, Chang CH, DiMauro et al (1978) *Neurology* 28: 147–151.
Ino T, Sherwood WG, Benson LN et al (1988) *J. Am. Coll. Cardiol.* 11: 1301–1308.
Kamikawa T, Suzuki Y, Kobayashi A et al (1984) *Jpn Heart J.* 25: 587–597.
Kosolcharoen P, Nappi J, Peduzzi P et al (1981) *Curr. Ther. Res.* 30: 753–764.
Matsuishi T, Hirata K, Terasawa K et al (1985) *Neuropediatrics* 16: 6–12.
Molstad P, Bohmer T and Eiklid K (1977) Specificity and characteristics of the carnitine transport in human heart cells (CCL 27) in culture. *Biochim. Biophys. Acta* 471: 296–304.
Patel AK, Kosolcharoen P, Thomsen J et al (1990) *Philipp. J. Cardiol.* 19: I-290 (abstract).
Pierpont MEM, Judd D, Godenberg IF et al (1989) *Am. J. Cardiol.* 64: 56–60.
Regitz V, Shug AL & Fleck E (1990) *Am. J. Cardiol.* 65: 755–760.
Reibel DK, Uboh CE & Kent RL (1983) *Am. J. Physiol.* 244: H839–H843.
Revis NW & Cameron AJV (1979) *Metabolism* 28: 601–613.
Rizzon P, Biasco G, Di Biase M et al (1989) *Eur. Heart J.* 10: 502–508.
Shug AL, Thomsen JH, Folts JD et al (1978) *Arch. Biochem. Biophys.* 187: 25–33.
Siliprandi N, Sartorelli L, Ciman M & Di Lisa F. (1989) *Clin. Chim. Acta* 183: 3–12.

Spagnoli LG, Corsi M, Villaschi, S et al (1982) Myocardial carnitine deficiency in acute myocardial infarction. *Lancet* i: 1419–1420.

Suzuki Y, Kamikawa T & Yamazaki N (1980) In Frenkel RA & McGarry JD (eds) *Carnitine Biosynthesis, Metabolism and Function*, pp 341–352. New York: Academic Press.

Suzuki Y, Masumura Y, Kobayashi A et al (1982) *Lancet* i: 116.

Tanphaichitr V & Broquist HP (1973) *J. Biol. Chem.* 248: 2176–2181.

Tein I, De Vivo DC, Bierman F et al (1990) *Pediatr. Res.* 28: 247–255.

Thomsen JH, Shug AL, Yap VU et al (1979) *Am. J. Cardiol.* 43: 300–306.

Treem WR, Stanley CA, Finegold DN et al (1988) *N. Engl J. Med.* 319: 1331–1336.

Tripp ME & Shug AL (1984) *Biochem. Med.* 32: 199–206.

Tripp ME, Katcher ML, Peters HA et al (1981) *N. Engl J. Med.* 305: 385–390.

Vary TC & Neely JR (1983) *Am. J. Physiol.* 244: H247–H252.

Waber LJ., Valle D, Neill C, DiMauro S & Shug A (1982) *J. Pediatr.* 101: 700–705.

Whitmer JT (1987) *Circ. Res.* 61: 396–408.

Wittels B & Spann JF (1968) *J. Clin. Invest.* 47: 1787–1794.

Wolf G & Berger CRA (1961) *Arch. Biochem. Biophys.* 92: 360–365.

York CM, Cantrell CR & Borum PR (1983) *Arch. Biochem. Biophys.* 221: 526–533.

18

PROFILE OF LONG-TERM L-CARNITINE THERAPY IN CARDIOPATHIC PATIENTS

C. Fernandez

With normal oxygen bioavailability, the most utilized energetic substrate employed by myocardial cells is represented by long-chain fatty acids (Opie, 1969). However their oxidation only takes place in the presence of carnitine at the mitochondrial level (Fritz et al, 1962). In acute or chronic myocardial ischaemia there is a marked reduction in the intramitochondrial carnitine content (Wood et al, 1973) causing an accumulation of acyl CoA and an inhibition of the intracytoplasmatic transport of high-energy compounds (i.e. ATP) (Shug et al, 1975) necessary to develop and guarantee normal myocardial contractility. Thus, it was thought that exogenous L-carnitine could be used to: (i) compensate for the post-ischaemic deficit; (ii) develop a cardioprotective effect; (iii) facilitate fatty acid metabolism and (iv) increase the intramitochondrial availability of ATP (Cherchi, 1985; Paulson, 1986). We thought it possible to postulate a protective role for carnitine in the ischaemic myocardium since, if present at the normal concentration and with the correct metabolism of mitochondrial fatty acids, L-carnitine would circumvent their cytoplasmic deposition.

The accumulation of fatty acids is highly toxic for the cardiac cell.

337

L-Carnitine and Its Role in Medicine:
From Function to Therapy. ISBN 0–12–253940–0

In fact free fatty acids (FFA), organized in lysophosphatides, damage cellular membranes, are arrhythmogenic, block certain enzymatic functions and eventually alter myocardial contractility. These physiopathological notions have established an ever widening use of L-carnitine under various pathological conditions whether the altered myocardial function causes direct, indirect, primary or secondary metabolic disturbances, but always in the presence of a reduced mitochondrial availability of carnitine.

SCOPE OF THE PAPER

Instead of evaluating the therapeutic efficacy of L-carnitine, already pointed out in numerous other clinical trials, we thought it opportune to investigate any eventual adverse reaction or collateral effect in cardiopathic patients who were given L-carnitine continuously for at least 12 months. (It must be kept in mind that L-carnitine is often administered concomitantly with cardiovascular drugs.)

The study population receiving this integrated therapy hailed from 410 different clinical centres. Such a wide study should not only make evident any remote effect, positive or negative, but also permit a comprehensive and specific insight into possible associations between cardioactive drugs and L-carnitine.

The geographic distribution of the researchers was uniform throughout Italy, with every province being involved. Great care was taken regarding the ratios between the number of centres and the number of inhabitants and between urban and rural areas. The aim was to obtain the most homogeneous set of patients possible.

The study was motivated by the constantly increasing use of L-carnitine. According to data furnished by the Ministry of Health, in 1989 over 8 million packages of levocarnitine were sold, a higher quota than that registered in 1988. Keeping with the trend, the statistics taken during the first 5 months of 1990 already showed an increase in use. It should be noted that, in Italy, levocarnitine is administered exclusively on the basis of diagnostic indications concerning cardiovascular pathologies.

MATERIALS AND METHODS

Four hundred and ten Italian doctors specialized in cardiology and working in the public health clinics chose, during a 24-month period,

3500 cardiopathic patients aged between 25 and 80 years. The patients were chosen on the basis of the confirmed and documented presence of the following cardiovascular pathologies:

1. stable effort angina;
2. ischaemic cardiomyopathy with signs of heart failure (2 and 3 class of NYHA).

These patients were not hospitalized and any eventual hospitalization caused their removal from the study.

The subjects affected by angina numbered 1225 of which 62% were males and 30% were females ranging in age from 25 to 80 years, with the highest peak between 55 and 60 years. Those patients suffering from ischaemic cardiomyopathy numbered 2230; 55% males and 49% females. In this group the age range was between 30 and 90 years, with the majority being between 65 and 70.

The patients considered suitable for the study were kept under observation for 30 days. During this time, all parameters relating to their subjective symptomatology and all types and doses of medications prescribed for them previous to their being considered for the trial were documented. At the end of the 30-day period, the subjects were entered into the study trial and underwent the routine analyses which were repeated every month.

Each patient's normal therapy was integrated with L-carnitine, 2.0 g day^{-1} orally, given in two doses following main meals. A chart was made for each patient noting all concomitant therapies, old or new, including the drug's trade name and dosage. Any eventual changes in dosage and the appearance of any collateral effect, characterized by type, intensity, duration, were recorded. The drugs commonly taken by these patients were: nitroglycerin, nitroderivatives (orally or transdermally), nifedipine, beta-blockers, cardioactive glucosides, diuretics, anti-arrhythmics (amiodarone, propafenone), ACE inhibitors, antiplatelet agents, oral antilipid agents and insulin. In both patient populations (angina/ischaemic cardiomyopathy), at least three drugs were taken simultaneously, to which was added L-carnitine.

The benefits attributed to this integrated therapy with L-carnitine, 2.0 g day^{-1} have been reported in other publications (Fernandez et al, 1985). Here we will limit ourselves to examining the pharmacological profile of L-carnitine exclusively in relation to its collateral effects and cases of intolerance during the course of therapy.

INTOLERANCE PHENOMENA AND COLLATERAL EFFECTS

Intolerance phenomena causing patient drop-out occurred uniformly during the 12-month therapy period at a rate of 0.3%. In these cases, suspension of L-carnitine abolished all subjective symptomatology consisting of gastralgia, nausea and diarrhoea. Upon readministration, the gastrointestinal disturbances returned. For this reason, four females and seven males were forced to abandon the trial.

The following list of collateral effects was composed: nausea, vomiting, gastralgia, insomnia, changes in appetite (increases and decreases), polyuria, diarrhoea, constipation, skin manifestations, astenia, hypotension, vertigine, tinnitus, headache, anxiety, excitation (nervous disturbances), rhythm changes, psychomotor hyperactivity, tremors, changes in urine odour, changes in breath odour (ammonaemia coma type), changes in perspiration odour and others. In all about 100 collateral effects were noted, although none were so intense as to merit treatment interruption. In many cases, they were linked to the concomitant administration of other drugs; in fact, an accurate history attested to their presence during the time preceding the administration of L-carnitine. The following is a list of those effects numerically relevant: *gastralgia*—6%, equal in both sexes and mainly encountered at the beginning of treatment (first to third month) and regressing from the second semester on; *nausea*—5%, more in women, disappearing from the fourth month on; *diarrhoea*—2%, equal in both sexes, present linearly, but in episodic fashion during the entire 12-month treatment period.

Based on this data, we think it possible to affirm that the collateral effects attributable to this integrated therapy arising during the entire 12-month period, foreseeable from the protocol and with the patients always kept under observation, were very modest both in intensity and number. It should be noted again that they caused a very limited number of patient drop-out. The most recent literature on this topic confirms our findings. Yakuri To Chiryo (1989) reports only four cases out of 127 (3.1%) in which moderate headache was encountered and which disappeared if L-carnitine was administered on alternate days. Other symptoms he reported were: diarrhoea, burning sensation in the extremities (only one patient), burning and inflammation of the tongue. None of these caused the cessation of treatment. Even in these cases, L-carnitine was given together with other cardioactive drugs, i.e. calcium antagonists, beta-blockers, nitrates, etc. Other authors have also reported extremely modest percentages of very slight and transitory collateral effects. In these cases, however, L-carnitine was administered for longer than 60 consecutive days of therapy.

CONCLUSIONS

The administration of L-carnitine, even for continuous and prolonged periods and with limited intolerance, only causes a very small percentage of patient drop-out (0.3%). The statistically insignificant occurrence of collateral effects, whether persistent or transitory, is, in our opinion, due to two main factors. One is that the drug under study is a natural substance which is easily absorbed and used immediately in cases of deficiency, without the need for metabolic processes requiring high-energy consumption. The second factor is that during the 12-month period, both the number of cardioactive drugs required and their dosages were reduced. Such a marked reduction could have a positive influence on the problem of tolerance and collateral effects. The administration of L-carnitine *per se* doesn't seem to cause serious tolerance problems, while its therapeutic benefit allows a progressive elimination, or at least a reduction, of many cardioactive drugs. Thus, there is a type of metabolic–parenchymal positive-feedback.

REFERENCES

Cherchi A (1985) *Clin. Pharm.* 23: 569–572.
Fernandez C, La Menza B & Pola P (1985) *J. Am. Med. Assoc.* (Italian edn) II: 2–9.
Fritz IB, Kaplan E & Yue KTM (1962) *Am. J. Physiol.* 202: 117–124.
Opie L (1969) *Am. Heart J.* 77: 100–122.
Paulson DJ (1986) *Cardiovasc. Res.* 20: 536–541.
Rizzon P (1989) *Eur. Heart J.* 10: 502–508.
Shug AL, Shrago E, Bittar N et al (1975) *Am. J. Physiol.* 228: 683–692.
Wood JM, Sordahe LA, Lewiss RM & Schwartz A (1973) *Circ. Res.* 32: 340–348.
Yakuri To Chiryo (1989) *Dis. Pharmacol. Ther.* 17: 5–9.
Yoshitoshi Y (1989) *Dis. Pharmacol. Ther.* 17: 561–583.

Part IIIb

Peripheral vascular disease

19

CARNITINE IN METABOLISM OF PACED CARDIAC AND SKELETAL MUSCLES: PREVENTION OF ACIDOSIS AND IMPROVEMENT OF VASCULAR FLOW

W.C. Hülsmann and M.-L. Dubelaar

INTRODUCTION

This chapter discusses the acute effects of L-carnitine on pre-ischaemic cardiac and skeletal muscles. The effects of carnitine on training will not be reported, as changes of muscle type and altered hormonal states may be involved. A comprehensive review of literature has not been attempted.

In 1959 Fritz reported that carnitine stimulates fatty acid oxidation.

345

Acetylcarnitine and fatty acid esters of carnitine are rapidly oxidized in isolated mitochondria. These carnitine derivatives can be transported through the mitochondrial inner membrane and oxidized after conversion to their coenzyme A (CoA) derivatives (for classical reviews see Fritz, 1961; Bremer, 1983). Figure 1 shows the involvement of carnitine in mitochondrial β-oxidation. The acyltransferase involved in the synthesis of long-chain acylcarnitine from fatty acyl CoA, carnitine palmitoyl CoA transferase-1 (CPT-1) is located in the outer membrane (Murthy and Pande, 1987). CPT-2, the inner membrane isoenzyme, converts long-chain acylcarnitine back to long-chain acyl CoA, then present in the inner membrane–matrix compartment, where β-oxidation of fatty acids takes place. This compartment also contains pyruvate dehydrogenase and the citric acid cycle activity. It is relatively rich in CoA, compared with the extramitochondrial cytosol, whereas the latter contains the bulk of cellular carnitine (Idell-Wenger et al, 1978).

Mitochondrial carnitine acetyltransferase is localized in the inner membrane, probably facing the matrix. Hence carnitine may liberate CoA from acetyl CoA by exporting acetylcarnitine from the mitochondria. In this way it would stimulate the citric acid cycle activity by the inhibition caused by a high acetyl CoA/CoA ratio (Hülsmann et al, 1964). This situation could occur during a shortage of cellular oxygen, as a decline in respiratory chain activity would limit citric acid cycle velocity and thus limit the use of respiratory substrates (such as pyruvate, ketone bodies and fatty acids). Fatty acids may be stored in the cytosol as triglycerides, whereas pyruvate (mostly after reduction to lactate) may diffuse out of the cell. Hence, if carnitine administration were able to delay metabolic disruption, by lowering the acetyl CoA/CoA ratio in the cell, it would probably be in a hypoxic or preischaemic state.

Carnitine could diminish lactic acidosis of tissues if it could stimulate citric acid cycle activity, as the resulting increased rate of ATP synthesis is known to inhibit glycolysis (cf. Randle et al, 1963). In addition, stimulation of pyruvate removal by acetylcarnitine formation may be expected. It must be stressed that this can only happen if at least some oxygen is available for respiratory chain and pyruvate dehydrogenase activities. Therefore, carnitine could operate in conditions of imminent ischaemia, but not once it was fully developed. To verify this assumption in vitro, the erythrocyte-free perfused and paced Langendorff heart is suitable. This preparation is borderline hypoxic, as judged by the continuous production of lactate from glucose or glycogen, particularly when the hearts are subjected to increased cellular Ca^{2+} turnover (Hülsmann and De Wit, 1990;

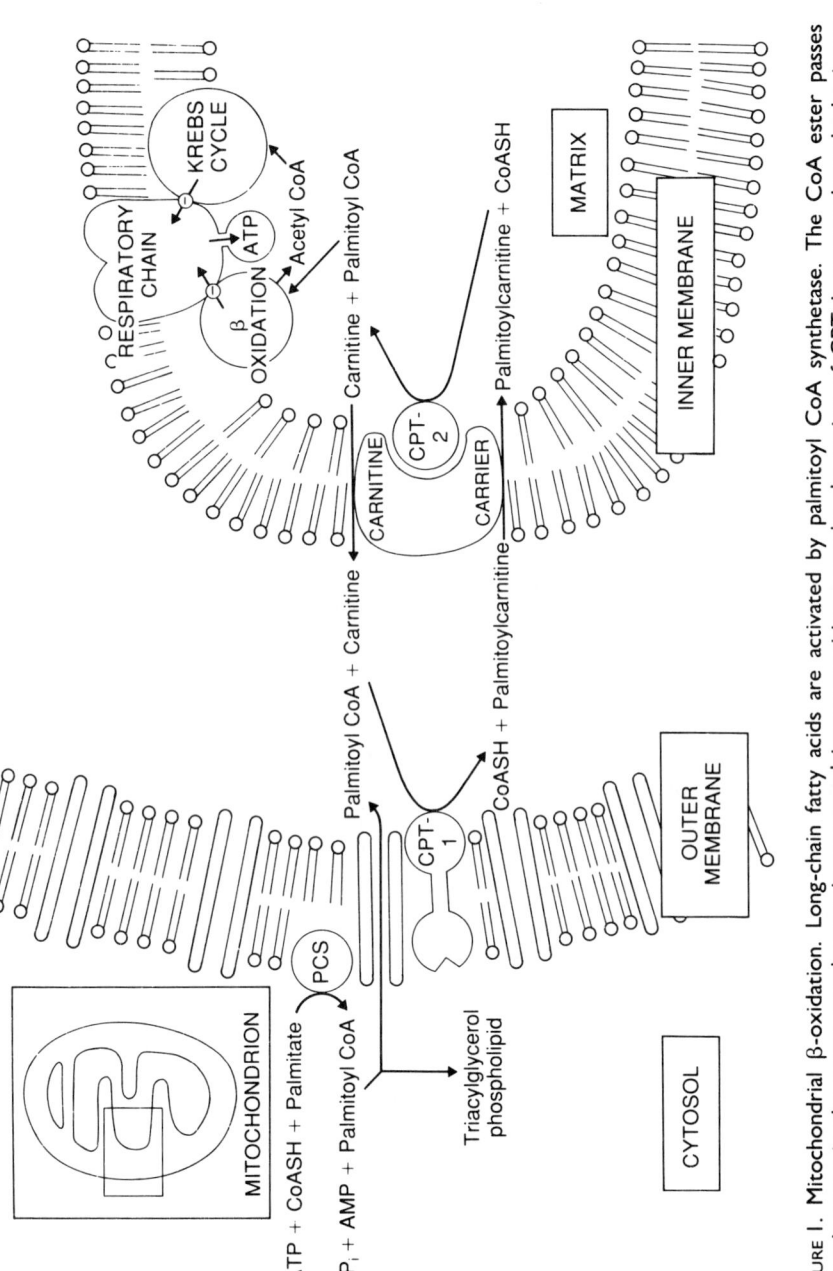

FIGURE 1. Mitochondrial β-oxidation. Long-chain fatty acids are activated by palmitoyl CoA synthetase. The CoA ester passes through pores in the outer membranes, is converted into a carnitine ester by the action of CPT-1, moves through the inner membrane via the carnitine carrier, and is reconverted into a CoA ester by CPT-2. Acyl CoA is oxidized by enzymes of β-oxidation and the respiratory chain to acetyl CoA, which is further oxidized by enzymes of the citric acid cycle and the respiratory chain. From Scholte and Jennekens (1988).

Hülsmann et al, 1990a, 1990b). The latter can be accomplished by including glucagon in the perfusion medium (Méry et al, 1990) or by brief acidification, known to cause release of plasmalemma bound Ca^{2+} into the cytosol (Hülsmann et al, 1990a; Vandeplassche and Borgers, 1990), and the release of noradrenaline (norepinephrine) into the interstitial space.

Before citing examples that indicate inhibition of lactic acidosis by carnitine, two types of experiment will be described, one with the paced Langendorff rat heart, as mentioned above, and one with paced dog skeletal muscle in vivo. The term lactic acidosis refers to acidosis caused by endogenous lactic acid production. This is different from lactate formed from added pyruvate, which may not be accompanied by acidosis. (By contrast, the lactate dehydrogenase reaction *per se* may consume protons, while forming lactate from pyruvate.)

EFFECT OF CARNITINE ON LACTIC ACIDOSIS IN THE LANGENDORFF HEART

Induction of acidosis by changing the pH of the perfusion medium during pacing from 7.5 to 7.0 results in dramatic alterations in the heart. After an initial increase of cardiac contractility (indicating increased cytosolic Ca^{2+} transients), accompanied by the release of Ca^{2+} from the cytosolic side of the plasmalemma, contractility decreased progressively (Hülsmann and De Wit, 1990; Hülsmann et al, 1990a). In approximately 60% of cases contractility ceased completely. The coronary flow initially increased after switching to pH 7.0 perfusion, but gradually decreased *after* contractility started to fall. This frequently resulted in complete cardiac arrest and strongly reduced flow after about 6 min of perfusion at pH 7.0. The addition of oleate to the perfusion medium minimized these phenomena and prevented irreversible changes, as judged by complete restoration of cardiac functions upon reperfusion with pH 7.5 medium (Hülsmann et al, 1990a). Perfusion with 5 mM L-carnitine instead of oleate did not protect against the pH 7.0-induced deterioration ($n = 3$, not shown). In these experiments we used hearts with normal (low) endogenous triglyceride content and no fatty acid in the perfusion medium. Therefore, no stimulation of fatty acid metabolism could have taken place.

The addition of 5 mM L-carnitine not only failed to improve cardiac function, but also failed to influence metabolism. In the absence or presence of added carnitine, lactate and acetylcarnitine levels in the hearts after 10 min perfusion at pH 7.0 were 8.9 ± 1.8 and 0.20 ± 0.03 μmol per g wet weight respectively (n = 3). In the presence of 5 mM L-carnitine, lactate and acetyl carnitine levels were 10.9 ± 1.9 and 0.25 ± 0.03 μmol per g wet weight respectively (n = 3). Hence, under the conditions of this test, there was no effect of carnitine in Langendorff perfused hearts subjected to acidosis. The absence of a positive effect of carnitine at low fatty acid supply has also been observed in skeletal muscle (see below). Hülsmann et al (1982) demonstrated that 5 mM carnitine prevented triglyceride accumulation during intralipid perfusion of rat Langendorff hearts. Thus, carnitine might only be effective when fatty acids are present in high concentrations.

ACUTE EFFECT OF CARNITINE ON SKELETAL MUSCLE FORCE IN VIVO

We have studied the effect of carnitine administration in an in situ fatigue test in the dog, using a pacemaker-stimulated latissimus dorsi muscle connected to a force-displacement transducer (Dubelaar et al, 1991a, 1991b). Intravenous carnitine injection increased muscular force by about one third in untrained dogs (n = 10); after training, the effect on the muscle was less pronounced. The acute effect of carnitine administration was unexpected as none of the dogs was carnitine-deficient and had average plasma concentrations of 23 nmol ml^{-1} prior to injection. The skeletal muscle concentrations were about 4700 nmol per g wet weight and not increased by carnitine administration. We explained the effect of L-carnitine as stimulation of oxidative phosphorylation. The effect of L-carnitine could not be mimicked by choline or by D-carnitine, which even inhibited force to some extent. Also, injection of insulin (while maintaining glycaemia) inhibited force production. Both D-carnitine (an inhibitor of CPT-1) and hyperinsulinaemia are known inhibitors of β-oxidation. L-Carnitine not only increased force of the stimulated muscle, but also improved vascular flow, which was demonstrated after injection of microspheres (Dubelaar et al, 1991b). Hence the acute effect of carnitine may be explained by increasing muscle aerobiosis by increasing flow (Dubelaar et al, 1991a, 1991b). The lesser effect of L-carnitine in trained muscle is in line with this hypothesis since the number of capillaries increases by 40% as a result of training.

These experiments did not reveal the mechanism by which carnitine injection increased flow in stimulated, untrained muscle. Carnitine may have decreased local acidosis, known also to be vasoconstrictive in skeletal muscle (Von Ardenne and Reitnauer, 1989). That carnitine probably does not act solely by accepting acetyl groups in the pyruvate dehydrogenase reaction is demonstrated during hyperinsulinaemia. In this situation, when pyruvate dehydrogenase may be expected to be activated, carnitine was found to be ineffective in stimulating muscle force (Dubelaar et al, 1991a). The explanation for this phenomenon could have been the expected low rate of β-oxidation of fatty acids during hyperinsulinaemia. In addition, acetyl L-carnitine was as good a stimulator of force as L-carnitine (Dubelaar et al, 1991b). Hence the carnitine effect must have a predominant catalytic character and not be solely caused by the trapping of acetyl groups in the pyruvate dehydrogenase reaction.

Stimulation of ATP generation by carnitine could be most effective in preventing local acidosis. This is substantiated by increasing fatty acid availability to the paced skeletal muscle instead of increasing carnitine. Figure 2 shows that increasing the circulating free fatty acid level (by infusion of Intralipid with heparin to stimulate lipolysis), results in a considerably higher force of the musculus latissimus dorsi during pacing, similar to the effect we observed after elevating the circulating carnitine concentration. During increased fatty acid supply, carnitine had no additional stimulatory effect in these experiments. Therefore we can conclude that L-carnitine or fatty acid supply may inhibit lactic acidosis and as such limit acidification of the interstitium, which is responsible for decline in vascular flow, as we have shown in the heart (Hülsmann and De Wit, 1990; Hülsmann et al, 1990a).

The beneficial effect of carnitine raised the question: Is there a carnitine-deficient compartment in muscle under the conditions of the tests? As the muscle cells are stores of carnitine in the body, it is unlikely that the sites of storage could be carnitine deficient. Perhaps subsarcolemmal or vascular sites could easily lose carnitine during local acidosis? In skeletal muscle and in heart two types of mitochondria can be distinguished (Hülsmann et al, 1968, 1969; Hülsmann, 1970): M-1 (superficial) and M2 (interfibrillar) mitochondria. The M-1 mitochondria have a relatively loose coupling of phosphorylation to oxidation, perhaps a reflection of higher vulnerability of the muscle compartment involved. This could also apply to mitochondria in cells of the blood vessels.

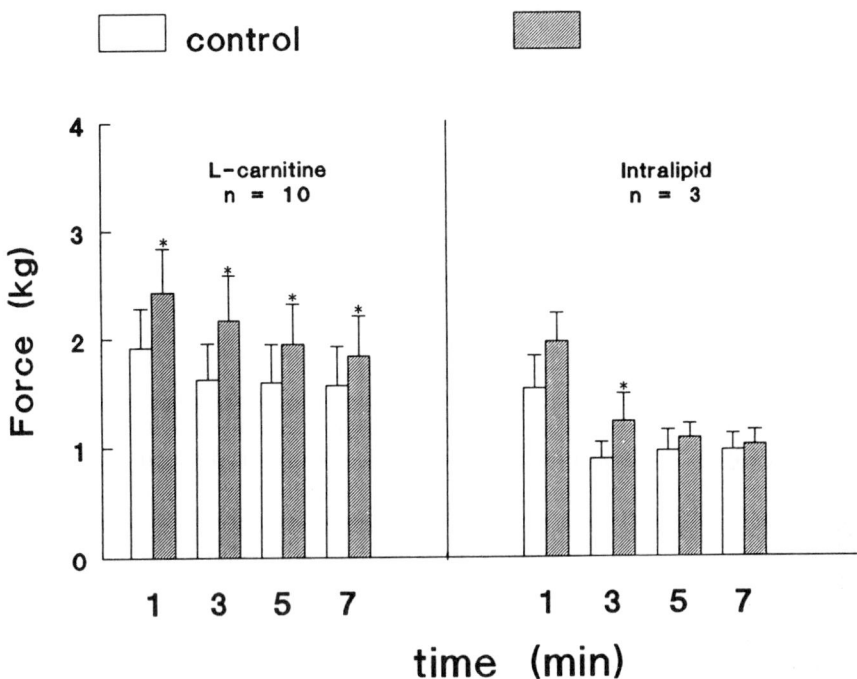

FIGURE 2. Effects of carnitine or high plasma fatty acid levels on muscle performance. Left: The effect of L-carnitine on latissimus dorsi (LD) force tests. The abscissa shows time in minutes after initiation of the pacing. Open bars represent the control test, hatched bars show force of the same muscle after a rest period of 30 minutes, during which 1 g of L-carnitine was infused intravenously. The experiment was carried out in ten dogs. Right: The effect of high plasma fatty acid levels on LD force tests. Open bars represent the control test, hatched bars show force of the same muscle after a rest period of 30 minutes, during which 75 ml 20% Intralipid together with 200 IU heparin per kg (to increase lipolysis) was infused. The experiment was carried out in three dogs. *, values significantly different from control values.

CARNITINE AND ENERGY SUPPLY IN BLOOD VESSELS

Both vascular endothelial and smooth muscle cells contain carnitine palmitoyl CoA transferases, as judged by the presence of (carnitine-dependent) fatty acid oxidation (Odessey and Chace, 1982; Hülsmann and Dubelaar, 1988). Van Hinsbergh et al (1983) observed that cultured endothelial cells occasionally contain lipid droplets, that disappear after carnitine addition. We observed that adding carnitine to endo-thelial cells in a glucose-containing culture medium strongly stimulates oxidation of oleate (Hülsmann and Dubelaar, 1988). By comparing the rates of oleate oxidation and lactate formation, we have been able to calculate that fatty acid oxidation may contribute much more than glycolysis to aerobic ATP synthesis. This conclusion is at variance with that of others (Mertens et al, 1990), who may have omitted carnitine from the culture medium.

In some species vascular endothelial cells may not be particularly sensitive to ischaemia (Buderus et al, 1989). In hypoperfused rat Langendorff hearts, however, we noted early leakage of the endothelial enzyme xanthine oxidase into the cardiac interstitium (Hülsmann and Dubelaar, 1987). The production of oxygen radicals, in the interstitial space, may have been partly responsible for the observed loss of cardiac contractility, as acute improvement of contractility was seen after addition of superoxide dismutase to the medium (Hülsmann and Dubelaar, 1987). Also, the addition of vasoxin, a strong α-adrenergic vasoconstrictor, increased cardiac contractility (Hülsmann and Dubelaar, 1987), which suggests increased cardiac performance by an increase of the perfusion pressure during perfusion by constant (low) flow instead of constant pressure.

High vascular vulnerability in dog hearts subjected to ischaemia has recently been observed by Dauber et al (1990). They noticed increased microvascular permeability and impaired endothelium-dependent vasodilatation. Early involvement of vascular endothelium in ischaemia has also been noted in humans as increased prostacyclin biosynthesis in obstructive arterial disease (FitzGerald et al, 1984). Therefore, in certain species, there is early vascular involvement in oxygen-deficient muscles which might lead to a lower carnitine concentration in endothelial cells. Whether vascular smooth muscle cells are as sensitive to ischaemia remains to be seen. They probably contain carnitine under normal conditions, as human arterial smooth muscle cells in culture oxidize added oleate, a process completely inhibited by the CPT inhibitor aminocarnitine (Hülsmann and Verkerk, unpublished data). Even if smooth muscle cells in vitro are as sensitive to ischaemia as endothelial cells, it need not be so in situ. Capillary endothelial cells may be more directly exposed to lactic acid (and perhaps also to long-chain acylcarnitine) produced by the bulk of striated muscle cells.

EXAMPLES OF IMPROVED FUNCTION BY CARNITINE IN PRE-ISCHAEMIC MUSCLES

Local deficiency of carnitine might occur in ischaemia followed by reperfusion. High intensity exercise has been shown to lead to a considerable loss of carnitine from skeletal muscle (Ferrannini et al, 1988; Brevetti, 1989; Hiatt, 1989; Siliprandi, 1990). This also occurs in heart due to pacing or infarction (Spagnoli et al, 1982). Carnitine could be lost from muscles by leakage through plasma membranes, together with other cytosolic compounds, as has been demonstrated after damage caused by the 'calcium paradox' (Scholte et al, 1986). Conversion of carnitine to acylcarnitines is another way to produce deficiency. Overall carnitine levels in muscle are high, both in white and red muscle fibres (Kerner and Bieber, 1983), but localized areas might be deficient under certain circumstances.

Brevetti et al (1989) recently showed a positive effect of carnitine administration on skeletal muscle function in humans, suffering from peripheral vascular disease. Walking distance improved, together with vascular flow. Ferrari et al (1984) observed, in patients with angina pectoris, a decline of lactate output during pacing, indicative of improved oxygenation of cardiac tissue. We observed acute improvement of force in stimulated musculus latissimus dorsi of the dog in situ, by carnitine injection, as has been discussed above. Siliprandi et al (1990) recently showed that, in seven out of ten humans subjected to physical exercise, a greater amount of work was carried out when exercise was started 1 hour after an oral dose of l-carnitine. The explanation given for this observation was stimulation of pyruvate removal in the form of acetylcarnitine, a phenomenon also observed by Ferrannini et al (1988).

MECHANISMS BY WHICH CARNITINE MAY IMPROVE BLOOD-FLOW

The vascular system appears to be vulnerable in pre-ischaemia (Hülsmann and Dubelaar, 1987; Dauber et al, 1990). One possible cause of this is a loss of carnitine, and another is altered signal transduction during acidification of interstitial spaces. This may result from glyco(geno)lysis, instead of fatty acid oxidation being the major source of ATP after an increase in noradrenaline release. Inhibition of glycolysis may be accomplished by stimulation of respiratory chain phosphorylation. Both limitation of metabolic acidosis and increased ATP synthesis might result from carnitine suppletion, particularly when it concerns a muscle compartment relatively deficient in carnitine. This need not be the vascular compartment itself, but may be an area of striated muscle cells. Limitation of local acidosis may be expected to increase flow, as lowering pH has been shown to cause the release of bound Ca^{2+} not only in striated, but also in vascular smooth muscle cells (Kwan and Daniel, 1989). In addition to this important phenomenon, other factors may be involved, such as alteration of intracellular ATP levels. High concentrations of ATP may stimulate the closure of plasmalemmal, ATP-dependent, K^+ channels (Lückhoff et al, 1988; Quast and Cook, 1989; Escande, 1989), and limit the loss of cellular K^+, generally seen in hypoxia/ischaemia. Both vascular smooth muscle and endothelial cells contain ATP-sensitive K^+ channels (Escande, 1989). Blocking these K^+ channels caused depolarization and reduction of Ca^{2+} influx, so that the cellular Ca^{2+} level decreases. Cytosolic Ca^{2+} increase in endothelial cells not only enhances EDRF, but also PG_{I2} release (Lückhoff et al, 1988). Both autacoids are vasodilators and inhibition of their secretion may result in increased perfusion pressure. Acidosis may also affect plasmalemmal $Na^+–Ca^{2+}$ exchange, as the exchanger may be strongly inhibited at pH 6 and stimulated at pH 9 (Philipson et al, 1982). The exchanger is present in arterial smooth muscle cells (Bingham-Smith et al, 1987) and may cause a rapid efflux of Ca^{2+} after increasing cytosolic Ca^{2+}.

From the above considerations we concluded that in the pre-ischaemic state protons play a central role in the mechanism of (Ca^{2+}-dependent) vasoconstriction. Proton excess may affect plasmalemmal signal transduction, in which increased noradrenaline release and stimulation of the phosphatidylinositol cycle (Bingham-Smith et al, 1989) could play an important role in the observed release of Ca^{2+} from the cytosolic side of plasma membranes (Hülsmann and De Wit, 1990; Hülsmann et al, 1990a; Vandeplassche and Borgers, 1990).

Acidosis may be prevented by inhibition of glyco(geno)lysis and by the stimulation of oxidative removal of pyruvate. Promotion of capillary flow is most important to remove metabolic products. Long-chain acylcarnitine can also flood the interstitium in the pre-ischaemic state. It might affect both vascular smooth muscle and endothelial cells (Dainty et al, 1990), as will be discussed below.

LONG-CHAIN ACYLCARNITINE AND LOSS OF CORONARY FLOW

From unpublished experiments we concluded, that in lipid-enriched Langendorff rat hearts, inhibition of β-oxidation by aminocarnitine does not lead to accumulation of long-chain acylcarnitine as long as glycogen is present (Hülsmann and Dubelaar, unpublished data). Apparently, fatty acid levels are kept low by the operation of the glucose/fatty acid cycle (Randle et al, 1963). This takes place at the surface of the endoplasmic reticulum, so that only small amounts of fatty acids can be converted to their carnitine derivatives in the mitochondrial CPT-1 reaction. In ischaemia, however, glycogen has disappeared and long-chain acylcarnitine can accumulate (Idell-Wenger et al, 1978; Shug et al, 1978). In pre-ischaemia, the retardation of acidosis by carnitine addition could delay the loss of flow, and as such limit long-chain acylcarnitine accumulation.

An acute effect of carnitine administration could only be visualized if it were to act in a carnitine-deficient compartment. The bulk of the muscle mass, which must be mainly responsible for interstitial flooding with long-chain acylcarnitine accumulation in pre-ischaemia, probably contains sufficient carnitine already. Therefore, it is not likely to ascribe the observed beneficial effect of carnitine addition to alteration of myocytal long-chain acylcarnitine production. However, by promoting flow, carnitine addition may be expected to lower interstitial long-chain acylcarnitine levels.

When, in the experiments mentioned above, the lipid-enriched rat hearts were depleted of glycogen by pre-perfusion with glucagon, prior to 60 min perfusion with glucagon and aminocarnitine, they were found to accumulate a large amount of long-chain acylcarnitine (0.3 μmol per g wet weight), while considerable amounts of long-chain acylcarnitine were secreted by the heart during perfusion. These hearts, paced at a rate of 300 beats per min, remained intact as judged by continued beating. There was no loss of myoglobin and coronary flow remained unaltered during constant pressure perfusion. These experiments (Hülsmann et al, 1991), indicate that cardiac membranes are not adversely affected by long-chain acylcarnitine during pH 7.5 perfusion as long as flow continues. Although long-chain acylcarnitine cannot be the initiator of metabolic and functional disruption, its occurrence during acidosis, resulting in a progressive decline of flow as in pre-ischaemia, may contribute to damage. We consider the beneficial effect of carnitine supplementation to be due to prevention of local acidosis and not to primary avoidance of interstitial flooding by long-chain acylcarnitine.

Finally, a possible cholinomimetic effect of carnitine requires discussion (although choline is not able to replace carnitine in stimulating force of paced dog latissimus dorsi muscle) (Dubelaar et al, 1991a).

CARNITINE AND ACUTE CHOLINOMIMETIC EFFECTS ON MUSCLE

Cholinomimetic effects of (acetyl)carnitine have been described by a number of authors (Bettini et al, 1987; cf. Fritz, 1959). We have observed that edrophonium chloride (Tensilon), a cholinesterase inhibitor, stimulated the force of the paced latissimus muscle of the dog in situ (Dubelaar et al, 1991b), as discussed above for carnitine. In the presence of Tensilon, carnitine did not have an additional effect. Both drugs may have promoted blood supply to the muscle, but cannot have the same mechanism of action. Carnitine is not an acetylcholinesterase inhibitor, and carnitine has no cholinergic action in the absence of ischaemia, whereas vasodilatory properties of true cholinergic agents may also be observed in the absence of ischaemia (Weinstock and McCarty, 1983; Coffmann and Cohen, 1987). It may be of interest to note that ischaemia impairs endothelium-dependent relaxation in response to acetylcholine (Dauber et al, 1990), which could be due to local acidosis and/or changes of membrane fluidity, caused by the accumulation of detergents (like long-chain acylcarnitine and lysophospholipids).

SUMMARY

During pacing of muscles, a considerable lowering of interstitial pH may occur. This is mainly due to secretion of lactic acid from pre-ischaemic, striated muscle cells. Local acidosis influences plasmalemmal changes, resulting in alterations of cellular ion fluxes, including Ca^{2+}. The resulting positive inotropy and limitation of vascular flow aggravates local acidosis. Continued pacing leads to further decline of flow and finally results in fully-developed ischaemia. Administration of L-carnitine in the pre-ischaemic state, has been shown to have a positive effect on muscle function by limiting lactic acidosis. The mechanism cannot only be the decline of the cellular acetyl CoA/CoA ratio, due to export of acetylcarnitine from the cells, but must be largely explained by inhibition of glyco(geno)lysis, as fatty acids or acetylcarnitine have been shown to delay loss of function during pacing as well.

Acknowledgements

The authors would like to thank Mrs C. Lucas and L.E.A. De Wit for help in some of the unpublished experiments mentioned. The Department of Cardiology of the University of Limburg, the Dutch Heart Foundation (The Hague, the Netherlands), and Sigma Tau, Pomezia, Italy, are thanked for financial support.

REFERENCES

Bettini V, Devarda E, Guerra B et al (1987) *Cardiologia* 32: 1039–1042.

Bingham-Smith J, Cragoe EJ & Smith L (1987) *J. Biol. Chem.* 262: 11988–11994.

Bingham-Smith J, Dwyer SD & Smith L (1989) *J. Biol. Chem.* 254: 8723–8728.

Bremer J (1983) *Physiol. Rev.* 63: 1420–1480.

Brevetti G, Attisano T, Perna S et al (1989) *Angiology* 40: 857–862.

Buderus S, Siegmund B, Spahr R et al (1989) *Am. J. Physiol.* 257: H488–H493.

Coffman JD & Cohen RA (1987) *Am. J. Physiol.* 252: H594–H597.

Dainty IA, Bigaud M, McGrath JC & Spedding M (1990) *Br. J. Pharmacol.* 100: 241–246.

Dauber IM, VanBenthuysen KM, McMurthy IF et al (1990) *Circ. Res.* 66: 986–998.

Dubelaar M-L, Lucas CMBH & Hülsmann WC (1991a) *Am. J. Physiol.* 260: E189–E193.

Dubelaar M-L, Lucas CMBH & Hülsmann WC (1991b) *J. Card. Surg.* 6 (supplement 2) 270–275.

Escande D (1989) *Pflügers Arch.* 414 (supplement 1): 893–998.

Ferrannini E, Buzzigoli G, Bevilaqua S et al (1988) *Am. J. Physiol.* 255: E964–E952.

Ferrari R, Cucchini F & Visioli O (1984) *Int. J. Cardiol.* 5: 213–216.

FitzGerald GA, Smith B, Pedersen AK & Brash ER (1984) *N. Engl. J. Med.* 310: 1065–1068.

Fritz IB (1959) *Am. J. Physiol.* 197: 297–304.

Fritz IB (1961) *Physiol. Rev.* 41: 41–52.

Hiatt WR, Regensteiner JG, Wolfel EE et al (1989) *J. Clin. Invest.* 84: 1167–1173.

Hülsmann WC (1970) *Biochem. J.* 116: 32–33.

Hülsmann WC & De Wit LEA (1990) *Cell. Biol. Int. Rep.* 14: 311–315.

Hülsmann WC & Dubelaar M-L (1987) *Cardiovasc. Res.* 21: 674–677.

Hülsmann WC & Dubelaar M-L (1988) *Biochimie* 70: 681–688.

Hülsmann WC, Siliprandi D, Ciman M & Siliprandi N (1964) *Biochim. Biophys. Acta* 93: 166–168.

Hülsmann WC, De Jong JW & Van Tol A (1968) *Biochim Biophys. Acta* 162: 292–293.

Hülsmann WC, Meyer AEFH, Bethlem J & Wijngaarden GK (1969) *Excerpta Medica Congress Series* 199: 319–322.

Hülsmann WC, Stam H & Maccari F (1982) *Biochim. Biophys. Acta* 713: 39–45.

Hülsmann WC, De Wit LEA, Scheydenberg C & Verkley AJ (1990a) *Biochim. Biophys. Acta* 1033: 214–218.

Hülsmann WC, De Wit LEA, Stam H & Schoonderwoerd K (1990b) *Biochim. Biophys. Acta* 1055: 189–192.

Hülsmann WC, Schneydenberg CTWM & Verkley AJ (1991) *Biochim. Biophys. Acta* (in press).

Idell-Wenger JA, Grotlohann LW & Neely JR (1978) *J. Biol. Chem.* 253: 4310–4318.

Kerner J & Bieber IL (1983) *Comp. Biochem. Physiol.* 758: 311–316.

Kwan CY & Daniel EE (1989) In Aoli MK & Frohlich ED (eds) *Calcium in Essential Hypertension*, pp 201–230. Japan: Academic Press.

Lückhoff A, Pohl U, Mülsch A & Busse R (1988) *Br. J. Pharmacol.* 95: 189–196.

Mertens S, Noll T, Spahr R et al (1990) *Am. J. Physiol.* 258: H689–H694.

Méry P-F, Brechler VE, Pavoine C et al (1990) *Nature* 345: 158–161.

Murthy MSR & Pande SV (1987) *Biochem. J.* 248: 727–733.

Odessey YY & Chace KV (1982) *Am. J. Physiol.* 243: H128–H132.

Philipson KD, Bersohn MM, Nishimoto AY et al (1982) *Circ. Res.* 50: 287–293.

Quast U & Cook NS (1989) *Trends Pharmacol. Sci.* 10: 431–435.

Randle PJ, Garland PB, Hales CN & Newsholme EA (1963) *Lancet* i: 785–789.

Scholte HR, Luyt-Houwen IEM, Dubelaar M-L & Hülsmann WC (1986) *FEBS Lett.* 198: 47–50.

Scholte, HR & Jennekens FGI (1988) *Neurology* 38: 60.

Shug AL, Thomsen JD, Folts JD et al (1978) *Arch. Biochem. Biophys.* 187: 4310–4318.

Siliprandi N, DiLisa F, Pieralsi G et al (1990) *Biochim. Biophys. Acta* 1034: 17–21.

Spagnoli LG, Corsi M, Villaschi S et al (1982) *Lancet* i: 1419–1420.

Von Ardenne M & Reitnauer PG (1989) *Biomed. Biochim. Acta* 4: 317–323.

Van Hinsbergh VMM, Emeis JJ & Havekes J (1983) *lst Int. End. Cell. Symp.*, pp 99–112. Basel: Karger.

Vandeplassche G & Borgers M (1990) *Cell Biol. Int. Rep.* 14: 317–334.

Weinstock M & McCarty R (1983) *Proc. Soc. Exp. Biol. Med.* 172: 194–201.

20

METABOLIC AND CLINICAL EFFECTS OF L-CARNITINE IN PERIPHERAL VASCULAR DISEASE

G. Brevetti and S. Perna

Peripheral vascular disease comprises many organic and functional vasospastic disorders, such as atherosclerosis obliterans, arterial thrombosis and embolism, thromboangitis obliterans, traumatic arterial occlusion and Raynaud's disease. The most frequent, however, is atherosclerosis obliterans; in patients over 50 years of age, this accounts for more than 95% of all arterial occlusions.

The term 'peripheral vascular disease' is generally used to indicate a condition of arterial insufficiency consequent to the localization of the atherosclerotic process in the lower limbs. Like coronary artery disease, the incidence of obliterative atherosclerosis of the lower limbs has increased considerably in the last 15 to 20 years, and its prevalence in the older population has been estimated at 12–16% (Criqui et al, 1985; Kannell and McGee, 1985).

As a consequence of obstructed peripheral arterial circulation, patients with peripheral vascular disease develop ischaemia in their legs. In the majority of cases, blood perfusion of the affected limb is within the normal range, under resting conditions, and patients

L-Carnitine and Its Role in Medicine:
From Function to Therapy. ISBN 0–12–253940–0

develop ischaemia only while walking, i.e. when the metabolic demand exceeds the supply of oxygen and substrate required for energy production. In others, however, resting blood flow is below critical levels and pain at rest and/or trophic lesions occur in the ischaemic limb. Except for the few cases requiring leg amputation, the spontaneous course of obliterative atherosclerosis of the lower limb is relatively benign. However, the disease assumes a great social significance because of the large number of patients affected and the chronic course of the disease. Patients with peripheral vascular disease have a reduced walking capacity that severely limits their range of activity, thus resulting in a high degree of disability. Indeed, patients with peripheral arterial insufficiency undergo a severe change in their quality of life. One third of affected individuals report decreased social participation and impaired sexual activity; more than 50% are forced to limit their recreational activities (Hunt et al, 1982).

In these patients, treatment aims to improve walking distance, and thus decrease the degree of disability. Until recently, treatment was limited to interventions aimed at increasing blood-flow to the ischaemic muscle. However, we have found that carnitine administration is able to increase walking ability in claudicant patients. This is probably a metabolic effect—it does not alter general or regional haemodynamics (Brevetti et al, 1988a). Apart from the therapeutic relevance of this finding, in that it represents a departure from current clinical practice, it also contributes to the understanding of the pathophysiology of peripheral vascular disease. In fact, our data strongly support the hypothesis that alterations in carnitine homeostasis may play a crucial role in the metabolic events that take place in the ischaemic skeletal muscle.

This chapter outlines present concepts on: (i) carnitine metabolism in peripheral vascular disease and (ii) metabolic and therapeutic effects of L-carnitine administration in patients with intermittent claudication.

CARNITINE METABOLISM IN PERIPHERAL VASCULAR DISEASE

Peripheral vascular disease is classified into four stages according to Fontaine (Table 1). Patients at stage I experience paraesthesias as the only symptom. Patients at stage II experience intermittent claudication, i.e. a cramping sensation in the affected leg which limits their performance. Stage III is characterized by pain at rest, and stage IV

TABLE I.
Fontaine's classification of peripheral vascular disease

Stage	Symptom
I	Paraesthesias
II	Intermittent claudication
III	Pain at rest
IV	Trophic lesions

by the occurrence of trophic lesions in the ischaemic limb. The progression in the severity of the clinical symptomatology reflects the progression in the severity of the ischaemic disease. Thus, to clarify the role of carnitine in peripheral vascular disease, we must first establish whether peripheral ischaemia induces alterations in carnitine metabolism, as occurs in myocardial ischaemia (Shug et al, 1978; Spagnoli et al, 1982). Second we must determine whether these alterations are related to the severity of the ischaemic process.

Carnitine is synthesized from two essential amino acids, lysine and methionine. In humans, the major sites of carnitine production are the liver and the kidney. The myocardium and skeletal muscle, which depend on fatty acid oxidation and thus require carnitine to maintain their normal energy metabolism, are highly dependent on carnitine transport from its sites of synthesis. In skeletal muscle, carnitine is taken up by a carrier-mediated system and its concentration is the result of several metabolic processes, i.e. carnitine uptake and synthesis, transport of carnitine in and out of the tissue, carnitine utilization and carnitine excretion. When one of these mechanisms is impaired, a condition of carnitine insufficiency takes place.

Primary carnitine insufficiencies are caused either by insufficient carnitine synthesis in liver or by impaired transport into extrahepatic tissues (see review by Ashbrook, 1986), whereas secondary carnitine insufficiencies are consequent to chronic disease states that imply an increased metabolic need for this amine (Rudman et al, 1977; Bohmer et al, 1978; Chalmers et al, 1984; Stumpf et al, 1985).

Carnitine transfers the acyl moiety from acyl CoA esters to carnitine, so producing free CoA and acylcarnitines that correspond to the original acyl CoAs (Bremer, 1980). Long-chain acylcarnitines (acylcarnitines whose acyl moiety consists of 10 or more carbon atoms) are generated to shuttle activated long-chain fatty acids across the inner mitochondrial membrane for subsequent β-oxidation. Short-chain acylcarnitines

(acylcarnitines whose acyl moiety is less than 10 carbon atoms) are formed from short-chain acyl CoAs. This latter function of carnitine is critically important in conditions that induce a noxious accumulation of short-chain acyl CoA esters into the mitochondria (Chalmers et al, 1984).

In normal muscle and plasma, the esterified fraction represents 15–30% of the total carnitine concentration, whereas the remainder is found as free carnitine. However, the ratio may be changed in various metabolic states. For example, an exercise of sufficient intensity to qualitatively alter muscle substrate metabolism (high-intensity exercise) produces, in normal subjects, a transient redistribution from free to short-chain acylcarnitine. This is indicated by the decrease in free carnitine in skeletal muscle and the concomitant increase in short-chain acylcarnitines in both plasma and skeletal muscle (Hiatt et al, 1989).

Changes in carnitine metabolism take place whenever oxidative metabolism is altered. Under these circumstances, the metabolic flux in the Krebs' cycle decreases and, consequently, acyl CoAs accumulate within the mitochondria. This leads to inhibition of the enzymes of the Krebs' cycle and of those involved in oxidative phosphorylation. In particular, accumulation of acetyl CoA (a short-chain acyl derivative) and the consequent increase of the acetyl CoA/CoA ratio inhibits pyruvate dehydrogenase and, thus, the oxidative utilization of glucose which cannot operate at the rate required by the metabolic demand. In such cases, carnitine is utilized to maintain a ratio of free to esterified CoA within the mitochondria that is optimal for oxidative phosphorylation (Harris et al, 1987).

Through the action of the enzyme carnitine acetyltransferase, which is very active in skeletal muscle (Alkonyi et al, 1975), carnitine may relieve the excess acyl CoA esters by forming short-chain acylcarnitines that can be transported out of the mitochondria and of the cell. It is conceivable that, in analogy with normal subjects performing a high-intensity exercise, patients with obstructive vascular disease may undergo similar changes in carnitine metabolism when claudication pain develops in the ischaemic muscle.

Patients with peripheral arterial insufficiency at stage II of Fontaine's classification show a significant increase in plasma short-chain acylcarnitines at maximally tolerated walking distance, compared with resting values (Hiatt et al, 1987). This implies that, in claudicant patients, the efficiency of the carnitine-linked system is preserved and is able, at least partially, to buffer the excess acyl CoA esters occurring during exercise-induced ischaemia. Such patients, however, also demonstrate a statistically significant correlation between the concentration of plasma short-chain acylcarnitines at rest and subsequent exercise performance (Figure 1). Therefore, patients who have the lowest walking capacity also have the greatest resting concentration of short-chain acylcarnitine. This suggests that the more severe the ischaemic disease, the greater the amount of carnitine required to remove the accumulation of acyl CoA esters produced by chronic ischaemia. This, although not affecting the muscle concentration of carnitine, may lead, in some cases, to a condition of relative carnitine insufficiency, i.e. insufficient free carnitine for the increased metabolic need produced by walking.

Because carnitine has the potential of enhancing, under certain conditions, aerobic and anaerobic metabolism, alteration of carnitine homeostasis may play a prime role in the pathophysiology of intermittent claudication. This is strongly supported by a recent report (Hiatt et al, 1990) demonstrating that, in claudicant patients, training-induced increase in walking ability is accompanied by a reduction in resting plasma concentrations of short-chain acylcarnitines. Exercise training has been shown to ameliorate physical performance in patients with peripheral vascular disease; this improvement has been attributed to increased blood-flow resulting from the development of collateral

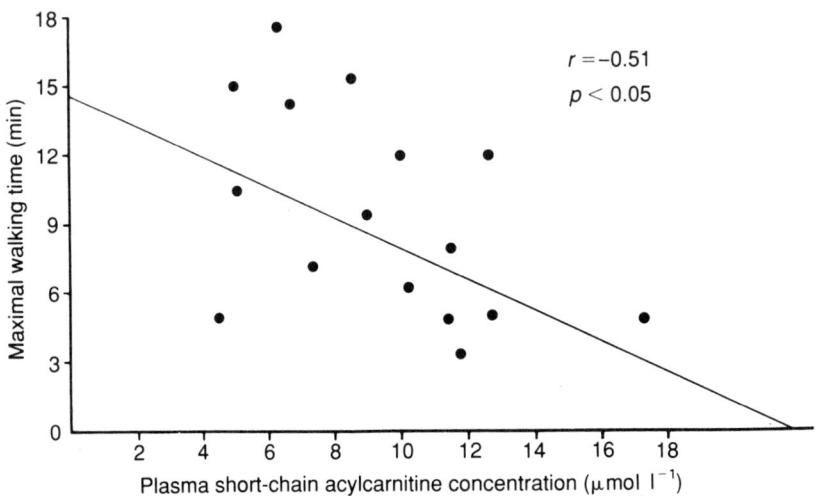

FIGURE 1. Plasma short-chain acylcarnitine concentration at rest correlated with maximal treadmill walking time in 16 patients with intermittent claudication. Pearson's $r = -0.51$, $p < 0.05$. (Hiatt et al, 1987. By permission of The American Physiological Society.)

circulation or reduced blood viscosity (Same and Sivertnoon, 1968; Ernst and Matrai, 1987).

Hiatt and coworkers also found that improvement in walking capacity was associated with a change in carnitine metabolism and not to a change in blood-flow. In fact, 12 weeks of exercise training reduced the plasma resting concentration of short-chain acylcarnitine from the control value of 12.5 ± 8.4 to 9.6 ± 8.8 μmol l^{-1} ($p < 0.05$).

Short-chain acylcarnitine is formed according to the formula:

$$\text{Short-chain acyl CoA} + \text{Carnitine} \rightarrow \text{Short-chain acylcarnitine} + \text{CoA}$$

Therefore, in patients with peripheral vascular disease at stage II of Fontaine's classification, a reduced short-chain acylcarnitine concentration at rest may reflect an increase in the availability of free carnitine for use during walking, i.e. when an increased yield of energy and a greater flux through the Krebs' cycle are required. This should result in an increase in walking distance. Indeed, Hiatt et al (1990) found that the plasma ratio of short-chain acylcarnitine concentration (an index of the distribution of total carnitine between free and acylated carnitine) decreased with training, and that change in this ratio from starting the training period to completion of it was inversely correlated to the change in peak walking time (Figure 2). Thus, subjects who had the greatest reduction in carnitine esterification with training, had

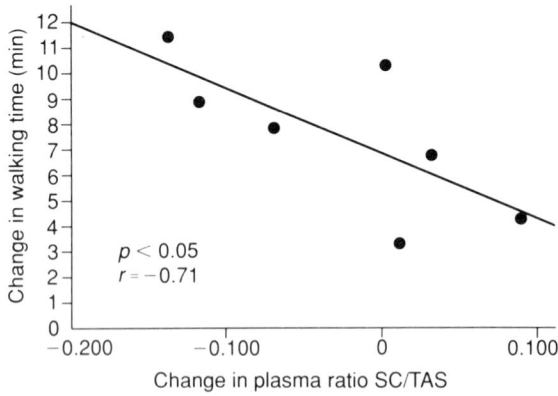

FIGURE 2. Plots of the relation between changes in peak exercise performance and changes in plasma carnitine metabolism. Change in the plasma ratio of short-chain acylcarnitine (SC) to total acid-soluble carnitine (TAS) from start of the training programme to its end negatively correlates with the change in peak treadmill walking time. Pearson's $r = -0.71$; $p < 0.05$. (Hiatt et al, 1990. By permission of the American Heart Association.)

the greatest improvement in exercise performance. From these results it may be hypothesized that, in patients with peripheral vascular disease, walking capacity depends, at least in part, on the carnitine availability to buffer the excess acyl CoAs that takes place with claudication.

Patients at stage II of Fontaine's classification have a normal concentration of carnitine in both plasma and skeletal muscle (Hiatt et al, 1987; Brevetti et al, 1988a). This implies that at stage II of the disease, the continued generation of acylcarnitines does not affect the content of carnitine in the ischaemic muscle. In other disease states, however, the chronic formation of acylcarnitines is followed by a fall in the concentration of carnitine in the active muscle that cannot be rapidly replenished by the normal nutritional and metabolic processes. For example, inherited disorders of organic acid metabolism are associated with export of carnitine from the tissue in the form of acylcarnitines, with consequent secondary carnitine insufficiency (Chalmers et al, 1984). Accordingly, it is conceivable that, in patients with peripheral vascular disease, the increase in the severity of the ischaemic process, by inducing a greater utilization of carnitine to remove the increased formation of acyl CoAs, may lead to a depletion of carnitine from the affected skeletal muscle.

To test this hypothesis, we measured the carnitine content of ischaemic skeletal muscles of patients with peripheral vascular disease at stages III and IV of Fontaine's classification (Brevetti et al, 1988b). As shown in Figure 3, compared with the normoperfused muscles of control subjects, the ischaemic muscles of these patients showed a significant reduction in total carnitine from 20.9 ± 5.2 to 11.6 ± 6.2 nmol per mg non-collagen protein ($p < 0.01$).

Patients with peripheral vascular disease can be divided into two groups, according to the alterations in their carnitine metabolism. Patients at Fontaine's stage II are characterized by normal levels of free and total carnitine in the ischaemic muscle and high levels of short-chain acylcarnitines in the plasma. Although an overt carnitine deficiency does not occur in these subjects, the increased ratio of acylcarnitine to free carnitine probably leads to a condition of relative carnitine insufficiency that may affect their performance. Indeed, reduction of resting values of short-chain acylcarnitines by increasing the availability of free carnitine for increased metabolic demand, may result in an improved walking ability in patients with intermittent claudication.

Patients at Fontaine's stages III and IV, on the other hand, are characterized by low levels of total carnitine in the ischaemic muscle.

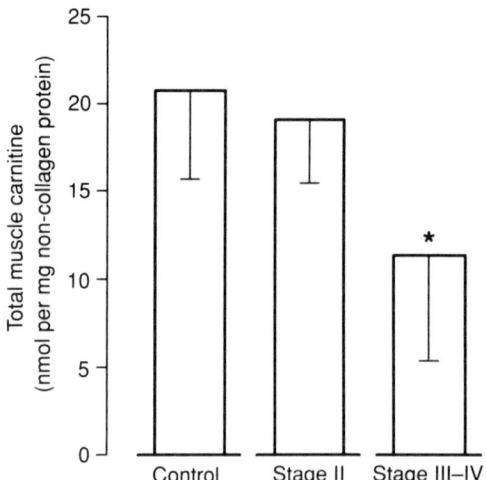

FIGURE 3. Total carnitine concentration in the skeletal muscle of control subjects ($n = 35$), patients with peripheral vascular disease at stage II of Fontaine's classification ($n = 4$) and patients at stage III and IV ($n = 5$). *, Significantly different from control $p < 0.01$.

In these subjects muscle carnitine deficiency develops as a consequence of an increased severity of the ischaemic disease, which leads to muscle carnitine depletion either because of increased utilization or because of loss through functionally-impaired cell membranes.

METABOLIC EFFECTS OF CARNITINE ADMINISTRATION

The capacity of the human body for work is dependent on energy-producing metabolic processes in the muscle cell. A continuing production of energy in the muscle cell is related to the supply of oxygen and energy-carrying substrates of which the most important are glucose, lactate, pyruvate, free fatty acids and amino acids.

The increased metabolic demand from skeletal muscles during exercise is normally almost exclusively met by an increase in the muscle blood-flow (Wahren, 1966). In patients with peripheral vascular disease, this compensatory mechanism is impaired because of arterial obliterations and thus metabolic alterations take place in the ischaemic muscles. It is important to clarify these metabolic changes so as to understand the pathophysiology of the disease. Moreover, they may be of practical importance in the management of patients unsuitable for surgery.

Biopsy studies of human claudicant muscles have demonstrated an increase in the proportion of type I (predominantly oxidative) fibres (Sjostrom et al, 1980) and in the number and size of mitochondria, suggesting an increased capacity for oxidative metabolism. Indeed, muscle oxygen extraction from blood is apparently increased in these patients (Carlson and Pernow, 1962), but measurement of lactate/pyruvate wash-out has suggested increased anaerobic metabolism (Hlavova et al, 1968). In any case, the resting metabolic balance between aerobic and anaerobic energy production within the cell of ischaemic muscles is unclear. On the contrary, there is an overt shift to anaerobic metabolism in the muscles of the affected leg during exercise. At a maximally tolerated walking distance, claudicant patients show a decline in the rate of ATP production, as indicated by the large decrease in phosphocreatine levels (Hands et al, 1986). As a consequence, glycolytic flux increases in an attempt to compensate for this shortfall in energy supply. However, the lack of oxygen inhibits the activity of Krebs' cycle and the metabolism of glucose can proceed only via anaerobic metabolism, which results in the accumulation of lactate (Maas and Alexander, 1982).

Carnitine, by functioning as an acetyl group buffer (Alkonyi et al, 1975), offers a number of potential advantages to cells functioning at or above their anaerobic threshold (Harris et al, 1987; Cerretelli and Marconi, 1990):

1. It stimulates the activity of pyruvate dehydrogenase by decreasing the acetyl CoA/CoA ratio, thus enhancing the oxidative utilization of glucose.
2. It enhances the metabolic flux in the Krebs' cycle by sparing free CoA.
3. It facilitates the transport of activated long-chain fatty acids into the mitochondria.
4. It activates the transport of adenine nucleotides across the inner mitochondrial membrane, by preventing adenylate translocase inhibition by long-chain fatty acid accumulation. This action may result in an increased ATP concentration in the muscle.

As a consequence of these mechanisms of action, carnitine may provide a more efficient regulation of the energy flow from the different oxidative sources, especially under ischaemic conditions when the reduction of blood-flow impairs delivery of substrates to the muscle and wash-out of metabolites.

In patients with peripheral vascular disease who are in a condition of relative carnitine insufficiency or even muscle carnitine deficiency this beneficial effect (optimization of the oxidative pathway) could be achieved through carnitine supplementation.

L-Carnitine administration to claudicant patients increases total carnitine concentration in the ischaemic muscles (Brevetti et al, 1988a). As shown in Figure 4, the increase of both free carnitine and short-chain acylcarnitine contributes to enhanced total carnitine concentration. These changes in the concentrations of muscle carnitine fractions indicate that part of the administered carnitine is taken up by the muscles of the affected leg and that a consistent portion is transformed into short-chain acylcarnitine, presumably acetylcarnitine (Bremer, 1980). This implies that a corresponding amount of short-chain acyl CoA, presumably acetyl CoA, is removed along with a concurrent release of free CoA (see equation above). The consequent decrease of the acetyl CoA/CoA ratio could stimulate pyruvate dehydrogenase, thus promoting an increase in the overall energy yield and a limitation of the adverse effects of increased lactic acid accumulation in the muscles. This assumption is supported by the finding that administration of carnitine reduces lactate production in the exercising ischaemic muscle (Brevetti et al, 1988a). The effect of

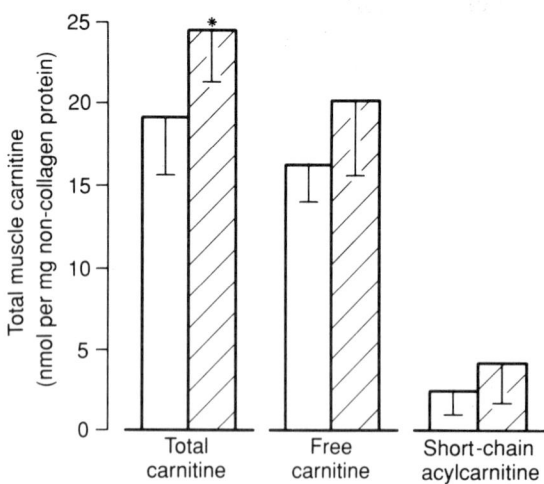

FIGURE 4. Changes in total, free and short-chain acylcarnitine induced by L-carnitine treatment in the ischaemic skeletal muscles of patients with intermittent claudication. *, Significantly different from pre-treatment value $p < 0.05$; □, before treatment; ▨, after L-carnitine administration.

L-carnitine administration on the arterial and venous lactate and pyruvate concentration in six patients affected by intermittent claudication as shown in Figure 5. In the absence of carnitine, maximally tolerated exercise increased popliteal venous lactate concentration by 107% ± 16%. After carnitine, lactate concentration in the venous blood leaving the ischaemic working muscle increased by only 54% ± 32% ($p < 0.01$ vs. controls). Moreover, after carnitine, at the same work-load as under control conditions, none of the patients experienced claudication pain. Furthermore, carnitine induced a quicker recovery to the resting values of the lactate/pyruvate ratio (Figure 6).

These data demonstrate that increased carnitine availability improves pyruvate utilization and oxidative phosphorylation efficiency in the exercising ischaemic skeletal muscle. Since glucose utilization in the anaerobic glycolysis yields 2 ATP, whereas its utilization in the aerobic pathway produces 36 ATP, the enhancement of pyruvate oxidation, and hence in energy production, may result in improved walking ability after treatment with L-carnitine.

An additional mechanism by which treatment with carnitine might

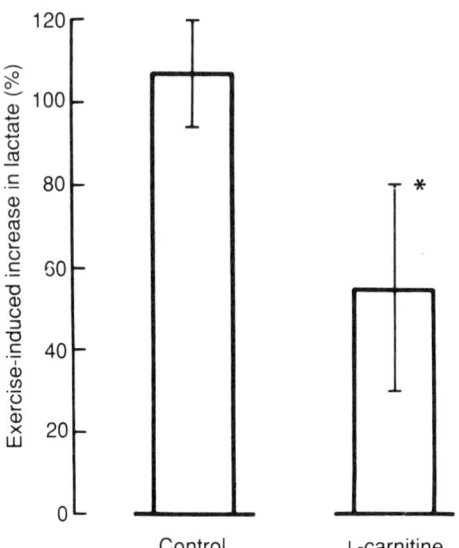

FIGURE 5. Exercise-induced increase in popliteal venous lactate concentration, before and after L-carnitine administration. *, Significantly different from placebo $p < 0.01$.

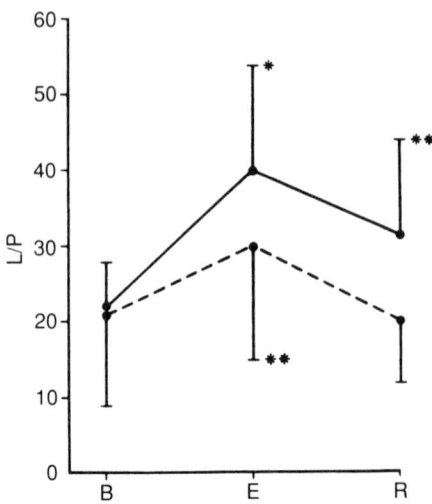

FIGURE 6. Popliteal venous lactate/pyruvate ratio at rest (B), during exercise (E), and during the recovery period (R), under control conditions (solid line) and after administration of L-carnitine (dashed line). *, Significantly different from rest value $p < 0.05$; **, Significantly different from rest value $p < 0.01$. (Brevetti et al, 1988. By permission of the American Heart Association.)

be beneficial in peripheral vascular disease is the removal of long-chain acyl CoAs and the consequent increase in the flow of adenine nucleotides across the inner mitochondrial membrane. This could generate a supply of ATP to the exercising muscle. In patients at stage II, however, better long-chain fatty acid use after L-carnitine supplementation seems to be ruled out: in the ischaemic muscles, even before carnitine administration, the concentration of total carnitine is above the value considered rate-limiting for optimal fatty acid oxidation (Long et al, 1982). On the other hand, this mechanism may operate in the more advanced stages of the disease, when the increased severity of the ischaemic process produces a marked reduction in total carnitine in the muscle.

CLINICAL EFFECTS OF L-CARNITINE IN PATIENTS WITH INTERMITTENT CLAUDICATION

Intermittent claudication is one of the commonest regional manifestations of degenerative arterial disease. It is also one of the major causes of disability in the middle-aged and elderly, because affected individuals become unable to meet the personal, social and occupational demands of daily life (Hunt et al, 1982). Nevertheless, treatment of this condition still represents a challenge. Apart from a small minority of individuals suitable for reconstructive surgery or transluminal angioplasty (Ruckley, 1986), patients with intermittent claudication are given conservative treatment, although so far no drug seems to be effective in improving walking ability. Cameron et al (1988) reviewed all trials of drug treatment for intermittent claudication published in English during the period 1965–1985. They concluded that: 'Despite 75 trials of 33 drugs it is still unclear whether any of these pharmacological agents has a clinically relevant effect on intermittent claudication, and it is probable that none of them has an important effect.'

The principal aim of treatment of obstructive vascular disease is to improve the balance between the energy supply and the metabolic demand in the affected muscle. Attempts to do this have relied on interventions aimed at increasing the blood perfusion to the affected limb, but no drug has yet been shown to increase muscle blood-flow during exercise. It would seem sensible to make more efficient use of the blood available to the exercising ischaemic limb in which an absolute increase in blood-flow is impossible. The untrained ischaemic limb may not be functioning at maximum metabolic capacity (Dahlof et al, 1984), and an agent able to improve metabolic efficiency may be beneficial to patients with intermittent claudication.

Carnitine is a crucial factor in regulating substrate flux and energy balance in the skeletal muscle and its dietary supplementation increases both the maximal aerobic (Marconi et al, 1985) and maximal anaerobic (Cerretelli and Marconi, 1990) power of trained subjects in the course of prolonged, heavy exercise. The use of this metabolic compound to treat patients with intermittent claudication is essentially justified by four considerations which have already been discussed in detail above:

1. walking capacity in these patients seems to depend, at least in part, on the carnitine availability to buffer the excess acyl CoAs occurring with claudication;
2. patients with intermittent claudication may be in a condition of relative carnitine insufficiency;
3. L-carnitine supplementation increases total carnitine content in the ischaemic muscle;
4. L-carnitine administration reduces lactate production in the exercising ischaemic skeletal muscle.

We evaluated the effect of L-carnitine (2 g b.i.d., orally) on the walking ability in 20 patients with intermittent claudication, according to a double-blind cross-over, placebo-controlled experimental design (Brevetti et al, 1988a). As shown in Figure 7, 3 weeks of carnitine treatment induced a marked increase in maximal treadmill walking capacity, from the placebo value of 174.7 ± 63.1 to 306.5 ± 121.8 m ($p < 0.01$). Compared with placebo, 12 of the 20 patients showed an increase in maximal walking capacity of 60% or more, four subjects had an improvement 25% to 59%, and only four showed no difference in walking ability between placebo and carnitine treatment. Changes in subjective symptoms such as sense of coldness, paresthesias, tiredness and pain during walking were also monitored. The intensity of each symptom was scored on a six-point scale: -3, total relief; -2, marked improvement; -1, slight improvement; 0, no change; $+1$, slight deterioration; $+2$, marked deterioration. As illustrated in Table 2, patients assigned to placebo showed slight changes after the first phase of treatment, while, when they crossed to carnitine, all symptoms improved significantly. Patients assigned first to carnitine reported improvements in all symptoms with respect to the wash-out period after the first phase of treatment; the improvement regressed when they crossed to placebo. The beneficial effects observed in this study could be attributable to the metabolic action of carnitine since the general and regional haemodynamics were not affected by treatment. Indeed, carnitine does not seem to have haemodynamic effects in the ischaemic skeletal limbs (Figures 8 and 9), but it does improve the blood perfusion to the affected muscle during reactive hyperaemia (Brevetti et al, 1989).

Reactive hyperaemia is the increase of blood-flow in a vascular district that occurs when a temporary ischaemia is released. This phenomenon is caused by an arteriolar dilatation induced by vasoactive

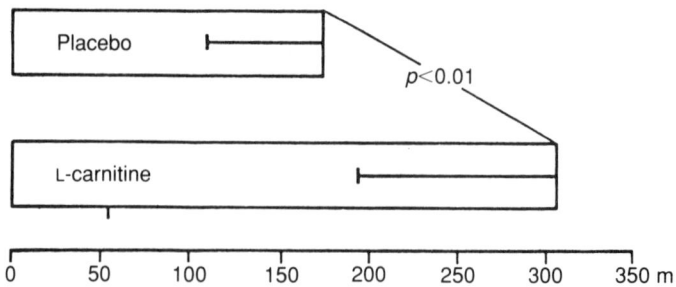

FIGURE 7. Effect of placebo and L-carnitine on maximal walking capacity.

TABLE 2.

Changes in subjective symptoms observed throughout the study in patients randomly assigned to receive placebo (top) and carnitine (bottom). (Brevetti et al, 1988a. By permission of the American Heart Association.)

Patient	Paraesthesias P vs WO	Paraesthesias C vs P	Tiredness P vs WO	Tiredness C vs P	Pain during walking P vs WO	Pain during walking C vs P	Coldness P vs WO	Coldness C vs P
1	0	-3	+1	-3	0	-2	0	-2
2	+1	-3	0	-3	0	-3	0	-2
3	-1	0	0	-1	0	-1	-1	0
4	0	-1	-1	-2	-1	-2	0	0
5	0	-2	0	-3	-1	0	0	0
6	+1	-2	-1	-3	0	-2	0	0
7	0	-2	0	-2	0	-3	0	0
8	0	-3	-1	-2	0	-1	0	-1
9	0	-3	-1	-2	-1	0	0	0
10	-1	-3	-1	-3	-1	-3	0	-1

Patient	Paraesthesias C vs WO	Paraesthesias P vs C	Tiredness C vs WO	Tiredness P vs C	Pain during walking C vs WO	Pain during walking P vs C	Coldness C vs WO	Coldness P vs C
1	-3	+2	-3	+1	-3	+2	-2	0
2	-3	+1	-3	+2	-2	+2	-2	+1
3	-2	+1	-3	+1	-2	0	-1	0
4	-3	+1	-3	+1	-3	+2	-1	0
5	-3	0	-2	+2	-2	+2	0	0
6	-3	+2	-1	+1	-1	-1	-1	0
7	-3	+2	-1	+2	-2	+2	-1	0
8	-2	+1	-2	+2	-2	+1	0	0
9	0	0	0	0	-1	0	0	0
10	-1	+1	-2	+1	-2	+1	-1	+1

WO = wash-out; P = placebo; C = carnitine.
All symptoms were significantly ($p < 0.01$) improved by carnitine (Mann–Whitney U-test).

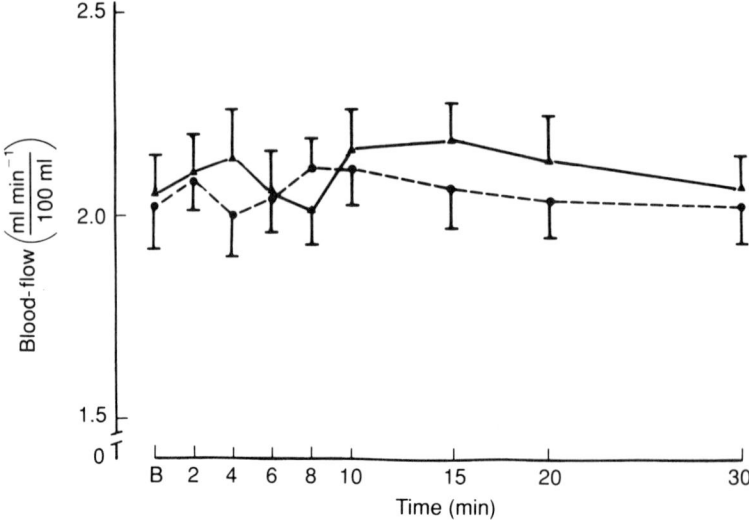

FIGURE 8. Effect of placebo and L-carnitine infusion on blood-flow to the affected limb. No significant difference was found between placebo ●——● and carnitine ▲——▲ treatment (Brevetti et al, 1989. By permission of Westminster Publications.)

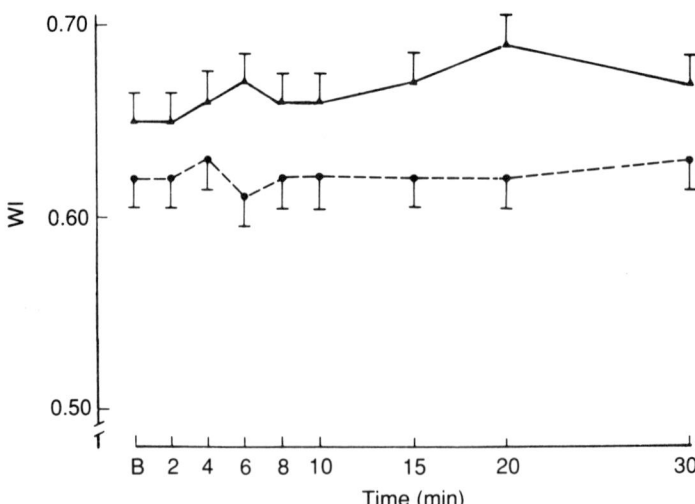

FIGURE 9. Effect of placebo ●——● and L-carnitine ▲——▲ infusion on ankle/arm systolic blood pressure ratio (WI) in the affected limb. No significant difference was found between treatments (Brevetti et al, 1989. By permission of Westminster Publications.)

substances released by the ischaemic tissue (Haddy and Scott, 1968; Berne et al, 1971), and its extent depends on the capacity of the circulation to respond to stress. Therefore, measurements of the blood-flow in the calf during reactive hyperaemia are widely used to evaluate the functional state of the arterial system in the affected limb of patients with obstructive peripheral arterial disease (Barnes, 1978). In such patients, the hyperaemic response is usually lower than in normal subjects (Strandell and Wahren, 1963) and a reduction in blood-flow during the post-ischaemic period may also be observed (Brevetti et al, 1977), as a consequence of the so-called 'steal phenomenon' (Sheperd, 1963). These abnormal responses have been found to be improved after L-carnitine administration (Brevetti et al, 1989).

Figure 10 shows the individual percentage changes in muscle blood-flow observed in 18 ischaemic limbs during reactive hyperaemia, before and after L-carnitine administration (3 g as a bolus followed by continuous intravenous infusion of 2 mg kg^{-1} min^{-1} for 30 min). Ten minutes after the release of ischaemia, in all but four patients, carnitine induced improvement in hyperaemic response, which in most cases was relevant. Furthermore, compared with resting values, 13 patients had either no change or even showed a reduction in muscle blood-flow, after placebo treatment, while, after carnitine, this was observed

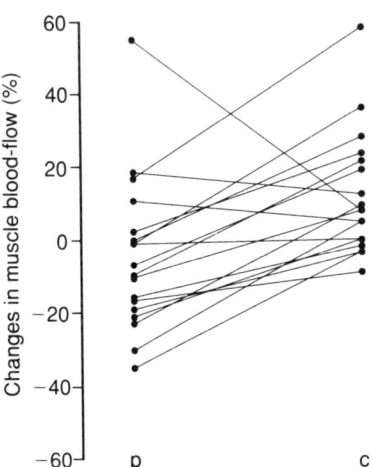

FIGURE 10. Changes in muscle blood-flow observed for 10 min during reactive hyperaemia, after placebo (p) and L-carnitine (c) treatment. Individual values represent percentage variation, using resting values as baseline.

only in five subjects. Figure 11 shows the effect of placebo and L-carnitine on reactive hyperaemia. With placebo, there was a significant increase in blood-flow at 2, 4 and 6 min after the release of ischaemia, whereas after carnitine administration blood perfusion to the affected limb rose significantly throughout the recording period. Moreover, the values of blood-flow at 2 and 10 min with carnitine were significantly higher than those recorded at the same times after placebo. These findings indicate an improvement of the functional circulatory reserve in the ischaemic limb and may contribute to the understanding of the mechanism by which L-carnitine ameliorates walking capacity in patients with intermittent claudication.

CONCLUDING REMARKS

L-Carnitine may be considered a potential aid for treating patients with peripheral vascular disease because: (i) carnitine is a natural component of muscle; (ii) carnitine has an important role in energy production in the skeletal muscle; (iii) carnitine homeostasis is altered in the ischaemic muscle; (iv) these alterations may be reversed by carnitine supplementation; (v) L-carnitine administration enhances the

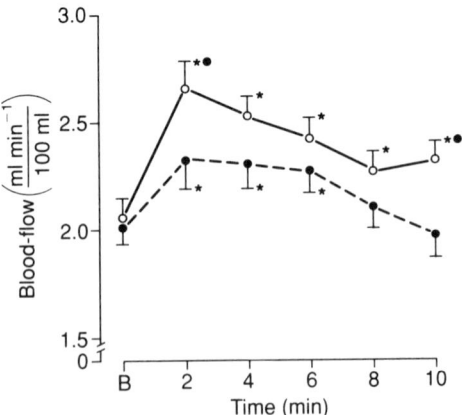

FIGURE 11. Effect of placebo ●——● and L-carnitine ○——○ on blood-flow to the affected limb under control conditions (B) and after 2, 4, 6, 8 and 10 min during reactive hyperaemia. *, Significantly different from basal value $p < 0.01$; **, Significantly different from placebo $p < 0.05$. (Brevetti et al, 1989. By permission of Westminster Publications.)

functional circulatory reserve; (vi) even an excessive intake of L-carnitine does not harm animals or man.

The finding of improved walking capacity after L-carnitine administration is encouraging. However, to confirm this observation, long-term studies in a larger population are needed, because the therapeutic response may be influenced by the size of the sample. In fact, in seven studies using pentoxifylline for treating claudicant patients, the larger the trial, the worse the outcome (Cameron et al, 1988).

In addition, comparative studies with other agents should be performed so as to permit the clinician to weigh the benefits and cost of the drug in the light of alternative therapies. In any case, because the mechanism of action of L-carnitine differs from that of other therapeutic agents, a combination of carnitine and more traditional drugs may be useful in treating intermittent claudication.

Studies should also be conducted to clarify the mechanism of action of carnitine in peripheral vascular disease. In particular, ^{31}P nuclear magnetic resonance spectroscopy is a useful non-invasive method with which to evaluate carnitine-induced changes in the metabolism of claudicating leg muscles. Finally, since evidence has been produced that propionyl-L-carnitine, a short-chain acyl-derivative, has greater effect than L-carnitine in protecting the ischaemic myocardium (Paulson et al, 1986), it seems worthwhile to investigate the efficacy of this new metabolic compound in peripheral vascular disease. Further studies should address this topic.

REFERENCES

Alkonyi I, Kerner J & Sandoz A (1975) *FEBS Lett.* 52: 265–268.
Ashbrook DW (1986) In Borum PR (ed.) *Clinical Aspects of Human Carnitine Deficiency*, pp 120–139. New York: Pergamon Press.
Barnes RW (1978) *Angiology* 29: 631–640.
Berne RM, Rubio R, Dobson JG & Curnish R (1971) *Circ. Res.* 28 (supplement): 115–119.
Bohmer T, Bergrem H & Eiklid K (1978) *Lancet* i: 126–128.
Bremer J (1980) *Physiol. Rev.* 63: 1420–1480.
Brevetti G, Rengo F, Chiariello M et al (1977) *Angiology* 28: 687–694.
Brevetti G, Chiariello M, Ferulano G et al (1988a) *Circulation* 77: 767–773.
Brevetti G, Angelini C, Marcialis A et al (1988b) *International Symposium on the Lipid Metabolism in the Normoxic and Ischemic Heart*, Maastricht, The Netherlands (abstracts), p 73.
Brevetti G, Attisano T, Perna S et al (1989) *Angiology* 40: 857–862.
Cameron HA, Waller PC & Ramsay LE (1988) *Br. J. Clin. Pharmacol.* 26: 569–576.

Carlson L & Pernow B (1962) *Acta Med. Scand.* 171: 311–323.
Cerretelli P & Marconi C (1990) *Int. J. Sports Med.* 11: 1–14.
Chalmers RA, Roe CR, Stacey TE & Hoppel CL (1984) *Pediatr. Res.* 18: 1325–1328.
Criqui MH, Franck A, Barrett-Connor E et al (1985) *Circulation* 71: 510–515.
Dahlof A, Bjorntrop P & Holm J (1985) *Eur. J. Clin. Invest.* 44: 9–15.
Ernst EE & Matrai A (1987) *Circulation* 76: 1110–1114.
Haddy FJ & Scott JB (1968) *Physiol. Rev.* 48: 688–707.
Hands LJ, Bore PJ, Galloway G et al (1986) *Clin. Sci.* 71: 283–290.
Harris RC, Foster CVL & Hultman E (1987) *J. Appl. Physiol.* 63: 440–442.
Hiatt WR, Nawaz D & Brass EP (1987) *J. Appl. Physiol.* 62: 2383–2387.
Hiatt WR, Regensteiner JG, Wolfel EE et al (1989) *J. Clin. Invest.* 84: 1167–1173.
Hiatt WR, Regensteiner JG, Hargarten HE et al (1990) *Circulation* 81: 602–609.
Hlalova A, Linhart J, Perovsky I & Ganz V (1966) *Clin. Sci.* 30: 377–387.
Hunt SM, McKenna SP, McEven J et al (1982) *Practitioner* 226: 133–136.
Kannell WB & McGee DL (1985) *J. Am. Geriatr. Soc.* 33: 13–18.
Long CS, Haller RG, Foster DW & McGarry JD (1982) *Neurology* 32: 663–666.
Maas V & Alexander K (1982) *Z. Kardiol.* 71: 39–43.
Marconi C, Sassi G, Carpinelli A & Cerretelli P (1985) *Eur. J. Appl. Physiol.* 54: 131–135.
Paulson DJ, Traxles J, Schmidt M et al (1986) *Cardiovasc. Res.* 20: 536–541.
Rudman D, Schwell CW & Arroley JD (1977) *J. Clin. Invest.* 60: 716–723.
Ruckley CV (1986) *Br. Med. J.* 292: 970–971.
Same H & Sivertnoon R (1968) *Acta Physiol. Scand.* 73: 257–263.
Sheperd JT (ed.) (1963) In *Physiology of the Circulation in Human Limbs in Health and Disease*, pp 1–416. London and Philadelphia: W B Saunders.
Shug AL, Thomsen JH, Folts JD et al (1978) *Arch. Biochem. Biophys.* 187: 25–53.
Sjostrom M, Angquist KA & Rais O (1980) *Ultrastruct. Pathol.* 1: 309–326.
Spagnoli LG, Corsi M, Villaschi S, Palmieri G & Maccari F (1982) *Lancet* i: 1419–1420.
Strandell T & Wahren J (1963) *Acta Med. Scand.* 173: 99–105.
Stumpf DA, Parker WD & Angelini C (1985) *Neurology* 35: 1041–1045.
Wahren J (1966) *Acta Physiol. Scand.* 67 (supplement): 269–274.

Part IIIc

Renal dialysis

21

CARNITINE, KIDNEY AND RENAL DIALYSIS

S. Ahmad

CARNITINE AND THE KIDNEY

Kidney is one of the major sites for the synthesis of carnitine from circulating 6-N-trimethyllysine (Rebouche, 1986). Beside intake and synthesis, carnitine metabolism largely depends on renal handling. Under normal conditions circulating carnitine is freely filtered at the glomeruli. Over 90% of the filtered free carnitine is reabsorbed by the renal tubules (Wanner and Hohl, 1988). The tubular reabsorption appears to be threshold-dependent and urinary loss increases as the filtered load exceeds the tubular threshold which is reported to be about 74 μmol dl^{-1} (Engel et al, 1981; Wagner et al, 1986; Wanner et al, 1988). Some tubular secretion of the carnitine synthesized by the kidney has also been reported (Engel et al, 1981). Compared with its esters, free carnitine is preferentially reabsorbed by the tubules, thus renal clearance of carnitine esters (acyl carnitine) is 4–8 times higher than that of free carnitine. This selected reabsorption of free carnitine and rejection of carnitine esters is important in the understanding of carnitine metabolism in conditions of renal failure. Normal urine contains about 46% free, 29% short-chain and 16% long-chain carnitine (Wanner and Hohl, 1988).

L-Carnitine and Its Role in Medicine:
From Function to Therapy. ISBN 0–12–253940–0

CARNITINE AND RENAL DISEASE

Tubular transport defects

Studies in selective tubulopathies such as cystinuria, Bartter's syndrome, phosphaturia, lysinuria and proximal tubular acidosis, have revealed variable but normal reabsorption of carnitine in the proximal tubule. Carnitine infusion in these patients does not result in increased urinary losses of either carnitine or that of the substance involved in the pathology (cystine, lysine, etc.). This suggests that these substances and carnitine do not share the same tubular transport mechanisms.

In patients with Fanconi's syndrome, more generalized defects of proximal tubule, decreased tubular reabsorption and increased urinary losses of carnitine have been reported (Steinmann et al, 1987). This suggests that carnitine and some amino acids may be handled in similar fashion by the proximal tubule. Steinmann et al (1987) observed good correlation between valine and carnitine tubular reabsorption, however authors concluded that these two substances did not share the same absorptive mechanisms. At this point it is unclear whether children with Fanconi's syndrome suffer from carnitine deficiency. Netzloff et al (1981), Bernardini et al (1985) and Gahl et al (1988) have reported cases with Fanconi's syndrome suggestive of carnitine deficiency. Gahl et al (1988) observed reduced muscle and plasma carnitine content in a group of patients with cystinosis and Lowe's syndrome. With carnitine supplement the plasma free fatty acid and lipid accumulation in muscle were significantly reduced. Netzloff et al (1981) also observed improved muscle strength after carnitine supplementation.

Acute renal failure

Patients with carnitine palmitoyl transferase (CPT) deficiency can present with acute renal failure secondary to rhabdomyolysis and myoglobinuria. The condition is usually precipitated when demand for energy is increased such as exposure to cold, stress, strenuous exercise and fasting. Under these conditions the availability of ATP is limited secondary to reduced metabolism of long-chain fatty acids due to CPT deficiency. ATP is necessary to maintain the integrity of sarcolemma and rhabdomyolysis can occur in its deficiency. It has been reported that L-carnitine administration is useful for this condition

(Bank et al, 1975; Roza et al, 1978; Brownell et al, 1979). The role of L-carnitine in the management of acute renal failure caused by other factors has not been well studied.

Chronic renal failure

With the declining glomerular filtration rate (GFR) the carnitine filtration also decreases leading to elevated plasma concentrations of carnitine. With progressive renal disease the tubular handling of carnitine and its esters becomes abnormal. The preferential reabsorption of free carnitine and rejection of acylcarnitine by the renal tubules is impaired. This leads to marked increases in blood concentrations of carnitine esters (Rodriguez-Segade et al, 1986a). In patients who are not on dialysis, both free carnitine and total carnitine concentrations are increased. However the ratio of free to acylcarnitine is quite abnormal (2.2 vs. 7.5 nmol ml^{-1} for uraemics and normals, respectively; Rodriguez-Segade et al, 1986a). Thus, in uraemia there is abnormal utilization of carnitine.

Peritoneal dialysis

Serum carnitine has been measured in a relatively small number of patients undergoing continuous ambulatory peritoneal dialysis (CAPD) and intermittent peritoneal dialysis (IPD). In both these groups serum total and free carnitine levels appear to be normal (Buoncristiani et al, 1981; Albright et al, 1982; Amair et al, 1982; Moorthy et al, 1983; Moorthy and Shug, 1985; Wanner et al, 1986). However, compared with normal controls, the acylcarnitine levels are significantly higher in both CAPD and IPD patients. Patients on IPD show the highest acyl-carnitine concentration when compared with either the CAPD or haemodialysis (HD) group. Thus the PD patients exhibit an abnormal carnitine profile. Buoncristiani et al (1981) reported a progressive decline in plasma carnitine levels in a group of PD patients over a 2-year period. Long-term peritoneal dialysis patients should be studied to clarify further the possibility of possible carnitine depletion.

Haemodialysis

Several factors affect the carnitine profile in patients on haemodialysis. Meat and dairy products are a rich source of carnitine and its precursors. Patients on dialysis have limited intake of these food items.

Being a small, water-soluble molecule carnitine is freely dialysed, resulting in as much as a 75% decline in plasma concentration during one haemodialysis session (Rumpf et al, 1983). As kidney is one of the major sites of carnitine synthesis, it was thought that endogenous synthesis might be impaired with the loss of renal parenchyma. It was proposed, therefore, that patients on the haemodialysis are carnitine-deficient. This contention has been disputed, however, for several reasons (Fagher et al, 1985; Nilsson-Ehle and Cederblad, 1985). The total normal urinary losses are comparable to, or exceed, the dialytic losses of carnitine; studies have shown that plasma concentration of total carnitine is either well within normal range or even slightly elevated (Golmer et al, 1990). It has also been argued that although the carnitine level during the dialysis declines quite significantly, a few hours after dialysis it is returned to predialysis levels. This repletion presumably occurs from the tissue stores.

Despite apparent evidence to the contrary, there are well-documented cases of significant dialytic loss of carnitine and presence of abnormal metabolism of carnitine in haemodialysed patients. Rodriguez-Segade et al (1986b) have reported that the carnitine levels significantly declined during dialysis session and were not restored before the next dialysis. The authors found that over a 25-week period there was an exponential decay of serum carnitine levels, leading them to conclude that the endogenous synthesis of carnitine is unable to replete the dialytic losses fully.

Several studies in dialysis patients have shown that the plasma concentration of total carnitine is normal or elevated. However the free carnitine concentration is subnormal (Table 1) whereas the concentration

TABLE I.

Plasma carnitine concentrations in haemodialysis patients as reported in three relatively large series. Values are presented in nmol ml^{-1}

Plasma carnitine	Golper et al (n = 82)	Rossle et al (n = 31)	Rodriguez et al (n = 54)
Free	31 ± 2	32 ± 12	39 ± 16
Total	61 ± 2	60 ± 19	62 ± 22
Free/Total	0.54	0.53	0.63
Acylated	26.3	27.7	23.4

In all three studies the free carnitine concentration was significantly lower and that of acylcarnitine was significantly higher than the healthy controls. Total carnitine concentration was not different from normals in Golper et al (1990) but were lower than normal in the other two studies (Rodriguez-Segade et al, 1986a; Rossle et al, 1986).

of carnitine esters (acylcarnitine), is markedly elevated (Bartel et al, 1981a; Leschke et al, 1983; Rodriguez-Segade et al, 1986; Wanner et al, 1986; Yderstraede et al, 1986; Golper et al, 1990). This results in a significant reduction of the free to total carnitine ratio as well as the free to acylcarnitine ratio (Guanieri et al, 1987; Golper et al, 1990). It has been suggested that a free carnitine to acylcarnitine ratio of less than 4 is indicative of carnitine deficiency. The free carnitine concentrations in muscle have also been reported to be subnormal in haemodialysis patients (Konig et al, 1978; Bellinghieri et al, 1983).

The factors contributing to these anomalies (Table 2) are the subject of considerable interest and debate. Fatty acid metabolism is impaired in uraemia, and could lead to production of large numbers of incompletely metabolized acyl moieties. Normally these acyl moieties are taken up by carnitine and the resulting acylcarnitine is removed by the kidneys. With the impairment of renal excretion short-chain and long-chain acylcarnitines accumulate in plasma (Table 1).

Figure 1 shows the effect of carnitine supplementation on its plasma concentration (Golper et al, 1990). With carnitine supplementation serum carnitine levels increased severalfold from baseline. However, the acylated carnitine increased more than free carnitine, as evidenced by a slight decrease in the short-chain acyl to free carnitine ratio, from 0.76 to 0.65 at 6 months (normal ratio 0.16). This suggests that administered carnitine became bound to acyl moieties, indicating that acyl groups are abundant in renal failure patients.

Acyl moieties are harmful to cellular metabolism because they inhibit several key enzymes (Table 3, Borum and Taggart, 1986). Abnormal acetyl oxidation (Ricanati et al, 1987; Guanieri et al, 1989) coupled with decreased renal excretion of acylcarnitine may result in its accumulation. Impairment of fatty acid oxidation would result in production of acyl moieties which utilize free carnitine and form carnitine esters.

TABLE 2.
The possible factors contributing to abnormal carnitine profile in the dialysis patients

1.	Abnormal fatty acid metabolism
2.	Abnormal renal excretion of acyl carnitine
3.	Increased free fatty acids (heparin-induced lipolysis)
4.	Incomplete mitochondrial fatty acid oxidation
5.	Enhanced long-chain fatty acid oxidation in peroxisomes

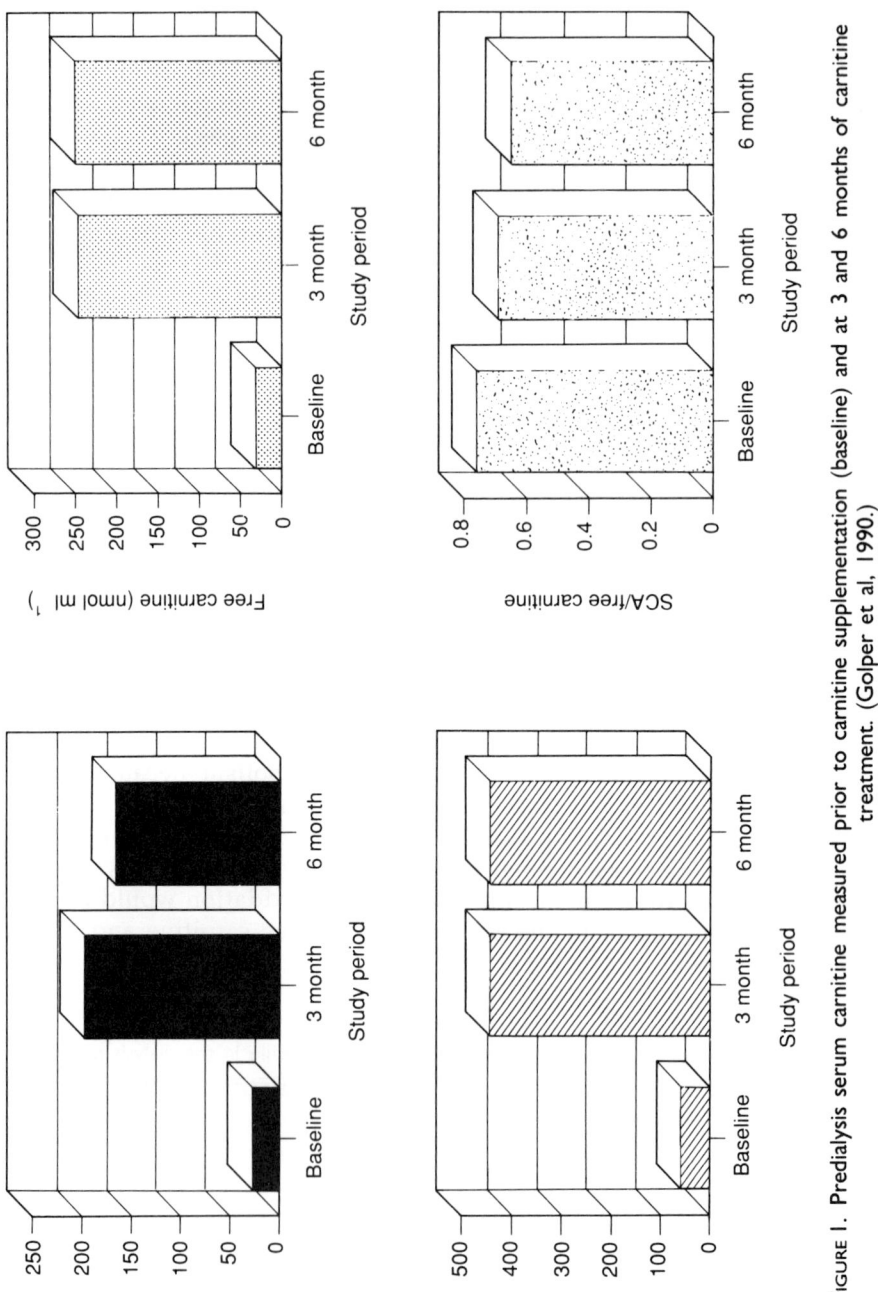

FIGURE I. Predialysis serum carnitine measured prior to carnitine supplementation (baseline) and at 3 and 6 months of carnitine treatment. (Golper et al, 1990.)

TABLE 3.
Enzymes inhibited by acyl CoA

Acetyl CoA carboxylase
Adenine nucleotide translocase
Citrate synthetase
Pyruvate dehydrogenase
Pyruvate carboxylase
N-Acetyl glutamate synthetase

As discussed above, normal urinary losses of carnitine appear to be similar to total dialytic losses. However, dialysis, unlike kidney function, is not a selective process and relatively more free carnitine is lost during haemodialysis than in the urine of a person without kidney disease. Wanner and Horl (1988) reported a 75% decrease in free carnitine after 4 hours of haemodialysis; decline in short-chain and long-chain acylcarnitine was about 65 and 50%, respectively. It has also been suggested that dialysis patients have decreased intake of carnitine and its precursors (Guanieri et al, 1987). Thus, the combination of excessive binding with acyl groups, excessive dialytic loss of free carnitine, decreased intake, and decreased renal excretion of acyl derivatives may be responsible for the abnormal pattern of carnitine concentrations (Table 4).

In summary, patients with renal failure, not undergoing dialysis, show elevated values of plasma carnitine concentrations. Patients

TABLE 4.
The possible causes for the abnormal pattern of plasma carnitine concentrations

I.	Decreased intake: meat and dairy products
	Precursors
	Carnitine
2.	Excessive dialytic losses
	Free carnitine
3.	Abnormal fatty acid metabolism
	? Incomplete metabolism
	Excessive acyl moieties
4.	Decreased glomerular filtration rate
	Decreased clearance of acylcarnitine
5.	Decreased renal parenchyma
	? Decreased synthesis

undergoing haemodialysis and peritoneal dialysis have markedly elevated acylcarnitine concentrations. Haemodialysed patients have subnormal plasma concentrations of free carnitine. With carnitine administration, all fractions of carnitine increase, but abnormal ratios of free to total carnitine remain abnormal.

Carnitine supplementation in haemodialysis patients

Certain clinical conditions which are common in dialysis patients have been suggested to be related to abnormal carnitine metabolism. These include: severe impairment of muscle function and metabolism, muscle weakness and myopathy, cardiac dysfunctions, cardiomyopathy and arrhythmias, and plasma lipid abnormalities. Intradialytic symptoms such as muscle cramps, cardiac arrhythmias and hypotension are often encountered and could be related to carnitine metabolism.

About 42 studies of L-carnitine supplementation in 600 dialysis patients have been reported (Table 5). Dose has ranged between 15 and 100 mg kg^{-1}—usually 20 mg kg^{-1} i.v. after each dialysis session. The supplementation is associated with a severalfold increase in plasma concentrations of free carnitine as well as acylcarnitine and total carnitine. As discussed above, the abnormal ratio of free to acylcarnitine tends to improve with carnitine supplementation. In the few cases where muscle carnitine levels have been measured, they increase with the supplementation (Aubia et al, 1980; Taggart et al, 1986).

TABLE 5.
Published studies ($n = 42$) reporting effect of L-carnitine supplementation on various parameters in haemodialysis patients ($n = 600$)

Parameters	Improvement	No improvement
Lipids	21	9
Dialytic morbidity	5	1
Skeletal function	5	0
Cardiac function	5	1
Haematocrit	6	1
Others	4	—

Lipid abnormalities

Raised plasma triglyceride with decreased HDL-cholesterol has been found in dialysis patients (Gutman et al, 1973; Bagdade and Albers, 1977; Brunzell et al, 1977). Studies with carnitine supplementation in dialysis patients have produced contradictory results. Of the 30 studies describing lipid profile, 21 reported improvement with the administration of L-carnitine, seven found no effect of the therapy and two observed even higher triglyceride concentrations. Recently it has been suggested that the dual response may be related to the administered dose of L-carnitine (Wanner et al, 1989). Most of the studies have used L-carnitine in the dose of 1–3 g i.v. after each dialysis session (Ahmad et al, 1987). Wanner et al (1989) used 1, 5 and 15 mg L-carnitine per kg body wt and found that the lower dose was more effective and prevented antiketogenic effects. It has been proposed that large doses of carnitine might remove the acyl groups from mitochondrial acyl CoA and transport it to the cytosol where fatty acids and triglycerides are synthesized. This would account for the worsening lipid profile. Depletion of mitochondrial acyl groups would also deplete the substrate supply for the β-oxidation of fatty acids. Support for this hypothesis comes from three published studies, one in rats (Bohles and Akcetin, 1987) and two using dialysis patients (Guarnieri et al, 1980; Chan et al, 1982). When rats were given small amounts of carnitine, ketogenesis occurred; with large doses antiketogenesis was observed. However, several studies utilizing a so-called larger dose (> 5 mg kg^{-1}) have reported improvement in lipid profile. In general, however, those studies which have reported no reduction in lipid concentrations have used higher doses of L-carnitine.

Recently, the dialysate anion has been implicated in the lipid-lowering effect of the carnitine treatment. Traditionally, acetate has been used as the basic anion in the dialysate in place of bicarbonate. In the past it has been suggested that acetate in the dialysate contributes to the lipid abnormality of these patients (Ahmad et al, 1980). A study in which acetate was replaced with bicarbonate reported an improvement in lipid profile (Ahmad et al, 1980). Similarly, Zilleruelo et al (1989) observed that patients undergoing acetate dialysis had higher triglyceride (TG) levels than those using bicarbonate dialysis. After 1 month of carnitine supplementation the triglyceride concentration decreased and that of HDL-cholesterol increased, but only in the acetate group. It was concluded that acetate dialysis patients who have hypertriglyceridaemia would benefit from carnitine supplementation. Guarnieri et al (1989) reported similar results with acetate dialysis patients. In a group of patients on acetate dialysis Maeda et al (1989) observed an increase in whole-body clearance of acetate after carnitine treatment. On the other hand, in a large multi-centre trial, no difference was detected in the effect of L-carnitine on lipids in acetate and bicarbonate patients (Golper et al, 1990).

A preliminary study of dialysis patients Ahmad et al (1989) found the fatty acid profile to be similar to that in essential fatty acid deficiency states (Figure 2). Lower proportions of linoleic, linolenic and arachidonic acids, along with higher proportions of oleic and eicosatrienoic acids were seen in patients not receiving carnitine treatment. In another haemodialysis group, treated with L-carnitine for more than 6 months, linoleic, linolenic and eicosatrienoic acids were comparable to normals. The ratio of saturated to unsaturated fatty acids was also higher in patients who were not on carnitine treatment. Maeda et al (1989) observed that, compared with untreated patients, carnitine treatment was associated with a lower free fatty acid concentration during haemodialysis; they concluded that this was a result of increased fatty acid oxidation with carnitine treatment.

Intradialytic complications

Between 10 and 40% of all dialyses are complicated by episodes of hypotension and/or muscle cramps. Cardiac arrhythmias are also encountered, though less frequently. These intradialytic symptoms are often very debilitating for the patients and their management is time-consuming for staff. Older patients and patients using acetate-containing dialysis solutions experience even higher incidences of intradialytic complications.

In a double-blind, controlled study (Ahmad et al, 1990) patients treated with carnitine had a significant reduction in hypotensive episodes and muscle cramps; no such reduction was seen in the placebo-treated patients (Figure 3). Similar beneficial effects of L-carnitine have been observed by others (Casciani and Caruso, 1982; Bellinghi-eri et al, 1983; Giorcelli and Corsi, 1983). Suzuki et al (1982) reported significant reduction in cardiac arrhythmias during dialysis in patients treated with carnitine. The reason for the improvement in intradialytic hypotension and muscle cramps is unclear. It is possible that carnitine metabolism improves with its supplementation which leads to improvements in skeletal muscle and cardiac muscle metabolism.

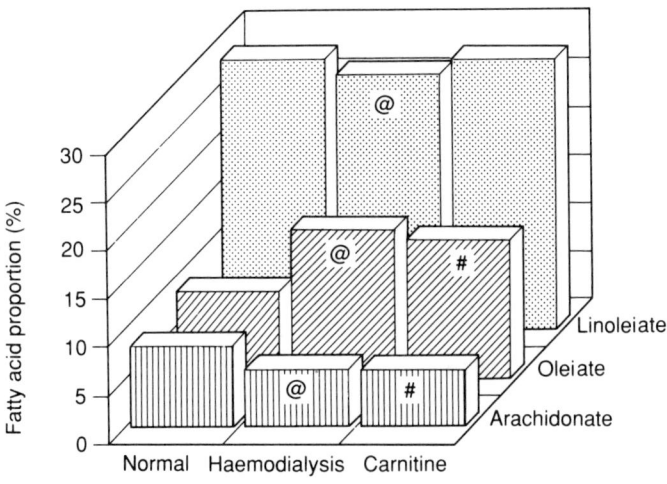

@Norm. vs HD, $p < 0.01$; #Norm. vs Carn., $p < 0.01$

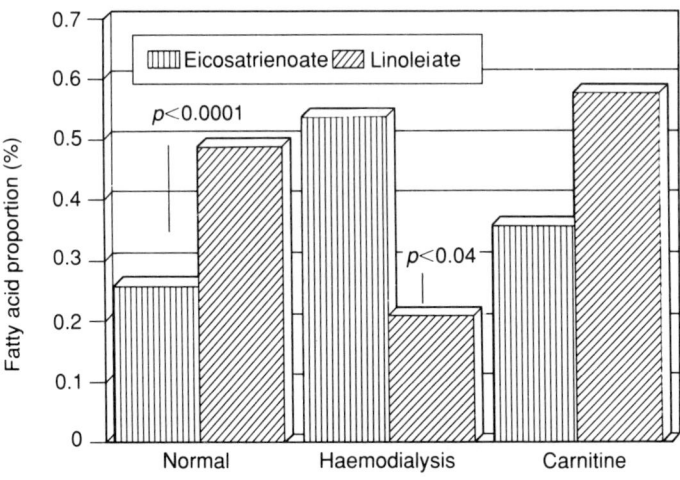

Carnitine vs normals, n.s.

FIGURE 2. Proportion of various fatty acids in plasma of haemodialysis (HD) patients not on carnitine, HD patients on carnitine and controls with normal renal function. (Ahmad et al, 1989.)

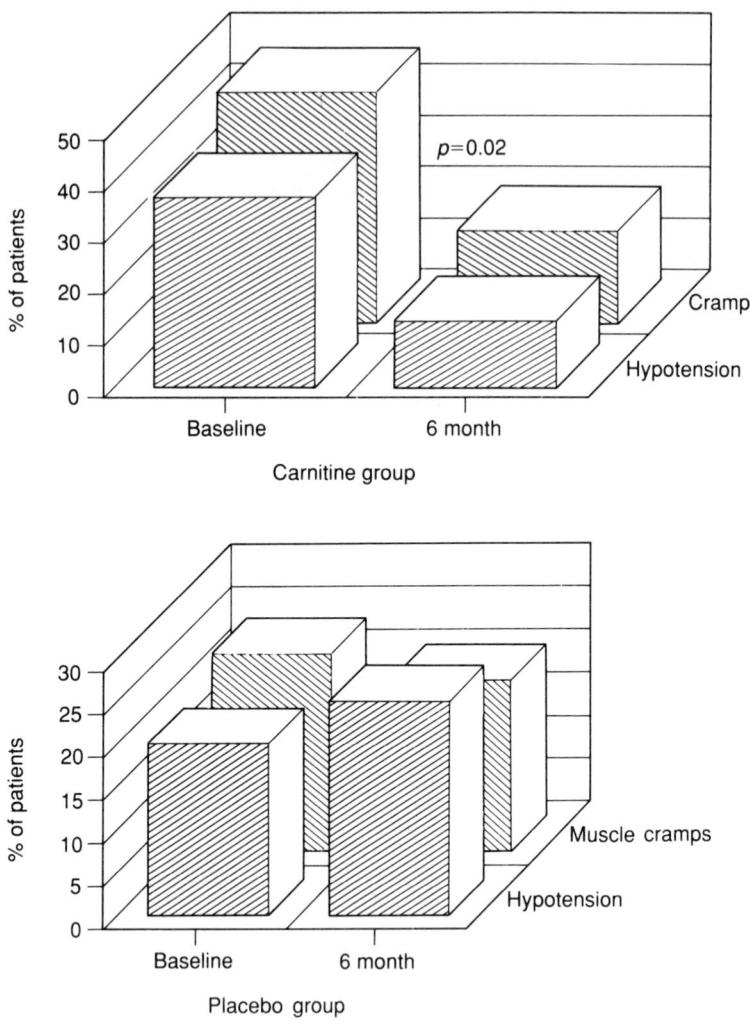

FIGURE 3. Number of patients with intradialytic hypotension and muscle cramps prior to carnitine or placebo administration (baseline) and after 6 months of study. (Golper et al, 1990.)

Patient well-being

Patients receiving carnitine have reported an improved sense of well-being and staff have commented on general clinical improvement. The physical endurance and ability to work also have been reported to improve with carnitine repletion. In a double-blind trial the investigators were asked to rate the clinical improvement in patients who either received carnitine or placebo. Significantly more carnitine patients were rated as improved clinically than those receiving placebo (Ahmad et al, 1990).

Muscle and cardiac problems

Energy derived from oxidation of fatty acids is used by both cardiac and exercising skeletal muscles. Administration of carnitine in non-uraemic patients has been reported to be associated with an improvement in left ventricular function, and a reduction in anginal attacks (Garzya and Amico, 1980; Giordani et al, 1983; Fernandez et al, 1985). Patients on maintenance dialysis have a significantly higher incidence of ischaemic heart disease, and accelerated atherosclerosis is the leading cause of death in this population (Lindner et al, 1974). In addition, cardiomyopathy and myopathy are also quite common among patients with chronic renal failure (Mielhac et al, 1977; Drueke, 1981; Albertazzi et al, 1980; Bellinghieri et al, 1983). Kudoh et al (1983) observed a reduction in cardiomegaly in patients receiving carnitine therapy. Significant reduction in cardiac arrhythmias and in the incidence and severity of anginal attacks have also been observed after the carnitine treatment (Trovato et al, 1983). Khoss et al (1989) studied the effect of carnitine supplementation on cardiac function in a small group of haemodialysed patients. Carnitine treatment was associated with a significant quantitative improvement in left ventricular function and performance (24% improvement at 6 months and 44% after 18 months).

It has been postulated that carnitine depletion in the myocardium may be responsible for the cardiac problems (Williams and Luft, 1978). Unfortunately the carnitine content of myocardium has not been well determined in humans. Peritoneally-dialysed rats were found to have very low cardiac carnitine content (Bartel et al, 1981b). Fagher et al (1985a) did not find any improvement in the left ventricular function with carnitine supplementation in a group of dialysis patients who had normal muscle carnitine level. It has been proposed that, with carnitine depletion, the acetate metabolism is altered and this might aggravate the cardiac effects of acetate as well as the dialytic morbidity (Wanner and Horl, 1988).

In two chronic dialysis patients with unexplained cardiomyopathy we measured the carnitine concentrations in the cardiac tissue. In both patients the free carnitine was almost unmeasurable while acylcarnitine was elevated. Carnitine supplementation in both patients was associated with remarkable improvement in clinical status as well as in cardiac function (ejection fraction).

Exercise limitation and oxygen consumption

Maximum exercise capacity, and maximum oxygen consumption are severely limited in haemodialysis patients (Goldberg et al, 1983; Robertson et al, 1985; Painter and Zimmerman, 1986). On average, these values are no better than 50% of age- and sex-matched controls with normal renal function. Associated with maximal exercise the maximum heart rate is also significantly lower in dialysis patients than is expected in age- and sex-matched normals. The abnormally low oxygen consumption, even in those who may have a normal haematocrit, with obviously normal pulmonary and cardiac function, suggest that the limitation is at the level of the skeletal muscle. Lack of carnitine might deprive the exercising muscle of its energy-providing substrate, fatty acids, thus causing these exercise limitations. In a double-blind study we observed a significant, albeit small, improvement in maximum oxygen consumption in patients treated with L-carnitine. No such improvement was noted in the placebo-treated group.

Carnitine seems to affect muscle structure as well as function. Fagher et al (1985b) in a well-controlled, double-blind study found a significant increase in the endurance of haemodialysed patients treated with L-carnitine. Giorcelli and Corsi (1983) observed an increase in arm circumference in haemodialysis patients on L-carnitine supplementation. Spagnoli et al (1990) reported a significant hypertrophy of type I muscle fibres in haemodialysis patients treated with carnitine for 12 months. When carnitine was discontinued there was a significant reduction in muscle fibre diameter.

Protein and muscle metabolism

Dialysis patients are in a state of accelerated protein catabolism and the process of haemodialysis appears to increase further the rate of protein catabolism (Borah et al, 1978). Similarly, muscle breakdown as well as loss of amino acids from the skeletal muscle seems to be enhanced by the dialytic process (Wassner et al, 1986). Myoglobin levels have been found to be elevated in azotaemic patients (Hallgren et al, 1978) and in patients on haemodialysis (Hart et al, 1982). It has been proposed that the myoglobinaemia is related to the myopathy which is prevalent among these patients. Feinfeld et al (1987) observed a drop in myoglobin concentration from 294 and 221 to 186 and 101 ng/ml, respectively, after the supplementation with L-carnitine. Since patients on peritoneal dialysis also exhibit hypermyoglobinaemia, this abnormality does not appear to be related to the haemodialysis process (Feinfeld et al, 1987). When two patients on peritoneal dialysis were given carnitine there was a marked decrease in myoglobin levels. Thus, there is good evidence that dialysis patients with end-stage renal disease suffer abnormal breakdown of muscle.

In a recent multicentre, controlled trial (Ahmad et al, 1990) one of the most significant findings was a drop in blood urea nitrogen, serum creatinine and phosphate concentrations only in those patients who were treated with L-carnitine (Figure 4). This reduction was not due to any change in dialysis treatment or dietary intake. There was no evidence of any decrease in muscle mass as judged by anthropometric evaluations. Thus, it appears that L-carnitine reduces the protein and muscle catabolism in dialysis patients. Further support for the anabolic effect of carnitine includes increase in muscle size, serum albumin, body weight and haematocrit with 1 year of L-carnitine treatment (Spagnoli et al, 1990).

Anaemia

Anaemia is one of the major problems of patients on dialysis, with average haematocrit typically in the range 18–24. Anaemia in uraemia is multifactorial: erythropoietin deficiency and reduced life-span of red blood cells are two major causes of anaemia. Significant increase in haematocrit with carnitine administration has been reported (Albertazzi et al, 1982; Trovato et al, 1982; Bellinghieri et al, 1983; Vacha et al, 1983; Labonia et al, 1987). Typical of these is the work of Trovato et al (1982) who observed an increase in haematocrit from a mean value of 25.5% to 37.3% in carnitine-treated and a decrease from 24% to 21.8% in placebo-treated patients. The duration of treatment may be important since most of the studies observing an increase in haematocrit have used carnitine for more than 9 months.

It has been proposed that L-carnitine stabilizes the erythrocyte membrane by improving the uptake of the lipids forming the structure of the membrane. Radiolabelled carbon of acetylcarnitine was shown to accumulate in the phospholipids and triglycerides, the major components of the erythrocyte membrane (Farrell et al, 1986). Donatelli et al (1987) observed a decrease in erythrocyte ATP associated with carnitine and proposed that carnitine reduces the inhibition of Na^+-K^+-ATPase which might increase the life-span of the red blood cells. Labonia et al (1987) found that the inhibition of Na^+-K^+-ATPase was

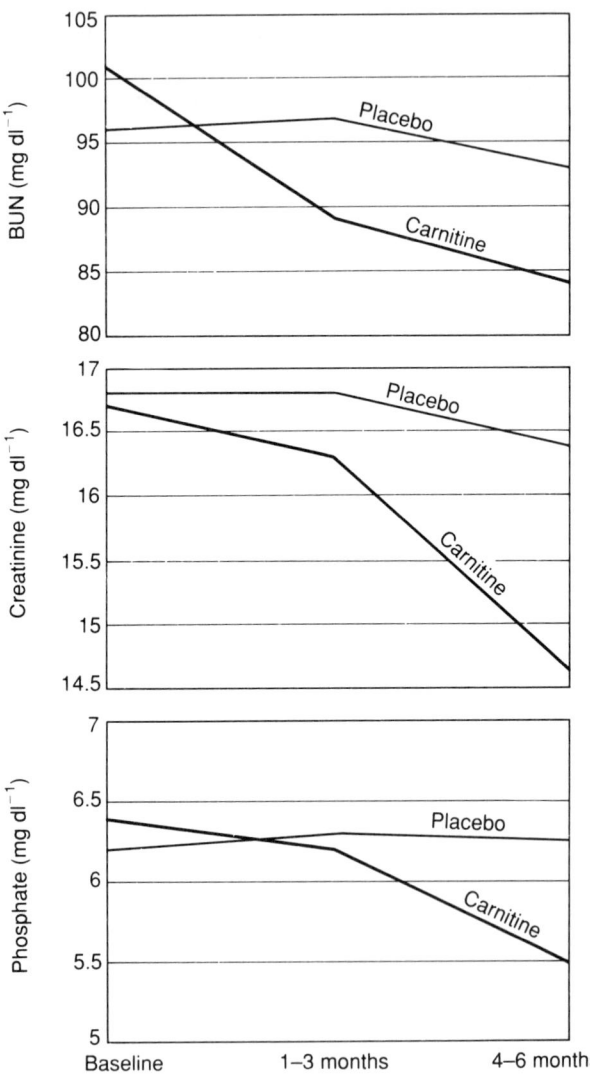

FIGURE 4. Predialysis concentrations of blood urea nitrogen (BUN), creatinine and phosphate at baseline and during treatment with carnitine and placebo. The decline in carnitine group was significant ($p < 0.004$). (Golper et al, 1990.)

significantly improved in uraemics treated with L-carnitine. Thus, administration of L-carnitine might result in decreased haemolysis and a consequent reduction in the dose of erythropoietin required for the correction of anaemia. If this proves to be true, a significant cost-saving would result.

Kidney transplantation

Not much is known about carnitine status after kidney transplantation. Kohse et al (1988) reported complete normalization of plasma carnitine in patients with normally functioning graft (normal serum creatinine). Patients with elevated creatinine had increased plasma carnitine concentrations similar to those observed in uraemics on conservative management. Wanner et al (1988) also observed normalization of plasma carnitine concentrations in patients with normal serum creatinine (< 1.3 mg dl^{-1}). Those with creatinine concentrations of > 2.0 mg dl^{-1} had an abnormal ratio of acyl to free carnitine. Patients in the latter group and receiving cyclosporin had higher plasma concentrations of total free carnitine and acylcarnitine than those treated with azathioprine. This indicated that immunosuppression might affect carnitine and/or fatty acid metabolism.

CONCLUDING REMARKS

Progressive renal failure is associated with abnormal profile of carnitine (increased acylcarnitine and a decrease in free carnitine relative to total or acylated carnitine). With the advent of dialysis this abnormality becomes more pronounced and the plasma free carnitine concentration becomes clearly subnormal. However more accurate and sensitive methods are needed so that a detailed profile of all carnitine esters can be worked out in patients with renal failure. This would enable the administration of the appropriate dose, route and time of administration with greater understanding.

REFERENCES

Ahmad S, Haas L, Pagel M & Sherrard D (1980) *Proc. Clin. Dial. Transplant Forum* 10: 186–189.

Ahmad S, Golper T, Hirschberg R et al (1987) *Kidney Int.* 31: 226 (abstract).

Ahmad S, Dasgupta A & Kenny MA (1989) *Kidney Int.* 36 (supplement): 243–246.

Ahmad S, Robertson HT, Golper TA et al (1990) *Kidney Int.* 38: 912–918.

Albertazzi A, Spisni C, Del Rosso G et al (1980) *Proc. Clin. Dial. Transplant Forum* 10: 1–6.

Albertazzi A, Capelli P, Di Paolo B et al (1982) *Proc. Eur. Dial. Transplant Assoc.* 19: 302–307.

Albright RK, Kram BW & White RP (1982) *Lancet* i: 218–219.

Amair P, Agis G, Rodela H et al (1982) *Peritoneal Dial. Bull.* 1: 11–12.

Aubia J, Masramon J, Lloveras L et al (1980) *Lancet* ii: 1028.

Bagdade JD & Albers JJ (1977) *N. Engl. J. Med.* 296: 1436–1439.

Bank WJ, DiMauro S, Bonilla E et al (1975) *N. Engl. J. Med.* 292: 443–449.

Bartel LL, Hussey JL & Shrago E (1981a) *Am. J. Clin. Nutr.* 34: 1314–1320.

Bartel LL, Hussey JL, Elson C & Shrago E (1981b) *Nutr. Res.* 1: 261–266.

Bellinghieri G, Savica V, Mallamace A et al (1983) *Am. J. Clin. Nutr.* 38: 523–531.

Bernardini I, Rizzo WB, Dalakas M et al (1985) *J. Clin. Invest.* 75: 1124–1130.

Bohles HJ & Akcetin Z (1987) *Am. J. Clin. Nutr.* 46: 47–51.

Borah MF, Schoenfeld PY, Gotch FA & Sargent JA (1978) *Kidney Int.* 14: 491–500.

Borum PR & Taggart EM (1986) *J. Am. Diet. Assoc.* 86(5): 644–647.

Brownell AKW, Severson DL, Thompson CD & Fletscher T (1979) *Can. J. Neurol. Sci.* 6: 367–370.

Brunzell JD, Albers JJ, Haas LB et al (1977) *Metabolism* 26(8): 903–910.

Buoncristiani U, Di Paolo N, Carobi C et al (1981) In Gahl GM, Kessel MW & Nolph KD *Advances in Peritoneal Dialysis*, pp 441–445. Amsterdam: Elsevier.

Casciani CV & Caruso U (1982) *Curr. Ther. Res.* 32: 116–127.

Chan MK, Persaud JW, Varghese Z (1982) *Nephron* 30: 240–243.

Donatelli A, Terrizzi C, Zummo G et al (1987) *Curr. Ther. Res.* 41: 620–624.

Drueke T (1981) *Medsche Klin.* 76: 560–562.

Engel AG, Rebouch CJ, Wilson DM et al (1981) *Neurology* 31: 819–825.

Fagher B, Cederblad G, Monti M et al (1985a) *Scand. J. Clin. Lab. Invest.* 45: 193–198.

Fagher B, Cederblad G, Eriksson M et al (1985b) *Scand. J. Clin. Lab. Invest.* 45: 169–178.

Farrell S, Vogel J & Bieber LL (1986) *Biochim. Biophys. Acta* 876: 175–177.

Fernandez C, La Menza B & Pola P (1985) *J. Am. Med. Assoc.* (Italian edn) 2: number 9.

Fienfeld DA, Verger C, Briscoe AM et al (1987) *Clin. Nephrol.* 28(3): 144–146.

Gahl WA, Bernardini I, Dalakas M et al (1988) *J. Clin. Invest.* 81(2): 549–560.

Garzya G & Amico RM (1980) *Int. J. Tissue React.* 2: 175–180.

Giorcelli G & Corsi M (1983) *Kidney Int.* 24 (supplement 16): 328 (abstract).

Giordani MP, Corsi M, Roncarolo P et al (1983) *Curr. Ther. Res.* 33: 305–311.

Goldberg AP, Harter HR, Patsch W et al (1983) *N. Engl. J. Med.* 308(21): 1245–1252.

Golper TA, Wolfson M, Ahmad S et al (1990) *Kidney Int.* 38: 904–911.

Guarnieri GF, Ranieri F, Toigo G et al (1980) *Am. J. Clin. Nutr.* 33: 1489–1492.

Guarnieri G, Toigo G, Crapesi L et al (1987) *Kidney Int.* 32 (supplement 22): 116–127.
Guarnieri G, Toigo G, Crapesi L et al (1989) *Kidney Int.* 27 (supplement): 247–255.
Gutman RA, Uy A, Shalhoub RJ et al (1973) *Am. J. Clin. Nutr.* 26: 165–172.
Hallgren R, Karlsson FA, Roxin LE & Vange P (1978) *J. Lab. Clin. Med.* 91: 246.
Hart PM, Fienfeld DA, Briscoe AM et al (1982) *Clin. Nephrol.* 18: 141.
Khoss AE, Steger H, Legenstein E et al (1989) *Wien. Klin. Wochenschr.* 101(1): 17–20.
Kohse KP, Dech E, Rossle C et al (1988) *Clin. Nutr* 29(4): 199–205.
Konig B, McKagney E, Conteh S & Ross B (1978) *Clin. Chim. Acta* 88: 121–125.
Kudoh Y, Shoji T, Oimatsu H et al (1983) *Jpn. Circul. J.* 47: 1391–1397.
Labonia WD, Morelli OH, Gimenez MI et al (1987) *Kidney Int.* 32: 754–759.
Leschke M, Rumpf KW, Eisenhauer TH et al (1983) *Kidney Int.* 24 (supplement 16): S143–S146.
Lindner A, Charra B, Sherrard DJ et al (1974) *N. Engl. J. Med.* 290: 697–701.
Maeda K, Shinzato T & Kobayakawa H (1989) *Nephron* 51(3): 355–361.
Mielhac B, Zingraff J, Koutoudis J et al (1977) *Br. Med. J.* i: 350–353.
Moorthy AV & Shug AL (1985) *Peritoneal Dial. Bull.* 5: 175–179.
Moorthy AV, Rosenblum M, Rajaram R & Shug AL (1983) *Am. J. Nephrol.* 3: 205–208.
Netzloff ML, Kohrman AF, Jones MZ et al (1981) *J. Neuropathol. Exp. Neurol.* 40: 351 (abstract).
Nilsson-Ehle P & Cederblad G (1985) *Scand. J. Clin. Lab. Invest.* 45: 179–184.
Painter P & Zimmerman SW (1986) (Review Art. 50 Refs.) *Am. J. Kidney Dis.* 7(5): 386–394.
Rebouch CJ (1986) In Borum PR (ed.) *Clinical Aspects of Human Carnitine Deficiency*, pp 1–15. New York: Pergamon Press.
Reza JM, Kar NC, Pearson CM & Kark RAP (1978) *Ann. Intern. Med.* 88: 610–615.
Ricanati ES, Tserng K-Y & Hoppel CL (1987) *Kidney Int.* 32 (supplement 22): 145–148.
Robertson HT, Rapoport DM, Goldberg L et al (1985) *Proc. Am. Soc. Nephrol.* 74-A.
Rodriguez-Segade S, Alonso de la Pena C, Paz JM et al (1986a) *Ann. Clin. Biochem.* 23: 671–675.
Rodriguez-Segade S, Alonso de la Pena C, Paz JM et al (1986b) *Clin. Chim. Acta* 159(3): 249–256.
Rossle C, Kohse KP, Kapp W et al (1986) *Clin. Nutr.* 5 (supplement) 136: (abstract).
Rumpf KW, Leschke M, Eisenhauer TH et al (1983) *Proc. Eur. Dial. Transplant Assoc.* 19: 298–301.
Spagnoli LG, Palmieri G, Mauriello A et al (1990) *Nephron* 55(1): 16–23.
Steinmann B, Bachmann C, Colombo JP & Gitzelmann R (1987) *Ped. Res.* 21(2): 201–204.
Suzuki Y, Narita M & Yamazaki N (1982) *Jpn. Heart J.* 23: 349–358.
Taggart EM, Siami G, Stone WJ et al (1986) In Borum PR (ed.) *Clinical Aspects of Human Carnitine Deficiency*, p 246. New York: Plenum Press.

Trovato GM, Ginardi V, Di Marco V et al (1982) *Curr. Ther. Res.* 31: 1042–1049.
Trovato GM, Ginardi B, Di Marco V et al (1983) *J. Mol. Cell. Cardiol.* 15: 25–30.
Vacha GM, Giorcelli G, Silliprandi N & Corsi M (1983) *Am. J. Clin. Nutr.* 38: 532–540.
Wagner S, Deufel T & Guder W (1986) *Biol. Chem.* 367: 75–79.
Wanner C & Horl WH (1988) *Nephron* 50: 89–102.
Wanner C, Forstner-Wanner S, Schaeffer G et al (1986) *Am. J. Nephrol.* 6: 206–211.
Wanner C, Schollmeyer P & Horl WH (1988) *Metabolism* 37: 263–267.
Wanner C, Wieland H, Waeckerle B et al (1989) *Kidney Int.* 27 (supplement): 264–268.
Wassner SJ, Bergstrom J, Brusilow SW et al (1986) *Am. J. Kidney Dis.* 7(4): 285–291.
Williams ES & Luft FC (1978) *J. Lab. Clin. Med.* 92: 548–555.
Yderstraede KB, Pedersen FB, Dragsholt C et al (1986) In *Proc. Int. Symp Trondheim, 1986* pp 209–213. Basel: Karger.
Zilleruelo G, Novak M, Hsia SL et al (1989) *Kidney Int.* 27 (supplement): 259–263.

Part IIId

Diabetes

22

EFFECTS OF CARNITINE AND CARNITINE ACYLTRANSFERASE INHIBITION ON ENERGY SUBSTRATE UTILIZATION IN THE INTACT HEART

G.D. Lopaschuk

Increasing the myocardial carnitine concentration can have a protective effect on the ischaemic myocardium (Folts et al, 1978; Liedtke and Nellis, 1979; Hulsmann et al, 1985; Molaparast-Saless et al, 1987; Nagao et al, 1987) and can increase heart function in cardiomyopathies associated with diabetes and carnitine-deficiency (Paulson et al, 1984, 1986; Pieper and Murray, 1987; Reinauer et al, 1990; Rodrigues et al, 1990). Studies have also demonstrated that carnitine palmitoyltransferase 1 (CPT-1) inhibitors can have a protective effect on the ischaemic myocardium (Hekimian and Feuvray, 1985; Paulson et al, 1986; Molaparast-Saless et al, 1987; Lopaschuk et al, 1988, 1990; Lopaschuk and Spafford, 1989) and can also improve mechanical function in diabetic hearts (Tahiliani and McNeil 1986; Wall and Lopaschuk, 1989;

403

L-Carnitine and Its Role in Medicine:
From Function to Therapy. ISBN 0–12–253940–0

Reinauer et al, 1990; Rodrigues et al, 1990). The mechanisms by which carnitine and CPT-1 inhibitors exert these effects have still not been completely delineated. The commonly proposed theories to explain the actions of carnitine, however, appear to contradict the commonly proposed mechanisms to explain the actions of CPT-1 inhibitors. Carnitine, by enhancing CPT-1 activity, has been suggested to enhance fatty acid oxidation and prevent the accumulation of potentially toxic levels of cytosolic long-chain acyl CoA. In contrast, CPT-1 inhibitors are thought to inhibit fatty acid oxidation and prevent the accumulation of long-chain acylcarnitine by inhibiting the transfer of acyl groups from long-chain acyl CoA to long-chain acylcarnitine (Tutwiler et al, 1978; Eistetter and Wolf, 1986). This, theoretically, should result in increased cytosolic concentrations of long-chain acyl CoA. In attempting to clarify this controversy, we directly determined the effects of carnitine and CPT-1 inhibitors on energy-providing substrate utilization in isolated working hearts perfused with relevant concentrations of fatty acids. Based on direct measurements of glucose and palmitate oxidation, we propose that the beneficial effects of carnitine and CPT-1 inhibitors can be explained by the effects of these agents on overcoming fatty acid inhibition of glucose oxidation.

PREFERRED ENERGY-PROVIDING SUBSTRATE IN MYOCARDIUM

Fatty acid oxidation is the primary source of ATP production in the aerobic heart (see Neely and Morgan, 1974 for review). The amount of fatty acid utilized varies, depending primarily on the workload of the heart, and the concentration of circulating fatty acids. We recently performed a series of experiments in which the relative proportion of ATP production from glycolysis, glucose oxidation, exogenous fatty acid oxidation, and endogenous triglycerides was determined (Saddik and Lopaschuk, 1991). In the presence of normal levels of fatty acids (0.4 mmol l^{-1} palmitate), 76% of total myocardial ATP production in isolated working hearts is obtained from fatty acids. In hearts perfused with high concentrations of fatty acids, 92% of total ATP production is obtained from fatty acid oxidation (Saddik and Lopaschuk, 1991). Even if hearts are perfused in the absence of added fatty acids, 42% of steady-state ATP production is derived from the oxidation of fatty acids originating from endogenous triglyceride hydrolysis. These results demonstrate the importance of fatty acids as an energy-providing substrate, and suggest that contractile function of the heart cannot be maintained by glycolysis or glucose oxidation alone.

INTERACTION OF FATTY ACIDS WITH GLUCOSE OXIDATION

A complex interaction exists between fatty acid and glucose utilization in the intact heart (Neely and Morgan, 1974; Pieper and Murray, 1987; Patel and Roche, 1990). A dramatic example of this regulation can be seen during periods of raised circulating fatty acid concentrations. Myocardial fatty acid oxidation rates increase with a concomitant decrease in both glycolysis and glucose oxidation. The decrease in glycolysis occurs primarily as a result of an increase in cytosolic citrate concentrations. Extensive studies by Randles laboratory (Bremer, 1983; Hansford and Cohen, 1978; Randle et al, 1986) have demonstrated that the major determinant of glucose oxidation in aerobically perfused hearts is flux through pyruvate dehydrogenase (PDH). During starvation or in diabetes, flux through PDH is markedly decreased. Following a carbohydrate-rich diet, the activity of PDH increases. These changes in PDH activity result in dramatic changes in glucose oxidation. Addition of palmitate (1.2 mmol l^{-1}) to the perfusate of isolated working rat hearts results in a decrease in glucose oxidation rates to 5–10% of the rates seen in hearts perfused in the absence of fatty acids (Lopaschuk and Spafford, 1989; Lopaschuk et al, 1990; Saddik and Lopaschuk, 1991). In comparison, glycolytic rates only decrease to 50% of the rates seen in the absence of fatty acids (Saddik and Lopaschuk, 1991).

Regulation of pyruvate dehydrogenase occurs via a phosphorylation–dephosphorylation cycle which is subject to both intrinsic and extrinsic effectors (see Randle (1986) and Patel and Roche (1990) for reviews). Phosphorylation of the PDH complex results in a decrease in activity, while dephosphorylation increases activity. Increases in intramitochondrial NADH/NAD$^+$, acetyl CoA/CoA, and ATP/ADP ratios will increase phosphorylation of PDH, resulting in a decrease in activity of the PDH enzyme complex. One of the effects of increasing fatty acid oxidation is to increase these ratios, particularly the intramitochondrial acetyl CoA/CoA ratio, thereby decreasing PDH activity. This is probably the key factor which results in the dramatic decrease in glucose oxidation observed in hearts perfused with high concentrations of fatty acids.

EFFECTS OF CPT-I INHIBITION ON MYOCARDIAL ENERGY SUBSTRATE USE

CPT-1 inhibitors are a class of compounds that inhibit the activity of carnitine acyltransferase 1, which is present on the outer side of the inner mitochondrial membrane. In isolated mitochondria, CPT-1 inhibitors cause marked decreases in the rate of oxidation of free fatty acids or acyl CoA (Tutwiler et al, 1978; Eistetter and Wolf, 1986). These compounds have been used in a number of intact heart or intact animal studies as agents to block fatty acid oxidation. Despite this, however, very few studies have directly measured the effects of CPT-1 inhibitors on fatty acid oxidation in the intact heart. In isolated working hearts, perfused in the presence of high concentrations of fatty acid, we have been unable to observe any inhibition of fatty acid oxidation with the CPT-1 inhibitor, etomoxir (Lopaschuk and Spafford, 1989; Wall and Lopaschuk, 1989; Lopaschuk et al, 1990). This is not surprising, since in these hearts over 90% of the steady-state ATP production originates from fatty acid oxidation (Lopaschuk and Spafford 1989; Saddik and Lopaschuk, 1991). As a result, in order to maintain ATP production (and presumably heart function), an inhibition of fatty acid oxidation would have to be accompanied by a parallel increase in ATP production from other sources. Etomoxir will increase glucose oxidation more than 100% in hearts perfused with high fat (from 75 to 192 nmol glucose oxidized per g dry wt per min). However, since glucose oxidation is providing less than 5% of total ATP production under these conditions (Saddik and Lopaschuk, 1991), a dramatic inhibition of fatty acid oxidation would not be expected. As a result, we suggest that in hearts perfused with high concentrations of fatty acids, the primary effect of CPT-1 inhibition is a decrease in the degree of fatty acid inhibition of glucose oxidation, rather than an actual large decrease in fatty acid oxidation. Etomoxir may act to lower intramitochondrial acetyl CoA/CoA ratios, thereby partially overcoming fatty acid inhibition of PDH activity. As discussed later, this increase in glucose may account for the beneficial effects of CPT-1 inhibitors observed in the diabetic and ischaemic heart.

CARNITINE EFFECTS ON GLUCOSE AND FATTY ACID OXIDATION

In isolated mitochondrial preparations, carnitine lowers intramitochondrial acetyl CoA levels (Snoswell and Koundakjian, 1972; Bremer,

1983). In heart mitochondria, carnitine increases both CoA levels and reduces acetyl CoA levels, resulting in a ten-to twentyfold decrease in the ratio of acetyl CoA/CoA (McGarry et al, 1975; Hansford and Cohen, 1978; Lysiak et al, 1988). The change in this ratio of acetyl CoA/CoA correlates with efflux of acetylcarnitine from the mitochondria, which is consistent with carnitine increasing the activity of carnitine acetyltransferase present on mitochondrial membranes.

As discussed above, the activity of the PDH complex is the major determinant of glucose oxidation in aerobically perfused hearts (Randle, 1986; Patel and Roche, 1990). This complex is regulated by a phosphorylation–dephosphorylation cycle that is responsive to changes in the ratio of intramitochondrial acetyl CoA/CoA. As would be expected therefore, carnitine, by decreasing the intramitochondrial acetyl CoA/CoA ratio, stimulates PDH activity (Uzeil et al, 1988). We were interested in determining if the carnitine-induced increase in PDH activity observed in isolated mitochondria also occurred in the intact heart. To perform these experiments, we initially perfused hearts for 60 min in the presence of L-carnitine (10 mmol 1^{-1}), followed by a 3 min wash-out period to remove any extracellular carnitine. These conditions were chosen since it has previously been demonstrated that carnitine is transported across the sarcolemmal membrane in slow Na^+-dependent manner (Vary and Neely, 1982). This 60 min perfusion resulted in an increase in myocardial carnitine content from 4376 ± 211 to 9496 ± 473 nmol per g dry wt (Broderick et al, 1991). Glucose oxidation was subsequently measured in hearts perfused either in the presence and absence of fatty acids (1.2 mmol 1^{-1} palmitate). Glucose oxidation rates in control hearts were markedly decreased if fatty acids were present in the perfusate (from 1817 ± 169 to 158 ± 21 nmol glucose per g dry wt per min). This probably occurred primarily as a result of an increase in the intramitochondrial acetyl CoA/CoA ratio (Randle, 1986). In hearts containing raised concentrations of carnitine, there was a significant increase in glucose oxidation (158 ± 21 and 454 ± 85 nmol glucose per g dry wt per min, in control and carnitine loaded hearts, respectively). This increase in glucose oxidation was accompanied by a parallel decrease in palmitate oxidation (from 728 ± 61 to 572 ± 111 nmol palmitate per g dry wt per min). The effects of carnitine loading on glucose oxidation did not occur in hearts perfused in the absence of fatty acids (1817 ± 169 and 2026 ± 171 nmol glucose per g dry wt per min, in control and carnitine-loaded hearts, respectively). This result would be expected since perfusing hearts in the absence of fatty acids or with carnitine should accomplish the same thing (i.e. decreasing the intramitochondrial acetyl CoA/CoA ratio).

CPT-I AND CARNITINE EFFECTS ON ISCHAEMIC AND DIABETIC HEARTS

A number of experimental studies have demonstrated that carnitine supplementation can have beneficial effects on ischaemic and diabetic hearts (Folts et al, 1978; Liedtke and Nellis, 1979; Paulson et al, 1984; Hülsmann et al, 1985; Molaparast-Saless et al, 1987; Nagao et al, 1987; Pieper and Murray, 1987; Rodrigues et al, 1990). Although the mechanisms by which this occurs are not known, it has been suggested that carnitine acts by stimulating fatty acid oxidation, or by decreasing the levels of long-chain acyl CoA. Long-chain acyl CoA is known to be a specific inhibitor of the adenine-nucleotide translocase located in the inner mitochondrial membrane (Shug et al, 1975; Shug, 1979). However, in the intact heart a good correlation between accumulation of long-chain acyl CoA and myocardial ATP levels has not been found (Ichihara and Neely, 1985; Hülsmann et al, 1985; Lopaschuk and Tsang, 1987; Wall and Lopaschuk, 1989; Lopaschuk et al, 1990). Furthermore, fatty acid oxidation is not impaired in either the diabetic heart or in the reperfused ischaemic heart (Lopaschuk and Spafford, 1989; Liedtke et al, 1988; Lopaschuk and Tsang, 1987; Wall and Lopaschuk, 1989). In fact, in both of these conditions fatty acid oxidation can provide 90–100% of myocardial ATP production (Garland et al, 1964; Lopaschuk and Spafford, 1989; Liedtke et al, 1988).

CPT-1 inhibitors have also been shown to exert a beneficial effect on ischaemic or diabetic hearts (Liedtke et al, 1984; Hekimian and Feuvray, 1985; Paulson et al, 1986; Tahiliani and McNeill, 1986; Molaparast-Saless et al, 1987; Lopaschuk et al, 1988; Lopaschuk and Tsang, 1987; Wall and Lopaschuk, 1989; Lopaschuk et al, 1990; Reinauer et al, 1990). This has been thought to occur as a result of an inhibition of fatty acid oxidation and a decrease in the accumulation of long-chain acylcarnitine within the myocardium (Corr et al, 1984; Liedtke et al, 1984; Hekimian and Feuvray, 1985; Paulson et al, 1986; Reinauer et al, 1990). However, we (Lopaschuk et al, 1988; Lopaschuk and Tsang, 1987; Lopaschuk et al, 1990) and others (Ichihara and Neely, 1985) have been unable to show a good correlation between the beneficial effects of CPT-1 inhibitors and a lowering of long-chain acylcarnitine levels. Similarly, we have also failed to find a correlation between the beneficial effects of CPT-1 inhibition and a decrease in palmitate oxidation.

SUMMARY

As discussed above, both carnitine and CPT-1 inhibition increase myocardial glucose oxidation in hearts perfused with high concentrations of fatty acids. It is our hypothesis that this increase in glucose oxidation may partly explain the observed beneficial effects of these agents. To date, we have yet to determine the effect of acute carnitine loading of hearts on glucose oxidation and function in diabetic hearts or in reperfused ischaemic hearts. We have shown, however, that a good correlation exists between reperfusion recovery of function, and stimulation of glucose oxidation during reperfusion in hearts perfused with high concentrations of fatty acids (Lopaschuk et al, 1988; Lopaschuk and Tsang, 1987; Lopaschuk et al, 1990; McVeigh and Lopaschuk, 1990). Our results also suggest that stimulation of glucose oxidation can improve function in the diabetic heart (Wall and Lopaschuk, 1989; Nicholls et al, 1991). We hypothesize, therefore, that stimulation of myocardial glucose oxidation by carnitine and CPT-1 inhibitors is part of the mechanism by which these agents exert their beneficial effect in diabetic and reperfused-ischaemic hearts, despite apparently opposing actions on CPT-1 itself. Further studies are required to determine if this hypothesis is correct.

REFERENCES

Bremer J (1983) *Physiol. Rev.* 63: 1421–1449.
Broderick T, Quinney HA & Lopaschuk GD (1991) *J. Biol. Chem.* (submitted)
Corr PB, Gross, RW & Sobel, BE (1984) *Circ. Res.* 55: 135–154.
Eistetter K & Wolf HPO (1986) *Drugs of the Future* 11: 1034–1036.
Ichihara K & Neely JR (1985) *Am. J. Physiol.* 249: H492–H497.
Folts JD. Shug AL, Koke JR & Bittar N (1985) *Am. J. Cardiol.* 41: 1209–1215.
Garland PB, Newsholme EA & Randle PJ (1962) *Nature* 195: 381–383.
Garland PB, Newsholme EA & Randle PJ (1964) *Biochem. J.* 93: 665–678.
Hansford RG & Cohen L (1978) *Arch. Biochem. Biophys.* 191: 65–81.
Hekimian G & Feuvray D (1985) *Diabetes* 35: 906–910.
Hulsmann WC, Dubelaar ML, Lamers JMJ & Maccari F (1985) *Biochem. Biophys. Acta* 847: 62–66.
Liedtke AJ & Nellis SH (1979) *J. Clin. Invest.* 64: 440–447.
Liedtke AJ, Nellis SH & Mjos OD (1984) *Am. J. Physiol* 247: H387–H394.
Liedtke AJ, Demaison L, Eggleston AM et al (1988) *Circ. Res.* 62: 535–542.
Lopaschuk GD & Spafford M (1989) *Circ. Res.* 65: 378–387.
Lopaschuk GD & Tsang H (1987) *Circ. Res.* 61: 853–858.
Lopaschuk GD, Wall SR, Olley PM & Davies NJ (1988) *Circ. Res.* 63: 1036–1043.

Lopaschuk GD, Spafford MA, Davies NJ & Wall SR (1990) *Circ. Res.* 66: 5346–5353.

Lysiak W, Lilly K, Di Lisa F et al (1988) *J. Biol. Chem.* 263: 1151–1156.

McGarry JD, Robles Valdes C & Foster DW (1975) *Proc. Natl Acad. Sci. USA* 72: 4385–4388.

Molaparast-Saless F, Liedtke AJ & Nellis SH (1987) *J. Mol. Cell. Cardiol.* 19: 509–520.

Nagao B, Kobayashi A & Yamazaki N (1987) *Jpn. Heart. J.* 28: 243–251.

McVeigh JJ & Lopaschuk GD (1990) *Am. J. Physiol.* 259: H1079–H1085.

Neely JR & Morgan HE (1974) *Annu. Rev. Physiol.* 36: 413–459.

Nicholls TA, Lopaschuk GD & McNeill JH (1991) *Am. J. Physiol* (in press)

Patel, MS & Roche, TE (1990) *FASEB J.* 4: 3224–3233.

Paulson DJ, Schmidt MJ, Traxler JS et al (1984) *Metabolism* 33: 358–363.

Paulson DJ, Noonan JJ, Ward KM et al (1986) *Basic Res. Cardiol.* 81: 180–187.

Pieper GM & Murray WJ (1987) *Biochem. Med. Metabol. Biol.* 38: 111–120.

Randle PJ (1986) *Biochem. Soc. Trans.* 14: 799–806.

Randle PJ, Newsholme EA & Garland PB (1964) *Biochem. J.* 93: 652–665.

Reinauer H, Adrian M, Rosen P & Schmitz F-J (1990) *J. Clin. Chem. Clin. Biochem.* 28: 335–339.

Rodrigues B, Ross JR, Farahbakshian S & McNeill JH (1990) *Can. J. Physiol. Pharmacol.* 68: 1085–1092.

Saddik M & Lopaschuk GD (1991) *J. Biol. Chem.* 266: 816–817.

Shug AL (1979) *Tex. Rep. Biol. Med.* 39: 409–428.

Shug AL, Shagro E, Bittar N et al (1975) *Am. J. Physiol.* 228: 689–692.

Snoswell AM & Koundakjian PP (1972) *Biochem. J.* 127: 133–141.

Tutwiler GF, Kirsch T, Mohrbacher RJ & Ho W (1978) *Metabolism* 27: 1539–1556.

Tahiliani AG & McNeill JH (1986) *Life Sci.* 38: 959–974.

Uzeil G, Garavaglia B & Di Donato S (1988) *Muscle Nerv.* 11: 720–724.

Vary TC & Neely JR (1982) *Am. J. Physiol.* 242: H5585–H5592.

Wall SR & Lopaschuk GD (1989) *Biochim. Biophys. Acta* 1006: 97–103.

23

BENEFICIAL EFFECTS OF L-CARNITINE AND DERIVATIVES ON HEART MEMBRANES IN EXPERIMENTAL DIABETES

N.S. Dhalla, I.M.C. Dixon, K.R. Shah
and R. Ferrari

It is now well known that L-carnitine is required for the transport of long-chain fatty acyl moieties across the mitochondrial inner membrane for β-oxidation and subsequent energy production (Bremer, 1983; Bieber, 1988). A deficiency of free carnitine in the cell thus can be seen to decrease the oxidation of long-chain fatty acids, depress the energy status of the cell and increase the accumulation of long-chain acyl esters in the cell. In fact, decreased carnitine concentrations have been shown to be associated with elevated concentrations of long-chain acyl esters in myocardial infarction (Suzuki et al, 1981) as well as in myocardial ischaemia (Piper and Das, 1987) and the mitochondrial β-oxidation of fatty acids is blocked during ischaemic injury (Liedtke et al, 1978; Neely and Feuvray, 1981). The long-chain acyl esters, including palmitoyl CoA and palmitoylcarnitine are considered to exert their toxic effects by detergent-like actions on heart membranes

411

(Idell-Wenger et al, 1978; Katz and Messineo, 1981). However, these long-chain acyl esters have also been shown to affect sarcolemmal Na^+-K^+-ATPase activities (Wood et al, 1977; Adams et al, 1979; Abe et al, 1984; Lamers et al, 1984; Pitts and Okhuysen, 1984; Kakar et al, 1987; Dhalla et al, 1991) and thus their direct action on the membrane cannot be ruled out. This view is further supported by the observation that palmitoylcarnitine has been reported to activate Ca^{2+}-channels (Spedding and Mir, 1987). Furthermore, sarcolemmal Na^+-Ca^{2+} exchange (Lamers et al, 1984; Ashavaid et al, 1985) and sarcoplasmic reticular Ca^{2+}-pump activity (Adams et al, 1979; Lopaschuk et al, 1983a; Dhalla et al, 1991) are altered by the long-chain acyl esters. Long-chain acylcarnitine was also found to decrease the maximal diastolic potential and action potential amplitude (Nakaya and Tohse, 1986). It is thus evident that adequate levels of L-carnitine in the myocardial cell are essential for proper functioning of the heart, whereas carnitine deficiency and/or accumulation of long-chain acyl ester in the cell may be intimately involved in the pathophysiology of ischaemic heart disease.

EFFECTS OF L-CARNITINE AND PROPIONYL-L-CARNITINE ON THE HEART

In addition to its effects on the transport of long-chain fatty acyl moieties across the mitochondrial membrane, L-carnitine has been shown to affect a wide variety of biological actions (Bremer, 1983). Experiments with perfused rat hearts have shown that carnitine exhibits a dramatic effect on fatty acid synthesis, uptake and esterification (Rodis et al, 1970a, 1970b). In particular, it has been shown that carnitine decreased the uptake of fatty acids by the myocardium. The addition of L-carnitine in the perfusion medium was also found to prevent the adverse electrophysiological actions of palmitoylcarnitine in papillary muscle (Hayashi et al, 1982). Likewise, changes in transmembrane potentials due to hypoxia were prevented by L-carnitine (Hayashi et al, 1984) and this agent was found to preserve mechanical function of the ischaemic hearts (Liedtke and Nellis, 1979; Liedtke et al, 1981). Although only seven of 51 patients with idiopathic dilated cardiomyopathy, coronary heart disease, myocarditis and rheumatic heart disease had low myocardial carnitine, plasma carnitine levels were elevated in all these patients with end-stage congestive heart failure (Pierpont et al, 1989). Whether the increased level of plasma carnitine in congestive heart failure serves as an adaptive mechanism for compensating the failing myocardium is not clear at present. Nonetheless, treatment of cardiomyopathic hamsters with L-carnitine was found to improve cardiac performance and restore the high-energy phosphate pool (Whitmer, 1987).

Since carnitine is converted to different acyl derivatives, including short-chain acyl esters such as propionyl carnitine (Brass and Beyerinck, 1987), it is not clear whether the effects of carnitine are due to carnitine *per se* or to propionylcarnitine. In this regard, it should be pointed out that propionyl-L-carnitine has been shown not only to affect the electrophysiological properties of myocardium but also to antagonize the deleterious effects of lysophosphatidylcholine and palmitoylcarnitine on the electrical and mechanical activities of the ventricular muscle (Aomine and Arita, 1987; Aomine et al, 1988, 1989). Propionyl-L-carnitine has also been shown to improve changes in mitochondrial function due to oxygen free radicals and myocardial ischaemia (Ferrari et al, 1988; Di Lisa et al, 1989). In fact, pre-treatment of myocardium in vitro (Ferrari et al, 1989) or in vivo (Liedtke et al, 1988) improved the recovery of mechanical function of the ischaemic reperfused hearts. These studies provide evidence that L-carnitine and propionyl-L-carnitine exert beneficial effects on the ischaemic heart but their exact mode of action remains to be investigated.

PATHOPHYSIOLOGY OF CARDIAC DYSFUNCTION IN DIABETES

It is becoming clear that diabetes is a complex disease in which several organs in the body are adversely affected, depending upon the severity and duration of the disease. Several investigators have observed heart dysfunction in both diabetic patients and experimental animal models of chronic diabetes; however, its mechanisms are poorly understood (Pierce et al, 1988; Nagano and Dhalla, 1991). Although coronary artery disease and atherosclerosis are generally considered to explain heart dysfunction in chronic diabetes, other lesions such as microangiopathy and cardiomyopathy have also been suggested to play a crucial role in its pathogenesis (Factor et al, 1980; Vadlamudi et al, 1982; Regan, 1983; Dhalla et al, 1985). In view of observations that heart dysfunction in chronic diabetes can be seen in the absence of atherosclerosis, it has been suggested that microangiopathy, cardiomyopathy, atherosclerosis and coronary artery disease may occur independently of each other and these factors individually or jointly, depending upon the type and stage of disease, may contribute to the development of cardiac pump failure in diabetes (Dhalla et al, 1985).

Although insulin deficiency and/or the ineffectiveness of insulin to promote glucose utilization are known to cause diabetes (Dhalla et al, 1985), the mechanisms responsible for the dysfunction of different organs, including heart, in chronic diabetes are essentially speculative. In view of the profound effects of insulin on myocardial metabolism (Dhalla et al, 1985), insulin deficiency itself can be seen to result in cardiac dysfunction. Insulin deficiency has also been observed to stimulate the sympathetic nervous system and thus the circulating levels of catecholamines are drastically elevated in diabetes (Ganguly et al, 1986, 1987). On the other hand, in some experimental models of diabetes, plasma levels of thyroid hormones are markedly reduced (Pierce et al, 1988). Although both catecholamines and thyroid hormones are known to affect several metabolic processes in the body and thus changes in these hormones and neurohormones can lead to the development of cardiac abnormalities (Buccino et al, 1967; Dhalla et al, 1977; Limas, 1978; Morkin et al, 1983; Rona, 1985), it should be recognized that changes in these hormones are not always seen in clinical and experimental diabetes and this may be due to differences in the type and stage of diabetes. It should also be pointed out that an excessive amount of circulating catecholamines may become available for oxidation and this process can be seen to generate oxygen free radicals, which are highly toxic (Singal et al, 1982).

Insulin deficiency, as well as changes in plasma levels of both catecholamine and thyroid hormones, can also affect the genetic apparatus of the cardiac cell and thus may restructure the myocardium in chronic diabetes. In this regard, some investigators (Dillman, 1980, 1982, 1984; Morkin et al, 1983) have reported changes in gene expression in diabetic animals, particularly with respect to contractile proteins. Thus it is evident that imbalance of hormones and neurohormones in diabetes may be responsible for producing metabolic derangements, oxidative stress associated with the formation of oxygen free radicals, and alterations in gene expression. These changes in turn may affect different membranes and contractile proteins of the myocardium and may result in contractile abnormalities in diabetic hearts. The pathophysiology of cardiac pump failure in diabetes is represented in Figure 1.

Extensive studies from our laboratory and by other investigators have shown that different membrane systems such as sarcolemma,

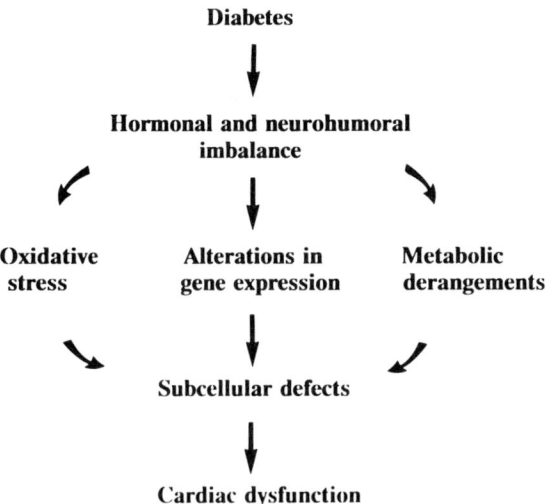

FIGURE 1. Pathophysiological events leading to heart dysfunction in chronic diabetes.

sarcoplasmic reticulum and mitochondria as well as myofibrillar proteins are altered in the diabetic heart (Dhalla et al, 1985; Ferrari et al, 1991). Abnormalities in both the rate of contraction and rate of relaxation of the diabetic heart (Fein et al, 1980) have been explained on the basis of defects in myofibrillar Ca^{2+}-stimulated ATPase and ATP-dependent Ca^{2+}-pump activity in the sarcoplasmic reticulum (Penpargkul et al, 1981; Pierce and Dhalla, 1981; Malhotra et al, 1981; Ganguly et al, 1983). The depressed myofibrillar ATPase activity in diabetic heart has been shown to be due to a shift in V_1 to V_3 form of myosin (Dillman, 1980; Rupp et al, 1989) whereas depression in the sarcoplasmic reticular Ca^{2+}-pump has been shown to be associated with an increase in the concentration of long-chain fatty acyl derivatives (Lopaschuk et al, 1983a, 1983b). Although sarcolemmal Na^+-K^+-ATPase and Na^+–H^+-exchange, Na^+–Ca^{2+} exchange and Ca^{2+}-pump activities have also been reported to decrease in the diabetic heart (Pierce and Dhalla, 1983; Heyliger et al, 1987; Kjeldsen et al, 1987; Makino et al, 1987; Pierce et al, 1990), the exact mechanisms of these alterations are poorly understood. Since marked changes in membrane phospholipid methylation occur during the development of diabetic cardiomyopathy (Ganguly et al, 1984; Panagia et al, 1990), it is likely that sarcolemmal defects in diabetic heart may be due to alterations in the phospholipid composition of the sarcolemmal membrane. Changes in phospholipid composition and increase in the cholesterol content in sarcolemma have also been reported in diabetic cardiomyopathy (Pierce et al, 1983). Such sarcolemmal changes can be seen to alter the cation content of the cell which may result in myocardial cell damage in chronic diabetes (Seager et al, 1984).

The diabetic heart has been shown to exhibit increased sensitivity to calcium (Bielefeld et al, 1983; Sauviat and Feuvray, 1986; Borda et al, 1988). This phenomenon has been explained on the basis of increased activity of the sarcolemmal Ca^{2+}-ATPase, which requires millimolar concentrations of Ca^{2+} for activity and has been suggested to serve as a calcium-gating mechanism for the entry of Ca^{2+} (Dhalla et al, 1982), in the myocardium from diabetic animals (Dhalla et al, 1986; Borda et al, 1988). In fact, increased binding of (^{3}H) PN 200-110 (a dihydropyridine derivative) to cardiac membranes in diabetic rats has been reported (Nishio et al, 1990) and this has been taken to indicate an increase in voltage-sensitive Ca^{2+} channels in the diabetic heart. These observations are consistent with the hypothesis that diabetic cardiomyopathy is associated with the occurrence of intracellular calcium overload (Dhalla et al, 1985). Depressed Ca^{2+}-pump and Na^+–Ca^{2+}-exchange activity in the sarcolemmal membrane as well as depressed Ca^{2+}-pump activity in the sarcoplasmic reticulum have also been suggested to contribute towards the intracellular Ca^{2+} overload (Ganguly et al, 1983; Makino et al, 1987). These alterations can be seen to result in mitochondrial Ca^{2+} overloading and subsequent impairments in energy production as well as Ca^{2+}-handling by mitochondria in the diabetic heart (Pierce and Dhalla, 1985a). The role of intracellular Ca^{2+} overload in the development of diabetic cardiomyopathy was further evident from the effects of a Ca^{2+}-antagonist, verapamil, in improving the ventricular performance, the status of myocardial metabolism and some of the subcellular defects in diabetic animals (Afzal et al, 1988, 1989). It should also be pointed out that Ca^{2+}-influx and its related mechanisms, including sarcolemmal superficial Ca^{2+} stores and phosphatidylinositol turnover have also been reported to be depressed in the diabetic myocardium (Pierce et al, 1983; Bergh et al, 1988; Horackova and Murphy, 1988). Although the exact reasons for conflicting results regarding the entry of Ca^{2+} into diabetic myocardium are not clear at present, the possibility of differences with respect to the stage and severity of diabetes cannot be ruled out. Nonetheless, all these studies indicate that heart membranes become defective with respect to their Ca^{2+}-handling properties and these changes may play a crucial role in the pathogenesis of contractile dysfunction in chronic diabetes.

EFFECTS OF L-CARNITINE TREATMENT ON THE DIABETIC HEART

In view of the decrease in the concentration of free L-carnitine in the diabetic heart (Vary and Neely, 1982), several investigators have attempted to identify the beneficial effects of L-carnitine treatment in diabetes (Ferrari et al, 1991; Rodrigues and McNeill, 1991). Treatment of rats with streptozotocin-induced diabetes with L-carnitine was not only shown to prevent the diabetes-associated changes in cardiac performance and plasma lipids (Rodrigues et al, 1988), but also partially reversed these alterations in diabetic animals (Rodrigues et al, 1990). Likewise, the beneficial effects of L-carnitine treatment were reported by Paulson et al (1984) indicating its action in preventing the decrease in myocardial carnitine content, lowering serum levels of glucose, ketones and lipids, as well as decreasing the vulnerability of the diabetic heart to ischaemia. Administration of L-carnitine to diabetic animals or perfusion of diabetic hearts with L-carnitine in the presence of elevated concentrations of fatty acids prevented the loss of ATP and the increase in long-chain acyl CoA (Pieper et al, 1984; Pieper and Murray, 1987). Chronic treatment of diabetic rats with L-carnitine also prevented the accumulation of long-chain acylcarnitines in addition to preventing the defect in Ca^{2+}-uptake in the sarcoplasmic reticulum (Lopaschuk et al, 1983a, 1983b). Thus, it appears likely that the beneficial effects of L-carnitine on cardiac performance may be due to its action on myocardial metabolism as well as its interaction with long-chain fatty acyl derivatives at the membrane level in the cell. Some of the effects of L-carnitine on streptozotocin-induced diabetes in rats, and the possible mechanisms of its action, are given in Tables 1 and 2.

EFFECTS OF PROPIONYL-L-CARNITINE TREATMENT ON THE DIABETIC HEART

Since propionyl-L-carnitine has been shown to be more effective than L-carnitine in preventing ischaemic changes (Paulson et al, 1986), it was considered worthwhile to test the actions of propionyl-L-carnitine on subcellular defects in the diabetic heart. Streptozotocin-induced diabetic rats were employed in this study and propionyl-L-carnitine (100 mg kg^{-1}; i.p.) was injected daily for 8 weeks in rats 3 days after

TABLE 1.
Effect of L-carnitine in streptozotocin-induced diabetes in rats

Parameter	Control	Diabetic	Carnitine-treated diabetic
Body weight (g)	400 ± 9	$298 \pm 6*$	$298 \pm 12*$
Plasma glucose (mg dl^{-1})	137 ± 3	$445 \pm 18*$	$215 \pm 38*$
Plasma insulin (μU ml^{-1})	55 ± 6	$20 \pm 2*$	$23 \pm 2*$
Myocardial free carnitine (nmol g dry wt^{-1})	287 ± 37	$131 \pm 25*$	324 ± 28
LVP (mmHg)	160 ± 5	$120 \pm 7*$	165 ± 7
+ dP/dt (mmHg s^{-1})	5300 ± 150	$4150 \pm 200*$	5200 ± 175
− dP/dt (mmHg s^{-1})	4600 ± 120	$3700 \pm 150*$	4800 ± 200

Diabetes was induced by a single injection of 55 mg kg^{-1} streptozotocin into the tail vein. The carnitine-treated diabetic group received 3 g L-carnitine per kg per day for 6 weeks; this treatment was started 3 days after streptozotocin injection. The isolated hearts were perfused according to the working heart perfusion procedure and the left ventricular developed pressure (LVP), rate of contraction (+ dP/dt) and rate of relaxation (− dP/dt) were measured. These data are based on the results reported in a study by Rodrigues et al (1988).
*, Significantly different ($p < 0.05$) from the respective control.

TABLE 2.
Mechanisms of the beneficial effects of L-carnitine on the heart

1. Increasing the transport of long-chain acyl CoA across the mitochondrial membrane (Bremer, 1983).

2. Modulating the acyl CoA to free CoA ratio in the mitochondria (Bieber, 1988).

3. Preventing the interaction of long-chain acyl esters with membranes (Hayashi et al, 1982; Lopaschuk et al, 1983a).

4. Removing the long-chain acyl esters from the body (Stumpf et al, 1985).

5. Lowering the blood concentrations of triglycerides by decreasing its synthesis and/or secretion by the liver (Brady et al, 1986).

6. Decreasing the uptake of free fatty acids in the cell (Rodis et al, 1970a; Liedke and Nellis, 1979).

7. Accelerating the rate of glycolysis by increasing the activity of pyruvate dehydrogenase (Opie, 1979).

inducing diabetes. The data in Table 3 indicate that propionyl-L-carnitine treatment failed to reverse the diabetes-induced changes in body weight, heart weight and plasma glucose concentrations. Furthermore, the yields of sarcolemma, sarcoplasmic reticulum and myofibrils were similar in control, diabetic and propionyl-L-carnitine-treated diabetic hearts. The depression in Na^+-K^+-ATPase in diabetic heart was prevented by propionyl-L-carnitine treatment in two different types of sarcolemmal preparations (Tables 4 and 5). As reported earlier (Pierce et al, 1990), the treatment of diabetic animals with propionyl-L-carnitine partially prevented the depressed Na^+-Ca^{2+}-exchange without affecting the decreased H^+-Na^+-exchange activity in the diabetic sarcolemmal vesicles (Table 5).

The depressions in sarcolemmal ATP-dependent Ca^{2+} uptake and Ca^{2+}-stimulated ATPase were not prevented upon the treatment of diabetic animals with propionyl-L-carnitine (Table 6). The diabetes-associated defects in sarcolemma were specific in nature because the non-specific Ca^{2+}-binding and Mg^{2+}-ATPase activities in the diabetic sarcolemmal preparations were not altered. Neither was any effect of propionyl-L-carnitine seen in preventing the diabetes-induced changes in sarcolemmal N-methylation (Ou et al, 1990). The exact mechanisms

TABLE 3.

Effect of propionyl-L-carnitine (PLC) in streptozotocin-induced diabetes in rats

Parameters	Control	Diabetic	PPLC-treated diabetic
Body weight (g)	435 ± 10	282 ± 7*	284 ± 8*
Heart weight (g)	1.2 ± 0.05	0.7 ± 0.06*	0.8 ± 0.04*
Plasma glucose (mg dl⁻¹)	141 ± 11	652 ± 23*	630 ± 15*
Sarcolemmal yield (mg protein g heart⁻¹)	1.2 ± 0.3	1.2 ± 0.3	1.2 ± 0.2
Sarcoplasmic reticular yield (mg protein g heart⁻¹)	1.34 ± 0.19	1.29 ± 0.17	1.42 ± 0.21
Myofibrillar yield (mg protein g heart⁻¹)	43 ± 2.1	37 ± 2.0	38 ± 2.2

Diabetes in rats was induced by a single dose of streptozotocin (65 mg kg⁻¹) injected into the femoral vein. PPLC was injected (100 mg kg⁻¹, i.p.) daily for 8 weeks in one group of animals 3 days after inducing diabetes. Plasma glucose concentrations were measured and sarcolemmal, sarcoplasmic reticular and myofibrillar fractions were isolated according to the procedures described earlier (Ganguly et al, 1983; Pierce and Dhalla, 1985b; Dixon et al, 1987). Each value is a mean ± SE of six to eight experiments. *, Significantly different ($p < 0.05$) from the respective control.

TABLE 4.

Na$^+$-K$^+$ activities in heart sarcolemma obtained from diabetic rats with or without propionyl-L-carnitine (PPLC) treatment

Time of incubation (min)	Na$^+$-K$^+$-ATPase activity (μmol P$_i$ mg^{-1})		
	Control	Diabetic	PPLC-treated diabetic
5	2.3 ± 0.3	1.2 ± 0.1*	1.8 ± 0.2
10	4.4 ± 0.6	2.5 ± 0.3*	3.7 ± 0.5
20	9.1 ± 1.0	5.3 ± 0.7*	7.9 ± 0.5

Values are means ± SE of six experiments. The protocol for inducing diabetes as well as for PPLC treatment is the same as described in Table 3. The procedures for the isolation of sarcolemma and measurement of Na$^+$-K$^+$-ATPase are described elsewhere (Dixon et al, 1987). *, Significantly different ($p < 0.05$) from the respective control.

TABLE 5.

Na$^+$-K$^+$-ATPase, Na$^+$–Ca^{2+}-exchange and Na$^+$–H$^+$-exchange activities in heart sarcolemma obtained from diabetic rats with or without propionyl-L-carnitine (PPLC) treatment

Activity	Control	Diabetic	PPLC-treated diabetic
Na$^+$-K$^+$-ATPase (μmol P$_i$ mg^{-1} h^{-1})	19.8 ± 2.1	10.7 ± 1.6*	15.7 ± 1.6
Na$^+$-dependent Ca^{2+} uptake (nmol Ca^{2+} mg 30 s^{-1})	8.8 ± 1.6	3.2 ± 1.4*	5.1 ± 1.2*
H$^+$-dependent Na$^+$ uptake (nmol Na$^+$ mg^{-1} 30 s^{-1})	0.35 ± 0.04	0.12 ± 0.03*	0.14 ± 0.03*

The protocol for inducing diabetes as well as for PPLC treatment is the same as described in Table 3. The procedure for the isolation of sarcolemma and measurements of biochemical parameters are described elsewhere (Pierce et al, 1990). *, Significantly different ($p < 0.05$) from the respective control.

of the beneficial effects of propionyl-L-carnitine on diabetic heart sarcolemma are not clear at present; however, it should be mentioned that propionyl-L-carnitine, under in vitro conditions, has been shown to depress site II of the phospholipid N-methylation process in the sarcolemmal membrane (Ou et al, 1990).

Because abnormalities in the sarcoplasmic reticular Ca^{2+}-pump and myofibrillar Ca^{2+}-stimulated ATPase were found to be prominent in

TABLE 6.

Heart sarcolemmal Ca^{2+}-pump activities in diabetic rats with or without propionyl-L-carnitine (PPLC) treatment

Activity	Control	Diabetic	PPLC-treated diabetic
Non-specific Ca^{2+} binding (nmol mg^{-1} 5 min^{-1})	4.3 ± 0.33	4.2 ± 0.54	4.3 ± 0.45
ATP-dependent Ca^{2+} uptake (nmol mg^{-1} 5 min^{-1})	26.8 ± 1.24	10.2 ± 0.52*	11.6 ± 0.47*
Mg^{2+}-ATPase (μmol P$_i$ mg^{-1} 5 min^{-1})	15.4 ± 0.75	13.9 ± 0.66	14.1 ± 0.71
Ca^{2+}-stimulated ATPase (μmol mg^{-1} 5 min^{-1})	1.4 ± 0.04	0.52 ± 0.03*	0.61 ± 0.05*

Values are means ± SE of five experiments. The concentration of Ca^{2+} was 10 μmol l^{-1}. The protocol for inducing diabetes as well as for PPLC treatment is the same as described in Table 3. The procedures for the isolation of sarcolemma and measurement of biochemical parameters are described elsewhere (Dixon et al, 1987). *, Significantly different ($p < 0.05$) from the respective control.

relation to other subcellular derangements in the diabetic heart (Ferrari et al, 1991), it was considered of interest to test if propionyl-L-carnitine treatment exerted beneficial effects on these parameters. The results shown in Table 7 indicate that depressions in both Ca^{2+} uptake and Ca^{2+}-stimulated ATPase activities in the diabetic heart were prevented by propionyl-L-carnitine treatment. Since this agent showed no action on the sarcoplasmic reticular Ca^{2+}-pump activities under in vitro conditions (Dhalla et al, 1991), it is unlikely that the observed beneficial effects of propionyl-L-carnitine in diabetic animals under in vivo conditions are due to any pharmacological action of this agent. It is possible that propionyl-L-carnitine may be affecting the diabetes-induced changes in Ca^{2+}-transport by acting on the sarcoplasmic reticular membrane whereby the accumulation of long-chain fatty acyl derivatives is prevented in a manner similar to that for L-carnitine (Lopaschuk et al, 1983a, 1983b). This view is further substantiated by our observation that diabetes-induced changes in myofibrillar Ca^{2+}-stimulated ATPase and myosin ATPase activities were not modified upon treating the diabetic animals with propionyl-L-carnitine (Table 8).

TABLE 7.

Effect of propionyl-L-carnitine (PPLC) on the sarcoplasmic reticulum Ca^{2+}-transport activities in diabetic rat heart

Activity	Control	Diabetic	PPLC-treated diabetic
Ca^{2+} uptake (nmol Ca^{2+} mg^{-1} 5 min^{-1})	224 ± 11	$135 \pm 15*$	205 ± 9
Ca^{2+}-stimulated ATPase (nmol P_i mg^{-1} 5 min^{-1})	814 ± 74	$428 \pm 50*$	784 ± 65

Each value is a mean $\pm$ SE of four experiments. The concentration of Ca^{2+} used in this study was 10 μmol l^{-1}. The experimental protocol for inducing diabetes as well as for PPLC treatment is similar to that described in Table 3. The procedures for the isolation of sarcoplasmic reticulum and measurement of Ca^{2+} uptake and Ca^{2+}-stimulated ATPase activities were identical to those described by Ganguly et al (1983). *, Significantly different ($p < 0.05$) from the respective control.

CONCLUDING REMARKS

It is evident that L-carnitine exerts some beneficial effects on heart performance, plasma lipids, energy status and accumulation of long-chain fatty acyl derivatives in the myocardium in experimental diabetes. Results in this study indicate that treatment of rats with streptozotocin-induced diabetes prevents (partially or completely) changes in sarco-

TABLE 8.

Effect of propionyl-L-carnitine (PPLC) on myofibrillar ATPase activities in diabetic rat heart

Activity	Control	Diabetic	PPLC-treated diabetic
Myofibrillar Ca^{2+}-stimulated ATPase (μmol P_i mg^{-1} 5 min^{-1})	0.48 ± 0.015	$0.33 \pm 0.025*$	$0.35 \pm 0.021*$
Myosin Ca^{2+}-ATPase (μmol P_i mg^{-1} 5 min^{-1})	4.25 ± 0.171	$1.76 \pm 0.142*$	$1.81 \pm 0.185*$

Each value is a mean $\pm$ SE of four experiments. The experimental protocol for inducing diabetes and for PPLC treatment is similar to that described in Table 3. The concentration of Ca^{2+} used for myofibrillar Ca^{2+}-stimulated ATPase was 10 μmol l^{-1}, whereas that for myosin Ca^{2+}-ATPase was 10 mmol l^{-1}. The procedures for the isolation of myofibrils and myosin as well as for the determination of ATPase activities were the same as described elsewhere (Pierce and Dhalla, 1985b). *, Significantly different ($p < 0.05$) from the respective control.

lemmal Na^+-Ca^{2+}-exchange and Na^+-K^+-ATPase activities without affecting the Na^+-H^+-exchange and Ca^{2+}-pump activities. Furthermore, the defect in the sarcoplasmic reticular Ca^{2+}-pump activity in diabetic heart was prevented without affecting the changes in myofibrillar and myosin ATPase activities. Although the mechanisms of the beneficial effects of propionyl-L-carnitine may be complex in nature, the data presented here support the view that this agent may act on heart membranes to prevent their dysfunction in some direct manner. These studies with an animal model of diabetes encourage clinical trials of propionyl-L-carnitine in the diabetic population, as an adjunct therapy to insulin for the prevention of heart dysfunction in chronic diabetes.

Acknowledgements

This research was partially supported by a grant from the Juvenile Diabetes Foundation International, New York. The authors wish to thank Professor E. Arrigoni-Martelli of Sigma Tau, Rome, Italy for his interest and helpful advice during the course of this study.

REFERENCES

Abe M, Yamazaki N, Suzuki Y et al (1984) *J. Mol. Cell. Cardiol.* 16: 239–245.
Adams RJ, Cohen DW, Gupte S et al (1979) *J. Biol. Chem.* 254: 12404–12410.
Afzal N, Ganguly PK, Dhalla KS et al (1988) *Diabetes* 37: 936–942.
Afzal N, Pierce GN, Elimban V et al (1989) *Am. J. Physiol.* 256: E453–E458.
Aomine M & Arita M (1987) *J. Electrocardiol.* 20: 287–296.
Aomine M, Arita M & Shimada T (1988) *Heart and Vessels* 4: 197–206.
Aomine M, Nobe S & Arita M (1989) *J. Cardiovasc. Pharmacol.* 13: 494–501.
Ashavaid TF, Colvin RA, Messineo FC et al (1985) *J. Mol. Cell. Cardiol.* 17: 851–861.
Bergh CH, Hjalmarson A, Sjorgren KG & Jacobsson B (1988) *Horm. Metabol. Res.* 20: 381–386.
Bieber LL (1988) *Annu. Rev. Biochem.* 57: 261–283.
Bielefeld DR, Pace CS & Boshell BR (1983) *Am. J. Physiol.* 245: E560–E567.
Borda E, Pascual J, Wald M & Sterin-Borda L (1988) *Can. J. Cardiol.* 4: 97–101.
Brady LJ, Kroeber CM, Hoppel CL et al (1986) *Metabolism* 35: 555–562.
Brass EP & Beyerinck RA (1987) *Metabolism* 36: 781–787.
Bremer J (1983) *Physiol. Rev.* 63: 1420–1480.
Buccino RA, Spann Jr, JF, Pool PE et al (1967) *J. Clin. Invest.* 46: 1669–1682.
Dhalla NS, Ziegelhoffer A & Harrow JAC (1977) *Can. J. Physiol. Pharmacol.* 55: 1211–1234.

Dhalla NS, Pierce GN, Panagia V et al (1982) *Basic Res. Cardiol.* 77: 117–139.
Dhalla NS, Pierce GN, Innes IR & Beamish RE (1985) *Can. J. Cardiol.* 1: 263–281.
Dhalla NS, Smith CI, Pierce GN et al (1986) In Rupp H (ed.) *Regulation of Heart Function—Basic Concepts and Clinical Implications*, pp 121–136. New York: Thième-Stratton.
Dhalla NS, Kolar F, Shah KR & Ferrari R (1991) *Cardiovasc. Drugs Therap.* 5: 25–30.
Dillman WH (1980) *Diabetes* 29: 579–582.
Dillman WH (1982) *Metabolism* 31: 199–204.
Dillman WH (1984) *Endocrinology* 114: 1678–1685.
Di Lisa F, Menabo R & Siliprandi N (1989) *Mol. Cell. Biochem.* 88: 169–173.
Dixon IMC, Eyolfson DA & Dhalla NS (1987) *Am. J. Physiol.* 235: H1026–H1034.
Factor SM, Okun EM & Minase T (1980) *N. Engl. J. Med.* 302: 384–388.
Fein FS, Korstein LB, Strobeck JE et al (1980) *Circ. Res.* 47: 922–933.
Ferrari R, Ciampalini G, Angoletti G et al (1988) *Pharmacol. Res. Commun.* 20: 125–132.
Ferrari R, Ceconi C, Curello S et al (1989) *Mol. Cell. Biochem.* 88: 161–168.
Ferrari R, Shah KR, Hata T et al (1991) In Nagano M & Dhalla NS (ed.) *The Diabetic Heart*, pp 167–181. New York: Raven Press.
Ganguly PK, Pierce GN, Dhalla KS & Dhalla NS (1983) *Am. J. Physiol.* 244: E528–E535.
Ganguly PK, Rice KM, Panagia V & Dhalla NS (1984) *Circ. Res.* 55: 504–512.
Ganguly PK, Dhalla KS, Innes IR et al (1986) *Circ. Res.* 59: 684–693.
Ganguly PK, Beamish RE, Dhalla KS et al (1987) *Am. J. Physiol.* 252: E734–E739.
Hayashi H, Suzuki Y, Masumura Y et al (1982) *Jpn. Heart J.* 23: 623–630.
Hayashi H, Suzuki Y, Abe M et al (1984) *J. Electrocardiol.* 17: 85–90.
Heyliger CE, Prakash A & McNeill JH (1987) *Am. J. Physiol.* 252: H540–H544.
Horackova M & Murphy MG (1988) *Pflügers Arch.* 411: 564–572.
Idell-Wenger JA, Grotyohann LW & Neely JR (1978) *J. Biol. Chem.* 253: 4310–4318.
Kakar SS, Huang W-H & Askari A (1987) *J. Biol. Chem.* 262: 42–45.
Katz AM & Messineo FC (1981) *Circ. Res.* 48: 1–16.
Kjeldsen K, Braendgaard H, Sidenius P et al (1987) *Diabetes* 36: 842–848.
Lamers JMJ, Stinis HT, Montfoort A & Hulsmann WC (1984) *Biochim. Biophys. Acta* 774: 127–137.
Liedtke J & Nellis SH (1979) *J. Clin. Invest.* 64: 440–447.
Liedtke AJ, Nellis S & Neely JR (1978) *Circ. Res.* 43: 652–661.
Liedtke AJ, Nellis SH & Whitesell LF (1981) *Circ. Res.* 48: 859–866.
Liedtke AJ, DeMaison L & Nellis SH (1988) *Am. J. Physiol.* 255: H169–H176.
Limas CJ (1978) *Am. J. Physiol.* 235: H745–H751.
Lopaschuk GD, Katz S & McNeill JH (1983a) *Can. J. Physiol. Pharmacol.* 61: 439–448.
Lopaschuk GD, Tahiliani AG, Vadlamudi RVSV, Katz S & McNeill JH (1983b) *Am. J. Physiol.* 245: H969–H976.
Makino N, Dhalla KS, Elimban V & Dhalla NS (1987) *Am. J. Physiol.* 253: E202–E207.
Malhotra A, Penpargkul S, Fein FS et al (1981) *Circ. Res.* 49: 1243–1250.
Morkin E, Flink IL & Goldman S (1983) *Prog. Cardiovasc. Dis.* 25: 435–463.

Nagano M & Dhalla NS (ed.) (1991) *The Diabetic Heart*, pp 1–533. New York: Raven Press.

Nakaya H & Tohse N (1986) *Br. J. Pharmacol.* 89: 749–757.

Neely JR & Feuvray D (1981) *Am. J. Physiol.* 102: 282–291.

Nishio Y, Kashiwagi A, Ogawa T et al (1990) *Diabetes* 39: 1064–1069.

Opie LH (1979) *Am. Heart J.* 97: 375–388.

Ou C, Majumder S, Dai J et al (1990) In Korecky B & Dhalla NS (eds) *Subcellular Basis of Contractile Failure*, pp 219–234. Boston: Kluwer Academic Publishers.

Paulson DJ, Schmidt MJ, Traxler JS et al (1984) *Metabolism* 33: 358–363.

Paulson DJ, Traxler J, Schmidt M et al (1986) *Cardiovasc. Res.* 20: 536–541.

Panagia V, Taira Y, Ganguly PK et al (1990) *J. Clin. Invest.* 86: 777–784.

Penpargkul S, Fein FS, Sonnenblick EH & Scheuer J (1981) *J. Mol. Cell. Cardiol.* 13: 303–309.

Pieper GM & Murray WJ (1987) *Biochem. Med. Metabol. Biol.* 38: 111–120.

Pieper GM, Murray WJ, Salhany JM et al (1984) *Biochim. Biophys. Acta* 803: 229–240.

Pierce GN & Dhalla NS (1981) *J. Mol. Cell. Cardiol.* 13: 1063–1069.

Pierce GN & Dhalla NS (1983) *Am. J. Physiol.* 245: C241–C247.

Pierce GN & Dhalla NS (1985a) *Can. J. Cardiol.* 1: 48–54.

Pierce GN & Dhalla NS (1985b) *Am. J. Physiol.* 248: E170–E175.

Pierce GN, Kutryk MJB & Dhalla NS (1983) *Proc. Natl Acad. Sci. USA* 80: 5412–5416.

Pierce GN, Beamish RE & Dhalla NS (ed.) (1988) *Heart Dysfunction in Diabetes*, pp 1–245. Boca Raton: CRC Press.

Pierce GN, Ramjiawan B, Dhalla NS & Ferrari R (1990) *Am. J. Physiol.* 258: H255–H261.

Pierpont MEM, Judd D, Goldenberg IF et al (1989) *Am. J. Cardiol.* 64: 56–60.

Piper HM & Das A (1987) *Basic Res. Cardiol.* 82 (supplement 1): 187–196.

Pitts BJR & Okhuysen CH (1984) *Am. J. Physiol.* 247: H840–H846.

Regan TJ (1983) *Ann. Rev. Med.* 34: 161–168.

Rodis SL, D'Amato PH, Koch E & Vahouny GV (1970a) *Proc. Soc. Exp. Biol. Med.* 133: 833–837.

Rodis SL, D'Amato PH, Koch E & Vahouny GV (1970b) *Biol. Med.* 133: 1070–1075.

Rodrigues B & McNeill JH (1991) In Nagano M & Dhalla NS (eds) *The Diabetic Heart*, pp 21–34. New York: Raven Press.

Rodrigues B, Xiang H & McNeill JH (1988) *Diabetes* 37: 1358–1364.

Rodrigues B, Ross JR, Farahbakshian S & McNeill JH (1990) *Can. J. Physiol. Pharmacol.* 68: 1085–1092.

Rona G (1985) *J. Mol. Cell. Cardiol.* 17: 291–306.

Rupp H, Elimban V & Dhalla NS (1989) *Biochem. Biophys. Res. Commun.* 164: 319–325.

Sauviat MP & Feuvray D (1986) *Basic Res. Cardiol.* 81: 489–496.

Seager MJ, Singal PK, Orchard R et al (1984) *Br. J. Exp. Pathol.* 65: 613–623.

Singal PK, Kapur N, Dhillon KS, Beamish RE & Dhalla NS (1982) *Can. J. Physiol. Pharmacol.* 60: 1390–1397.

Spedding M & Mir AK (1987) *Br. J. Pharmacol.* 92: 457–468.

Stumpf DA, Parker Jr, WD & Angelini C (1985) *Neurology* 35: 1041–1045.

Suzuki Y, Kamikawa T, Kobayashi A et al (1981) *Jpn. Circ. J.* 45: 687–694.

Vadlamudi RVSV, Roger RL & McNeill JH (1982) *Can. J. Physiol. Pharmacol.* 60: 902–911.

Vary TC & Neely JR (1982) *Am. J. Physiol.* 243: H154–H158.

Whitmer JT (1987) *Circ. Res.* 61: 396–408.

Wood JM, Busch B, Pitts BJ & Schwartz A (1977) *Biochem. Biophys. Res. Commun.* 74: 677–684.

INDEX